The Caregiver's Encyclopedia

A Johns Hopkins Press Health Book

THE
Caregiver's
Encyclopedia

A Compassionate Guide to Caring for Older Adults

MURIEL R. GILLICK, MD

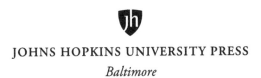

JOHNS HOPKINS UNIVERSITY PRESS
Baltimore

Note to the Reader: This book is not meant to substitute for medical care, and treatment should not be based solely on its contents. Instead, treatment must be developed in a dialogue between the individual and his or her physician. Our book has been written to help with that dialogue.

Drug dosage: The author and publisher have made reasonable efforts to determine that the selection of drugs discussed in this text conform to the practices of the general medical community. The medications described do not necessarily have specific approval by the US Food and Drug Administration for use in the diseases for which they are recommended. In view of ongoing research, changes in governmental regulation, and the constant flow of information relating to drug therapy and drug reactions, the reader is urged to check the package insert of each drug for any change in indications and dosage and for warnings and precautions. This is particularly important when the recommended agent is a new and/or infrequently used drug.

© 2020 Johns Hopkins University Press
All rights reserved. Published 2020
Printed in the United States of America on acid-free paper
9 8 7 6 5 4 3 2 1

Johns Hopkins University Press
2715 North Charles Street
Baltimore, Maryland 21218-4363
www.press.jhu.edu

Library of Congress Cataloging-in-Publication Data

Names: Gillick, Muriel R., 1951– author.
Title: The caregiver's encyclopedia : a compassionate guide to caring for older adults / Muriel R. Gillick, MD.
Description: Baltimore : Johns Hopkins University Press, 2020. | Series: A Johns Hopkins Press health book | Includes index.
Identifiers: LCCN 2019015992 | ISBN 9781421433578 (hardcover : alk. paper) | ISBN 1421433575 (hardcover : alk. paper) | ISBN 9781421433585 (pbk. : alk. paper) | ISBN 1421433583 (pbk. : alk. paper) | ISBN 9781421433592 (electronic) | ISBN 1421433591 (electronic)
Subjects: LCSH: Geriatric nursing—Encyclopedias. | Older people—Home care—United States—Encyclopedias. | Older people—Medical care—Encyclopedias. | Older people—Care—United States—Encyclopedias.
Classification: LCC RC954 .G55 2020 | DDC 618.97/023103—dc23
LC record available at https://lccn.loc.gov/2019015992

A catalog record for this book is available from the British Library.

Images on pages 13, 72, 74, 115, 136, 160, 162, 170, 179, 180, 187, 192, 193, 198, 201, 207, 220, 254, 256, 280, 336, 344, and 378 are © iStockphoto.com. Images on pages 14 and 15 are © Shutterstock .com. Image on page 110 is © Dreamstime.com. Image on page 224 is © Alamy. All other images were created for this book unless otherwise noted.

Special discounts are available for bulk purchases of this book. For more information, please contact Special Sales at specialsales@press.jhu.edu.

Johns Hopkins University Press uses environmentally friendly book materials, including recycled text paper that is composed of at least 30 percent post-consumer waste, whenever possible.

Contents

Part IV. Going to the Rehabilitation Facility 125

Part V. Chronic Care at Home 157

Part VI. Acute Care at Home 241

Part VII. Care in the Nursing Home 297

Part VIII. Getting Additional Help 319

The Caregiver's Encyclopedia

What This Book Is (and What It Is Not)

Dear Caregiver,

Caregiving is one of the loneliest jobs, even though it's performed regularly by forty-five million people in the United States, most of whom are caring for an aging parent. Usually that means the person you are helping is over age sixty-five but, in practice, she is probably over seventy-five, quite possibly over eighty.

You will find many authorities telling you what to do in your role: exhorting you to take care of yourself, urging you to join a support group, instructing you how to manage distressing symptoms such as belligerence or incontinence. I'm not going to tell you what to do. Rather, the idea behind this book is to provide a kind of tour guide to the land of medicine. Based on my experience as a physician, I will tell you what I think you need to know about the lay of the land, about the local customs, and the relevant background. For the tourist using a travel guidebook, the background might be history, geography, and politics; for you, the background might be geriatric medicine, Medicare regulations, and health services research. I'll share with you some important information about basic "geriatric

syndromes" such as delirium, dementia, and falls; I'll discuss what Medicare covers and what it doesn't; and I'll bring you up to date on different approaches to care such as PACE (Program of All-Inclusive Care for the Elderly) and Guided Care that you might want to explore for your family member. Sometimes, I will make a strong recommendation—just as the tour guides tell you about "can't miss" sites—but much of the time my goal is to inform you of your options and let you choose the one that makes most sense to you. I will tell you what is fact and what is my opinion, and when I offer a personal perspective, I will tell you why I think what I do. For example, I will tell you that the hospital is a perilous environment for a frail, older person. That's a fact, not an opinion. I will then go on to say that it is often better to be cared for at home than in the hospital—but that's my opinion since we don't have much information on how home care (even with physician and nursing involvement) compares to hospital care in terms of either beneficial outcomes or hazards, except in a few select cases. Finally, I'll suggest that whether you choose home or hospital care should depend both on the services available and the particular kinds of risks your relative is willing to take.

The reason for providing you with information is twofold: first, so that you can better manage the medical problems your family member has, both acute and chronic problems; and second, to help you think through medical decisions. With respect to managing diseases, you are likely to find yourself playing an increasingly large role in dealing with everyday issues such as taking medications, going to medical appointments, monitoring health indicators (for instance, blood pressure), and administering treatment (for example, changing dressings on a wound). Ideally, your relative will be engaged in her own health care, but various disabilities may prevent her from doing everything herself. You will also need a partner in your family member's physician—or the nurse practitioner or physician assistant who works with her physician—but you will be an effective partner only if you are knowledgeable about your relative's medical conditions.

With respect to medical decision-making, you and your relative will have to make all sorts of choices: whether to get care in the hospital or at home, whether to enroll in hospice, whether to sign a "do not attempt cardiopulmonary resuscitation" order, and whether—and how—to fill out a POLST form (Physician Orders for Life-Sustaining Treatment). You will be involved in decisions about whether to perform screening examinations such as colonoscopy and mammography and whether to use potentially burdensome but possibly life-prolonging treatment such as dialysis

or chemotherapy. The list goes on and on. I hope to equip you to engage in the complex process of decision-making, recognizing that it will often appear daunting. I will spend a good bit of time talking with you about your relative's *goals of care* and how figuring out her priorities can shape the decisions you make together. You will soon discover that managing your family member's medical problems is intimately related to making medical decisions: dealing with a problem, whether it's acute or chronic, necessitates making decisions about what strategy is best in a given situation.

One of my first dilemmas in setting out to write this guide was figuring out what to call you. Technically, you are an "informal caregiver," which is a euphemism for saying you are not paid and you are probably not a professional. Some people refer to you as a "care partner" to emphasize the collaborative nature of your work; in England you would be called a "carer." I have decided to stick to the term commonly used in the United States, which is "caregiver," because in this book I focus on all that you are *giving*. You may well be receiving as well as giving, and you may be partnering with a physician or social worker in what you do, but the aspect of the role I'm going to address is what you *do*.

The next problem, which is considerably harder, is deciding what to call the person to whom you provide care. Many people refer to this person as "your loved one." I confess I don't like this term. For me, it conjures up someone who has died. I also realize there's the possibility you are acting out of duty, filial or otherwise, not out of love. Finally, the phrase is awkward. Others who have written books about providing care to an older individual use the word *parent* in a sort of generic sense. That makes statistical sense, but it assumes a particular relationship between the giver and receiver of care that may not be applicable. I thought about the more neutral term, *charge*, but that makes you sound like a legally appointed guardian. I tried coining a new word, *caree*, where *caree* is to care-giver as donee or recipient is to donor, but everyone to whom I suggested this option thinks it sounds too much like *carry* or like *caries* (dental cavities). Instead, I'm going to refer to the person for whom you provide care as your *family member* or *relative*, recognizing that this person may not literally be your kin but is certainly related sym-bolically. I also had to find a suitable pronoun to use for your relative. While there's a two in three chance that your family member is a woman, you might find it jarring if I always use the femi-nine when in fact your relative is male, so I compromise by alternating the pronouns I use by chapter. Likewise, I alternate the pronouns used to refer to your relative's physician.

A few words about me. I'm a phy-sician who specializes in geriatrics (the medical care of older people) and palliative care (an approach to care for people with advanced illness that em-phasizes symptom management, ad-vance care planning, and psychosocial support). I have more than thirty years of experience as a practicing doctor, working in a community health center, several hospitals and long-term care facilities, and in a multi-specialty group practice. I also have an academic side—I've published numerous articles in medical journals addressing various as-pects of care in the last phase of life. I've written five books about medical care for a general audience, each of which included stories about real people I've cared for as a jumping-off point for dis-cussing topics such as choosing where to live and making decisions near the very end.

Because I'm a physician, this book is strongly weighted toward the medical aspect of caregiving. That doesn't mean that other aspects of caregiving don't deserve attention; they do. Financial planning is crucial. Addressing legal matters is often important. But these topics won't come up except insofar as they relate to managing acute illness or chronic disease. For instance, I address advance care planning—thinking about what to do in the event of serious ill-ness and incapacity—and mention the importance of appointing a health-care surrogate (which entails completing a legal document, though it doesn't require a lawyer to do so) as well as of making sure that the surrogate is well-informed. The reason I want to devote a whole book to matters medical, aside from the fact that I know about such things, is that while you as a caregiver have many roles, the responsibilities for which you are perhaps least well pre-pared are your medical ones.

Understanding what congestive heart failure is and what the treatments involve is a good deal more complicated than learning how to contact Meals on Wheels or finding an adult day care program. Nonetheless, you will likely find yourself immersed in administering sophisticated medical care and making life-altering medical decisions. Just under half of all family caregivers provide medical or nursing care for relatives with complex chronic conditions. That care is not just administering pills, though many caregivers do help with oral medications; in addition, it includes giving intravenous medicines, dressing wounds, providing artificial nutrition through a tube, and using complicated machines such as a ventilator or dialysis machine. I cannot teach you how to perform all the tasks you might be faced with as a caregiver, but I can familiarize you with the most common medical conditions your family member is apt to have. Once you have some basic knowledge, you will find learning a new technique or procedure much easier.

Despite my medical background, this volume is far from a textbook on geriatrics. While I want to help you feel comfortable with some basic medical concepts and medical lingo, I also want to familiarize you with the institutions (the hospital, the doctor's office, the rehab facility) where your relative will be treated for medical problems, as well as with the people who do the treating (primary care physicians, specialists, hospitalists, nurse practitioners, registered nurses, physical therapists, and so forth). Just as you need to be passably conversant with the language of medicine, so, too, do you need to be comfortable finding your way around in the halls of medical institutions and interacting with their inhabitants.

A word about the organization of the book. I realize that for many of you, this will serve as a reference book rather than a narrative that you read through from beginning to end. While there are multiple discrete sections, each of which can stand alone, and some of the symptom-oriented and disease-oriented chapters within a section are also independent of the remaining text, I encourage you to read part I, "Underlying Health State," straight through to give you a framework for thinking about the issues that will repeatedly crop up. My view is that you as the caregiver need to understand your family member's underlying health state in order to be able to manage any of her medical conditions. It's very important that you know what I mean by this if you are to be maximally effective as a caregiver. The next three parts address the three most common sites of medical care for older individuals outside the home: the office, the hospital, and the rehabilitation facility. Part II, "Going to the Doctor," is relevant for just about everyone, and interacting with physicians is a crucial part of your role, so I encourage you to read this section next. You might want to hold off on part III, "Going to the Hospital," until your relative needs hospital care. However, several chapters deal with avoiding hospitalization altogether and with how to choose a hospital, issues you might want to think about *before* your relative finds herself hospitalized. It's time to think about part IV, "Going to the Rehabilitation Facility," when your family member is in the acute care hospital—although for growing numbers of people, a rehab stay can take place without going to the hospital first or can *substitute* for, rather than follow, hospitalization.

The next chunk of the book, part V, "Chronic Care at Home," may be the part you consult most frequently. It is meant to help you address problems as they arise in the home setting, whether "home" is your relative's house or apartment, your house or apartment, or a different type of environment, such as an assisted living facility. I begin by talking about your "medical bag," various supplies that you might want to keep on hand. These range from a blood pressure cuff and thermometer to bandages and a scale. Then I go through the ten most common chronic conditions afflicting older people, focusing not on the biology or the prognosis but rather on what you need to know to help manage your relative's illness. I also pay special attention to decisions you might need to be involved in such as whether your family member should have a pacemaker or whether she should sign an out-of-hospital do-not-resuscitate (DNR) form. I will talk with you about tailoring your decision depending on what matters most to your relative, or what I call her "goals of care." Part V concludes with a chapter on prevention, discussing strategies that may be relevant to many of the other chapters (for example, exercise is a topic in the chapters on heart disease) as well as other strategies, such as promoting good nutrition and getting vaccinations, that don't fit anywhere else.

While much of your medical role involves chronic management, some may entail addressing acute issues. Part VI, "Acute Care at Home," recognizes that you may be the first line of defense when your relative develops a new problem. Since she is far more likely to develop "shortness of breath" than to be able to assert with confidence that she has "a flare of congestive heart failure" or "an exacerbation of chronic obstructive lung disease," this part of the book is organized by symptom. Here is where a disclaimer is in order. Reading a chapter about "chest pain" or "nausea" does not make you a physician and is not intended to substitute for professional guidance. But just as new parents learn when to call the pediatrician and when to take matters into their own hands, or wait and see before calling, you, as a caregiver, may benefit from some advice on how to think about various symptoms. Sometimes the answer to the question of whether to call or to wait depends on the *severity* of the symptom; sometimes it depends on your family member's *goals of care*. I will also suggest types of additional information that you can collect that could be very helpful to the physician who is deciding on a treatment strategy. I am going to focus on ten of the most common symptoms that your relative may develop. For a more comprehensive list and more elaborate medical information, you may want to consult a resource such as the Merck manual, *Family Caregiving for the Elderly*.

The next section, part VII, "Care in the Nursing Home," is only relevant if your family member is headed for a nursing home. I include it because you may have been functioning as a caregiver for some time, and you may think that your role is coming to an end because your relative is going into a nursing home—when, in fact, your role is merely changing. In some ways, the move allows you to step back, to let the staff at the facility provide direct care. But you are an invaluable source of information about your relative: you know what works and what doesn't if, for example, she is depressed or constipated. You know that the last three times she became confused, it was because she had a bladder infection, and the last time she got constipated the only thing that helped was sorbitol. You have discussed her goals of care with her and know when she would want to go to the hospital and when she wouldn't. And on and on. To be effective, you need to know a bit about how nursing homes operate and who the important players are. You want to be able to leverage your expertise without overburdening yourself—or stepping on the toes of the nursing home employees.

The last part of the book, part VIII, "Getting Additional Help," is my opportunity to share with you some thoughts about community, family, and other resources that can help you manage your relative's medical problems. My goal here is not to talk about all the nonmedical dimensions of caregiving such as the legal, financial, or religious aspects, but rather to give you some guidance on enlisting help with health care. Making sure your family member has the best possible health insurance plan for her is clearly directly related to her health. Availing yourself of nutritional resources in the community, for example, and engaging in advance care planning for *future* illness are useful steps. Sharing the medical caregiving responsibilities with other family members can help take some of the burden off your shoulders and assures backup if you are unavailable. I will mention caregiver support, not so much because it's good for you, though it is, but because it's good for your family member—her health and well-being may be dependent on yours.

The epilogue, "Rest in Peace," addresses the medical issues that arise even after death, questions about organ donation and autopsy. It's also my chance to acknowledge that if you have been involved in even a fraction of the caregiving tasks I discuss, you have performed a remarkable service.

I hope that this book will serve as a companion to you on your caregiving journey. Consult its pages as you see fit, allowing me to share with you what I know and what I've seen and to help you figure out how to be the best caregiver you can be.

PART I

Underlying Health State

Whealth hen you go for a routine checkup, you expect your physician to sit down at the end of the visit and go over each of your medical problems. For every new problem, along with all your chronic problems, your physician will say something about how you are doing, what tests or treatments he recommends, and what you should expect next. The same is true when your family member goes to the physician. But what's missing from this review, and what is especially important for your relative, is a general sense of how he is doing *as a whole.*

The view of how your relative is doing *overall*, the big picture, is what I mean by the underlying health state. If you are going to be an effective caregiver, you need to hear that general assessment. The chapters in this section will help you understand why health state matters and the components that go into it. It turns out that health state is determined not just by diseases but also by function (how well your relative can attend to his personal care, how well he can get around, and how well he can take care of other basic necessities such as preparing meals or paying bills). Health state is also crucially affected by the presence or absence of several disorders that are neither diseases nor functions, conditions such as incontinence and falling that physicians refer to as "geriatric syndromes." Once I've spoken with you about both function and geriatric syndromes, you'll be able to get a good handle on the spectrum of health states. At one extreme are people who are very vigorous (whom I call *robust*); at the other extreme are those who are dying. In between are people who are physically fairly tenuous (*frail*) or mentally tenuous (individuals with *dementia*). When you appreciate what each of these varieties looks like, you may be able to see where your relative fits in.

CHAPTER 1

Why Health State Matters

You should start your caregiving journey by knowing your family member's underlying health state. Where your relative stands along the spectrum of health matters because it shapes *prognosis*. Moreover, it affects how well he is likely to tolerate a new medication, a new treatment, or even hospitalization.

What most people think of when they hear the word *prognosis* is life expectancy. Life expectancy matters to people for social reasons: If they want to accomplish certain things during their lifetime and they know they don't have much time left, they can plan accordingly. It also matters for medical reasons: there are decisions to be made about whether to undergo a screening test—say, a stool test looking for colon cancer or a prostate-specific antigen (PSA) test looking for evidence of prostate cancer—and deciding rationally depends on life expectancy. It makes sense for men to be screened for prostate cancer if they can expect to live another twenty years; it doesn't make sense if they can expect to live only five years. The rationale for screening is that early detection makes a difference

in terms of outcomes; if your family member isn't likely to live much longer, then he stands to suffer all the potential risks of treatment—in the case of treatment for prostate cancer, these include incontinence, impotence, and diarrhea—without any of the benefits.

When I say that understanding your family member's health state matters for purposes of prognosis, I mean it matters beyond knowing his life expectancy. How well your relative will fare if he undergoes standard medical treatments depends crucially on his overall condition. He can be said to fare well if he suffers few or no side effects from the treatment and if the treatment achieves its desired goal; he can be said to fare poorly if he develops complications or if the treatment is ineffective. And it's important to realize that your family member is likely to come down with one or more acute medical problems each year, problems related to underlying conditions—like cancer or heart failure or Parkinson's disease— that collectively produce his health state and also new problems—such as pneumonia or an ulcer. What kind of medical care he should get when he has an acute issue depends on how well he will do with each option along with his own willingness to tolerate potential risks in exchange for potential benefits.

Health State and Planning for the Future

Health state also matters if you and your family member are to plan for the future rather than deal with each new medical problem when it arises. I'm not talking about very elaborate scheming, about developing complex decision trees in advance. Too much is unpredictable and unknowable to engage in extremely detailed planning. But suppose your family member has been hospitalized several times for shortness of breath and each time he became very confused and left the hospital much weaker than when he entered. Suppose you would really like to treat the next episode of shortness of breath at home, and you're fairly confident there will be a next time because your family member has chronic heart failure, which is marked by periodic flares and which will become progressively more severe over time. If home treatment is to be feasible you are best off laying the groundwork in advance. That entails making sure the primary care physician knows you want to keep your family member at home; it may be useful to fill out a special form that indicates to emergency medical technicians that your family member does not, under any circumstances, want a breathing tube inserted; you may want to obtain an oxygen tank and mask in advance of actually needing them; you might even want to have appropriate medications on hand to be able to initiate treatment promptly.

Finally, health state matters because it can influence where your family member lives. If he's very frail, for example, and at high risk of needing considerably more help in the face of the flu or a simple bladder infection, he may be best off living in an environment with some degree of supervision and assistance on site. If he's dying or very likely to die within a matter of months, living alone may be inadvisable even if he is doing all right for the moment.

What Your Physician Doesn't Tell You

Maybe you're thinking that you already know your family member's health state. After all, the last time you went with him for a checkup the doctor probably went over each medical problem and said something about how well each one was coming along. Dad has diabetes? Yes, but it's under excellent control with that medication he takes for it, metformin (or glipizide or insulin or some other drug). That record you brought in of all his blood sugars? It shows that, for the most part, his level isn't too high or too low. It's just right. How was his hemoglobin A1C test, a measure of his average sugar over the last couple of months? It confirms that he's taking the right amount of medication. He has high blood pressure? Well, his blood pressure was a bit high today and last time it was on the high side, too, but that might be what's called "white coat hypertension," anxiety in the doctor's office that results in the blood pressure shooting up. His kidney function was a little off on his last blood test? Just a laboratory test, not really anything significant, but we'll monitor his numbers every few months, to be sure. And you said he was forgetful? That's normal for eighty-five-year-olds, nothing to worry about. He seemed fine today. He has a chronic cough? What do you expect after smoking a pack of cigarettes a day for fifty years? But he stopped smoking now, so it isn't really an issue. After that litany or something like it, you were left with the impression that your family member is in good health; his underlying health state is fine.

But is that true? Is that kidney malfunction evidence of early chronic renal failure? Is the forgetfulness normal aging or is it due to mild cognitive impairment? Maybe it's even early dementia. Is the cough indicative of chronic obstructive lung disease (COLD)? How much do all those problems interfere with your relative's ability to function day to day? Has his elevated blood pressure led to very small strokes that affect his thinking? Does the memory problem interfere with his social life—his weekly card game, his monthly book club? Does the cough make him short of breath, limiting how far he can walk? And even if he is still able to get by day to day, does the combination of all those different medical conditions put him at risk of a major decline or multiple complications if he gets a new problem such as the flu? You will want to know more than how well-controlled each isolated medical problem is: you want the big picture.

This may come as a surprise, but doctors aren't very good at giving you the big picture. For the past fifty years, medical schools have taught students to use the "problem-oriented medical record." This was an approach advocated by a physician named Lawrence Weed in the 1960s and it caught on big time. The best way to think about medical problems and, therefore, the best way to organize a medical record, Weed and others felt, was by diagnosis or, if you didn't have a diagnosis, by symptom. Every office visit, or for that matter hospital visit or skilled nursing facility visit, could be broken down into the specific problems that the doctor addressed. And each problem that came up in a visit or, as it came to be called, an "encounter" between a patient and physician, would be immortalized in the "problem list," a kind of table of contents for the medical record. Weed also promoted using the "SOAP" format for each note, where "SOAP" stands for subjective, objective, assessment, and plan. If your family member comes to see his doctor because he's worried about his memory, the physician will write a single SOAP note in his medical chart recording what he said about the kinds of things he forgets, what she found on examination, what she thinks is wrong, and what she plans to do about it.

If your family member goes in for a checkup, the medical record will document his "chief complaint" (his main concern), summarize the "history" (when the problem started, what makes it worse, what makes it better), itemize the "review of systems," record a "physical examination," and if the physician is very thorough, a "family history" (which isn't a history at all but a list of the medical problems of close relatives) and a "social history" (which also isn't really history but rather a few comments about the highest grade your family member attended in school, his occupation, whether he's married, and whether he has any children). Finally, the record will enumerate each problem with a brief "assessment and plan," or a statement of what the diagnosis is and what the recommended action steps are, such as getting a lab test or starting a new medication. Nowhere is there space for putting all the problems together, for saying something about the patient's overall condition. At most, another doctor reading the medical record might get a hint from the very first line of the "chief complaint," which might read "healthy appearing eighty-five-year-old man here for a checkup and expressing concerns about his memory." Or maybe it would say "pale seventy-five-year-old man who appears older than his stated age."

Physicians are trained to be reductionists, to break health into pieces, typically organized by organ system. The "assessment and plan" might include an overall evaluation of each of the components, describing the overall status of the heart under the problem "congestive heart failure" with words like "moderately severe heart failure," or "NY Heart Class IIIC heart failure," which is the same thing. It might then go on to provide an overall assessment of the next major organ system, such as the lungs, and so forth, producing what some have referred to as the "organ recital."

What you probably want to know, and what the doctor isn't likely to come out and tell you, is where your family member lies along the continuum from vigorous to near-the-end-of-life. You'll want to know if he's *robust, frail, has dementia, or is dying.*

The Different Health States and Why They Make a Difference

Someone with a long list of diagnoses on his problem list who's taking one or more medications for each of them could still be *robust*. If all those disorders, issues such as arthritis and cataracts, high blood pressure and elevated cholesterol, don't interfere with every day activities, he's robust. Being robust implies that certain procedures, such as bypass surgery, may be quite reasonable, if recommended based on technical considerations, and shouldn't be rejected out of hand on the basis of age alone. An example of a *robust couple* can be seen in figure 1.1.

Someone else who has the same list of diagnoses might be in a different situation if the medical disorders are severe enough to get in the way of everyday life. If his problems require him to have a fair amount of assistance and if they interact in such a way as to make him vulnerable to still more problems, then he's in the state of *frailty*. Frailty is a condition of decreased reserves, a diminished ability to fight off an infection, recover from a fall, or heal after a cut. A *frail woman* is depicted in figure 1.2.

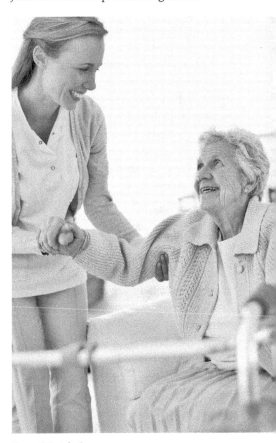

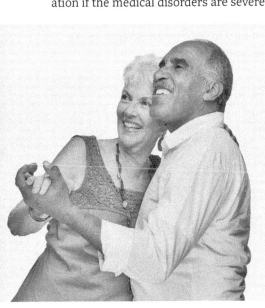

Figure 1.1. A robust couple

Figure 1.2. A frail woman

Being frail has implications for how well a person will tolerate an operation, a long trip, or even hospital care itself. You might think your family member will benefit from hospital treatment for a flare of heart failure, for example, much as your car would benefit from periodic tune-ups. What you don't realize, however, is that being frail means being tenuously balanced between barely making it and disaster. Hospitalization sometimes unleashes an entire cascade of problems among frail people (see chapter 10, "The Perils of Hospitalization"). That strong intravenous medication you are expecting your family member to get in the hospital, the medicine that always used to work so well, might worsen his slightly impaired kidney function, with the consequence that he will have trouble excreting another medication he is getting, a pill he takes against the nerve pain he experiences from diabetes, resulting in his having too much pain medication in his system, producing drowsiness, leading his food to go down the wrong way, causing pneumonia . . .

Whether or not your family member has physical frailty, he might have a kind of mental frailty, or *dementia* as shown in figure 1.3. Not all memory problems are due to dementia or to mild cognitive impairment, a condition that sometimes but not always progresses to full blown dementia (for more on dementia, see chapter 29, "Alzheimer's Disease and Other Dementias"). Over the last few years, researchers have started to

talk about "cognitive aging," or the memory lapses and slower reflexes that are characteristic of normal aging. You'll find it reassuring to learn that your family member's forgetfulness is just part of normal cognitive aging. But if it isn't, you'll probably want to know that, too. Alzheimer's disease is by far the most common form of dementia, but all varieties of dementia are progressive, incurable, and ultimately fatal. Because people with dementia have a disease involving the brain, they are exquisitely sensitive to medications that may affect the central nervous system. Translation: If your family member has dementia, many ordinary medications are apt to exacerbate his memory and judgment problems. Some of these medicines are available over-the-counter, such as diphenhydramine (brand name Benadryl), an antihistamine used to treat allergies, itchy rashes, and insomnia. If you don't realize your family member has dementia and what that means for taking medication, you might inadvertently make matters worse.

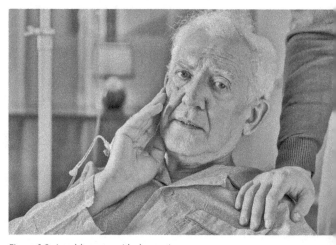

Figure 1.3. An older man with dementia

You might also want to understand just how advanced your relative's dementia is. That information can influence your choice of how aggressively to treat a new, acute medical problem. Just as it doesn't make a lot of sense to repair a broken hip in a person whose death is imminent, it doesn't make sense to treat a condition that won't cause any problems for at least five years if your family member is already in the advanced stage of Alzheimer's disease. Tight control of blood sugar in a person newly diagnosed with diabetes, for example, which is important to prevent vision problems (retinopathy) and kidney abnormalities (nephropathy), is only effective if the individual lives the ten years it takes to develop those problems.

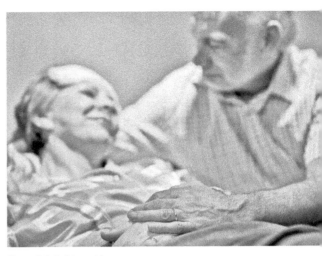

Figure 1.4. A dying older woman

Eventually your family member will approach the end of life and you will also want to know when that time has come. Sometimes there is little or no advance warning, but in many instances the physician will be reasonably certain the end is imminent. Cancers that have metastasized and for which there is no good treatment, heart failure that is extremely advanced, or dementia that is in its final stage are all situations where the physician can say that not much time remains. You will want to know that your family member is dying, however painful this knowledge, because you might not want to subject him to very uncomfortable or anxiety-producing treatments if death is near (figure 1.4). You might want to think about enrollment in home hospice. At the very least, you may decide to alert other family members so they can visit.

How do you know whether your family member is robust, frail, has dementia, or is dying? It's not your job to make the diagnosis—any more than it's appropriate for you to conclude that your family member who is coughing has congestive heart failure or pneumonia. You will need to ask your family member's doctor. (For a more detailed discussion of these four states, see chapter 4, "Determining Your Family Member's Health State.")

Pinning Down the Doctor

I'm not advocating that you march into the doctor's office and demand to know whether your family member is robust, frail, has dementia, or is dying. But since most physicians aren't going to tell you, you ought to be ready to ask some leading questions. You can try asking how your family member is doing "overall." The idea of a summary rating or statistic is, after all, very common: Kids in school have their grade point average, not just individual grades; restaurants and hotels get ratings as well as reviews, as do colleges and graduate schools. In fact, you can look up ratings for just about every consumer good you might be considering purchasing; many of us wouldn't think of buying a computer or a television or even a toaster or an electric shaver without checking which products win four or five stars from their customers. I'm sure I don't have to explain to you that five stars is the highest rating or that it's very rare for hundreds of people to independently award five stars to a particular consumer item. You also know that four stars is above average and often the best you can hope for, but three stars should cause you to have second thoughts. The concept of an overall assessment is ubiquitous in nonmedical settings. By analogy, you know what it means to ask how your family member is doing "overall" and so will the physician.

Since your relative needs a caregiver, he probably isn't robust—people in vigorous health who are fully independent don't typically need caregivers, though your robust family member might temporarily appear frail after a long, complex illness. If you've been pulled in to provide caregiving following a lengthy hospitalization and are not sure whether your family member is likely to recover, you can ask his physician. The physician may not know, but she should be able to tell you if there's a good chance your relative will return to his baseline level of function or not. If you're pretty sure your family member wasn't robust, even before the recent illness, you've just reduced the options for underlying health state to three: is your family member frail or dying, or does he have dementia?

Frailty is often the trickiest of the three to get at because many physicians aren't good at diagnosing it. Frailty, unlike pornography, is not something that people know when they see it—even doctors. The reason is that frailty usually arises from multiple different diseases that interact to produce impaired function and limited reserves, but both physicians and the general public are accustomed to thinking in terms of individual diseases. Unless frailty stems from a single disease such as Parkinson's or multiple sclerosis that affects many different bodily functions, it often goes undetected. Moreover, while there are some simple screening tests for frailty, most American physicians (other than specialists in geriatrics) don't know about them. The tests are easy to administer: one is a seven-item questionnaire that patients can answer in writing or on the telephone and another involves timing how long it takes to get up from a chair and walk a few yards across the room (the "get up and go" test). The British Geriatrics Society has recommended that general practitioners use one of these tests whenever they encounter a high-risk patient. Someday, perhaps, American primary care doctors will use the tests regularly and start diagnosing frailty. In the meantime, you can ask about your family member's overall condition.

Dementia is another health state that often goes unrecognized. Early in the course of dementia, your relative will likely still have his social graces. He is able to cover up his deficits and if he doesn't remember the names of his medications, he might make a joke of it, saying he has private nicknames for his pills. The physician may not probe further if your relative seems to be mentally intact. When she performs a routine neurological examination, she often pays scant attention to the mental function, asking only if your family member knows who he is, where he is, and what the date is. She then writes in the record "oriented times three" and assumes, based on an insufficient evaluation, that there's no dementia.

Many physicians are unfamiliar with doing a more comprehensive evaluation themselves. They feel uncomfortable diagnosing dementia since there's no blood test or x-ray to clinch the diagnosis. But if you're worried about your family member's mental function, you should ask about it, giving specific examples of episodes you found worrisome. If the physician isn't able to address your concerns, she will probably refer your family member to someone who can, whether a psychiatrist, a neurologist, or a geriatrician.

The last of the possible underlying health states is dying. Many doctors aren't comfortable talking about the end of life and resort to euphemisms when discussing the seriousness of a patient's condition. But there's nothing wrong with you asking, "How much time do you think he has?" If the physician tries to avoid answering by telling you that everyone is different and some people live for years this way, you can ask what happens to *most* people in your relative's situation. Or you can explain that you need to know how bad things are because you have to know what to tell other family members, or you have to decide whether this is the time to take a family leave from work. The physician may be vague because of her own discomfort but may also be trying to protect you. If you want to know the truth, you can make it clear that shielding you from bad news is not protecting you. I can't remember any family members who came right out and asked me whether their relative was dying, but perhaps that's because I tend to tell things as I see them. Often, to make clear that my prediction comes with considerable uncertainty, I'll say something like, "I would be surprised if your mom were still here at Christmas." And then I might qualify this further, saying "I'd be happy to be wrong."

Once you have the big picture, you're ready to home in on the different components of the overall health state. This is where specific diseases come in. But it's also where physical functioning enters the picture (the capacity to do things such as walk, dress, and bathe); it's where mental functioning plays a role (not just the presence or absence of dementia but also normal aging and that in-between state, mild cognitive impairment); and it includes the emotional state (anxiety, depression, paranoia, and other psychological conditions). See a list of the reasons that the big picture is important in box 1.1.

Box 1.1

Why the Big Picture Matters

- Health state affects prognosis
- Health state shapes the response to treatment
- Health state is the starting point for advance care planning

CHAPTER 2

Ingredients of the Underlying Health State

When she reached age ninety, my mother always used to tell me she was in excellent health because all her major organ systems were working well. In some ways, she was absolutely right. She was correct that her heart and her lungs and her brain were all functioning normally for a ninety-year-old. She didn't have any major diseases such as coronary heart disease or asthma or Parkinson's. She took only a couple of medications on a regular basis. She hadn't been hospitalized in five years. In many respects, she was doing astonishingly well. And yet, if you asked her how her health was compared to the way it had been ten years earlier, she would have complained bitterly. She would have told you that she used to walk several miles a day—in rain or shine, no matter how cold it was, and she lived in New England—but now she could walk only a few yards before developing severe back pain. She pushed herself, so she still walked. But she took along a walker, not so much for balance, although the walker did help steady her, as for the built-in seat it provided. She would tell you she used to have a terrific memory: she remembered names and faces and life histories. Now she found she was constantly forgetting common words and she was hopeless with names. Ten years ago, she drove everywhere by car, and not only to common haunts such as the local senior center. She delivered library books to "shut-ins," providing both reading material and companionship, and thought nothing of going to an unfamiliar location. Now, she went only very short distances and when she thought about it—though she tried not to—she was a bit concerned about all the dings on her car, not to mention all the damage that she'd had repaired. Evaluating my mother's health solely in terms of organs or diseases just didn't seem entirely accurate.

The Role of Diseases in Determining Health

My mother thought of her health as determined by her diseases and you probably think of your family member's health the same way. That's what most people believe. It's what *anyone* would think after a typical visit to the doctor because doctors generally take a disease-by-disease approach to their patients. They may generally start by asking the patient how she's doing but then quickly organize the visit into disease or symptom categories. Ideally—from the physician's perspective—each symptom is caused by a discrete medical problem: shortness of breath might result from congestive heart failure or chronic obstructive lung disease or pneumonia, or any of a variety of other specific entities, rather than from the interaction of several different problems. After the doctor has taken a history and examined your family member and is ready to summarize all the issues and formulate a plan, you probably noticed that, in the wrap-up at the end of the outpatient visit, the doctor usually goes over each of the disorders on the "problem list"—the itemized list of all the active medical conditions—again, taking things disease by disease.

You're perfectly correct that your family member's overall health is *partly* determined by the sum of all the diseases on the problem list. It's true that it's important to understand the nature of each medical problem your family member has. You also need to know something about its severity and its likely trajectory. It's not enough to know, for example, that she has breast cancer. There are different types of breast cancer. Some tumors have estrogen receptors, which means they depend on estrogen to grow and can, therefore, be treated with medications that starve the tumor of estrogen; other tumors have progesterone receptors; and still others have yet a different type of receptor. Each receptor has different implications for treatment and prognosis. Some breast cancers are localized at the time of diagnosis and can be entirely removed surgically; others are metastatic, affecting organs as remote as the brain, the lungs, or the liver. After several years of treatment, some cancers are almost certainly cured, others are being kept in check by medication and might continue in that state for years to come, and still others have progressed to the point where they are no longer responsive to disease-focused treatment.

Other diagnoses are also highly variable in what they mean for your family member, depending on the type and stage of the disorder. Take another condition common in old age, heart failure, the leading cause of hospitalization in people over age sixty-five. If your family member has heart failure, her heart doesn't pump as efficiently and effectively as it once did. As a result, relatively minor disturbances such as the flu or eating a can of salt-laden soup can put more stress on the heart than she's able to handle, resulting in fluid backing up into places it doesn't belong. Sometimes that means the ankles, sometimes the fluid builds up in the belly, other times in the lungs (see chapter 28, "Heart Failure"). What doctors don't always mention is that heart failure is usually a chronic, progressive disorder. Early on, when the heart function is still fairly good, one or two medications may suffice to keep your family member breathing comfortably. As the condition deteriorates, sometimes after a heart attack (or two or three), sometimes for other reasons, smaller and smaller additional medical problems can produce dramatic effects. Sometimes your family member has a flare of her disease without any obvious provocation at all. Early in the course of the disease, taking an extra fluid pill by mouth might be enough to get rid of any excess fluid; later on, your family member may need intravenous medication in the hospital to treat her. And in the most advanced stage of the disease, your family member will find she is weak and tired all the time; she gets short of breath just from putting on her shoes or going from the sofa in the living room to the bathroom; and nothing short of a heart transplant can truly fix her problems.

So yes, diagnoses matter. And clearly, it's not enough to know *what* diseases your family member has, you also have to know *how far along* she is in the disease—and you have to have some idea of the overall road map. But other factors figure into the determination of the overall health state as well.

The Role of Physical Function in Determining the Health State

First and foremost is *physical function*, how well your family member can walk, hear, and see. When I mentioned my mother earlier, I said she wasn't quite as healthy as she thought she was because she suffered from limitations in her ability to do the things she used to do, despite the relatively good performance of her major organs. If your relative has mild dementia, she might be able to get by reasonably well if all her senses are intact. If she is both very hard of hearing and has visual difficulties, she will have trouble compensating for the memory deficit.

What exactly goes into physical function? I said earlier that it's an area that physicians today tend to ignore. That was true historically, as well, with one important exception. A doctor named Sidney Katz stumbled into the area of rehabilitative medicine and quickly grasped the importance of mobility on the one hand and measuring the severity of any limitations on the other. Katz, by the way, was an interesting fellow. He was born in Cleveland, Ohio, in 1924, the son of a storeowner. His education was interrupted by World War II, but during his time in the navy, he had his first major exposure to medicine and surgery. After the war, he attended college and then medical school, only to rejoin the armed forces during the Korean War. At the end of the war, he got a job at a rehabilitation hospital in Cleveland, where he studied the effect of vitamins on the elderly. He found that the relevant "effect," relevant that is to his subjects' getting along in life, had a great deal to do with whether a person was able to be independent. And being independent, in turn, was related to a variety of fundamental tasks, from feeding oneself to dressing. He ended up devising a scale that he called the "index of activities for daily living." Published in the *Journal of the American Medical Association* in 1963, it is still used today.

You should have a look at the Katz Activities of Daily Living (ADL) scale (see table 2.1). It includes six fundamental domains that are the areas on which your family member's degree of independence depends. First, there's bathing. This can be taking a bath or a shower; it can be sponge bathing; but whatever the strategy, your family member is *independent* if she can wash her entire body. If your family member needs help reaching a few body parts, or can't get out of the shower or tub unassisted, then she's *dependent*. Next comes dressing. To be considered independent, your family member has to be able to pick out clothes from drawers or

a closet and put them on. The only exception is tying shoelaces. Then there's toileting. That entails getting to the bathroom, disrobing sufficiently to use the toilet, doing what needs to be done, wiping, and then getting dressed again.

Transferring is the next item in the scale. It means getting out of bed or up from a chair without any human assistance. Help from a cane or a walker or some other device is permissible, but anyone who needs another person to get up is considered *dependent*. Then there's continence, which refers to both bladder and bowel function. The Katz ADL scale doesn't address how many slip-ups it's legitimate to have and still be deemed continent, but a good rule of thumb is that anyone who leaks at least once a month has an incontinence problem. Finally, there's feeding. This refers to getting food from the plate into the mouth, chewing, and swallowing. Your family member doesn't have to do the food shopping or the cooking, but she has to be able to eat without help to be considered independent in this domain.

That's it: just six very basic activities. The degree of impairment is typically quantified, so since every area of independence is awarded one point and every area of dependence is awarded zero points, the best possible score is 6 and the worst possible score is 0. As a point of reference, about two-thirds of nursing home residents are impaired in at least four domains.

Table 2.1

Katz Index of Independence in Activities of Daily Living

Activities (Score 0 or 1)	Independent *No supervision or personal assistance needed (1 point)*	Dependent *Requires supervision, personal assistance or total care (0 points)*
Bathing: Points: _____	Bathes completely or needs help bathing only 1 part of body such as back or genitals	Needs help with bathing more than 1 body part, getting in or out of tub or shower
Dressing: Points: _____	Takes clothes from drawers or closets; puts on and fastens clothes; may need help tying shoes	Needs help dressing
Toileting: Points: _____	Goes to bathroom; gets on and off toilet; cleans genital area without help	Needs help getting on or off toilet or uses bedpan or commode
Transferring: Points: _____	Gets in and out of bed or chair without help of person	Needs help going from bed to chair
Incontinence: Points: _____	Has control over urination and defecation	Partially or totally incontinent of bladder or bowels
Feeding: Points:___	Gets food from plate or bowl without help	Needs help with feeding or requires tube feeding

Score of 6 is independent; score of 0 is very dependent

Sources: S. Katz, T. D. Down, H. R. Cash, and R. C. Grotz, "Progress in the development of the index of ADL," *The Gerontologist* 10, no. 1 (1970): 20–30; copyright © The Gerontological Society of America. Reproduced [Adapted] by permission of the publisher.

The Role of Cognition in Determining Health State

Cognitive function is another important ingredient of the overall health state. If your family member has diabetes, for instance, she is apt to be much worse off if she cannot recognize symptoms of low blood sugar or cannot draw up the right amount of insulin in a syringe because of dementia. But cognitive dysfunction doesn't necessarily equal dementia. There's "cognitive aging," which typically means some degree of forgetfulness and a lower processing speed. It accounts for the phenomenon that I'm sure you've observed when talking to your family member or some other older person: you ask a question and there's silence. You think maybe she didn't hear you, so you repeat the question. Or you think she didn't understand you so you re-phrase the question. Of course, it might be that your family member really didn't hear you or understand you. But it might also be that she is just slow in figuring out what you meant or reason-ing out a response. It could also be that she couldn't find the word needed for the answer.

There's also *mild cognitive impair-ment* (MCI), a condition that is more severe than normal aging, but not severe enough to qualify as dementia. Sometimes it progresses to dementia but sometimes it doesn't. If your family member's doctor checks her cognitive function with a mental status exam-ination, he will find that it's normal in both cognitive aging and mild cognitive impairment—but with MCI, families and sometimes patients *know* something isn't right. That something just isn't severe enough to significantly interfere with everyday activities.

Finally, there's dementia, which is a disease state but which can be due to a variety of causes ranging from Alz-heimer's disease, the most common form, to vascular disease, the next most common form, to more obscure mal-adies, many of which are named after nineteenth or early twentieth century neurologists, like Binswanger's disease, Lewy body dementia, and Creutzfeldt-Jakob disease. Regardless of the type of dementia, it will produce abnormal-

ities on your relative's mental status examination and the more advanced the dementia, the greater the degree of abnormality.

You will learn about the ingredients of the most common mental status examinations if you accompany your family member to the doctor, especially if the appointment is with a neurolo-gist, psychiatrist, or geriatrician. But it's helpful to get a sense of what the questions are as well as what areas of cognition they are testing. One of the most popular mental status examina-tions is the Folstein Mini-Mental State Exam (MMSE), which asks eight ques-tions and is scored from zero to thirty. It tests orientation to time and place, attention, calculation, recall, language, and visuospatial skills. Even though the test has been around since 1975, it is still copyright protected. Technically, clinicians must pay a fee to administer the exam and document the results. Because of the financial obstacles and because of concerns that the MMSE is not valid in people with limited ed-ucation, many doctors prefer other tests. One widely used alternative is the Montreal Cognitive Assessment tool, or MoCA. Like the MMSE, this is a ten-minute test scored from zero to thirty. It tests slightly different domains from the MMSE: it also tests language, short-term memory, attention, and concentration, but, in addition, it tests the ability to process and understand visual information, along with higher functions (so-called executive function, or problem-solving ability).

You may be well aware that your family member has some degree of im-pairment, but her physician does not.

Or, you may know your relative is not as sharp as she once was but not be aware just how profoundly off-kilter her cognitive function is. For example, many people compensate for their deficits by using circumlocutions when they can't remember a name or they change the subject when they don't know the answer to a question. I find it very useful to have the caregiver in the room when the patient has a mental status exam. You may find seeing what areas your family member has difficulty with extremely illuminating.

The Role of Psychological Factors in Determining Health

Another neglected but equally important ingredient of the overall health state is the *emotional state*. Anxiety is common and can get in the way of adhering to even simple recommendations for healthy behavior. If your relative is afraid of falling, a specific form of anxiety, she may deliberately limit her own mobility. If she has agoraphobia, she is likely to avoid public transportation and may end up a recluse. Perhaps the most common and most significant mental health problem in older people is depression. Depression can make the treatment of other physical conditions very challenging; it can worsen the symptoms of dementia; and it has a profound effect on overall well-being.

As with dementia, you may think you know if your family member is depressed or not. Sometimes you will be right and, in fact, you may pick up on subtle clues long before the doctor does. Other times you may miss the telltale symptoms, perhaps attributing your family member's passivity to normal aging, to fatigue, or to dementia. When the diagnosis is unclear, it's useful for the doctor or nurse to perform a screening test for depression.

One of the most widely used screening tools is the Geriatric Depression Scale, created by Dr. Jerome Yesavage, a psychiatrist at Stanford University (box 2.1). Because its development was supported by federal government research grants, the scale is in the public domain, which means it can be used freely by clinicians everywhere. It consists of fifteen yes/no questions. A score of five or more suggests your relative has depression and a score of ten or more is diagnostic. Anyone who tests in the suggestive range should be evaluated more fully and anyone who is diagnosed with depression should be treated.

The good news is that depression can often be effectively treated—we now have antidepressant medications that work in most people. Moreover, the side effects are often minimal, or at least it is usually possible to find a drug that is both effective and well-tolerated. Since your family member may attach a stigma to a mental health diagnosis and prefer to avoid psychiatric medication, your job will be to convince her that taking an antidepressant doesn't mean she's crazy but does offer possible relief from debilitating symptoms.

I'll talk more about the symptoms of depression later (see chapter 31, "Depression"). Suffice it to say that depression has a profound effect on the quality of life. Depression makes people apathetic: they may be so apathetic that they are mistakenly thought to have dementia. Depression interacts with physical problems such as difficulty with vision or mobility to diminish the social

Box 2.1

Geriatric Depression Scale: Short Form

Choose the best answer for how you have felt over the past week:

1. Are you basically satisfied with your life? YES/**NO**

2. Have you dropped many of your activities and interests? **YES**/NO

3. Do you feel that your life is empty? **YES**/NO

4. Do you often get bored? **YES**/NO

5. Are you in good spirits most of the time? YES/**NO**

6. Are you afraid that something bad is going to happen to you? **YES**/NO

7. Do you feel happy most of the time? YES/**NO**

8. Do you often feel helpless? **YES**/NO

9. Do you prefer to stay at home, rather than going out and doing new things? **YES**/NO

10. Do you feel you have more problems with memory than most? **YES**/NO

11. Do you think it is wonderful to be alive now? YES/**NO**

12. Do you feel pretty worthless the way you are now? **YES**/NO

13. Do you feel full of energy? YES/**NO**

14. Do you feel that your situation is hopeless? **YES**/NO

15. Do you think that most people are better off than you are? **YES**/NO

Answers in bold indicate depression. Score 1 point for each bolded answer.

A score > 5 points is suggestive of depression.

A score ≥ 10 points is almost always indicative of depression.

A score > 5 points should warrant a follow-up comprehensive assessment.

interactions that are the main source of meaning and satisfaction for many people. And depression is a killer. The suicide rate among white men over age sixty-five is three times that of the national average. The suicide rate among white men over age eighty-five is higher than in any other group in the United States, causing more than fifty out of every one hundred thousand deaths, most commonly due to guns.

What you also need to remember is that, although depression is common in older people and takes a heavy toll, as many as 60 percent of cases go undiagnosed. Your role as an advocate means you have to be alert to any possible symptoms of depression and report them to your family member's physician. Don't let the doctor dismiss telltale signs as due to dementia or hearing loss or any of a host of other medical problems. They *might* be due to concomitant illnesses, but they *might* be due to depression. It's worth investigating.

Determining the Overall Health State

Physical functioning, cognitive functioning, and *emotional functioning* all come together with medical conditions or diseases to determine the overall health state. They also interact to affect how well your family member carries out the somewhat more sophisticated functions—more sophisticated than those measured with the Katz ADL scale—that are also essential for a person to get by. Not surprisingly, there's another scale that measures this sort of activity and quantifies just how needy your family member is. The best known of these scales, tools that measure the "instrumental activities of daily living" (IADLs), is the Lawton scale, devised by the behavioral psychologist, M. Powell Lawton, together with his colleague E. M. Brody, in 1969 (see table 2.2). Lawton was the director of research at a teaching nursing home, the Philadelphia Geriatric Center, for thirty years and was well aware of what makes older people dependent. This scale is more complex than the Katz ADL scale. It has eight items, rather than six, and while each domain is scored as zero or one, like on the ADL scale, the definition of what constitutes independence is more complicated. Take the first item, the ability to use the telephone. This measure is going to need to change now that push-button phones have replaced dial phones, and cell phones and smart phones are increasingly superseding landlines altogether. But you can get an idea of how the scale works: *Any* kind of phone use counts as independence, even though this could mean the ability to look up a phone number and place a call, it could mean using speed dial, or it

Table 2.2

Lawton Instrumental Activities of Daily Living Scale

1. Telephone Use
Can look up and call some or all telephone numbers independently 1
Answers telephone but cannot make calls 0
Can never use telephone without help 0

2. Shopping
Can shop independently for small or large items 1
Needs assistance shopping 0
Unable to go shopping, even with help 0

3. Food Preparation
Plans, prepares, serves meals independently 1
Can prepare meals but intake inadequate 0
Needs meals prepared, served 0

4. Housekeeping
Maintains home independently, except heavy work 1
Does light housework such as washing dishes 1
Needs partial or complete help with all housework 1

5. Laundry
Does laundry independently 1
Can wash small items such as socks, underwear 1
Unable to do personal laundry 0

6. Transportation
Uses public transportation or drives own car 1
Can arrange for taxi or shared ride but does not use public transportation 1
Cannot travel, or travels only with help 0

7. Medication Use
Takes medications correctly 1
Needs help preparing or dispensing medication 0

8. Handling of Finances
Manages all finances independently, including paying bills and writing checks 1
Takes care of small purchases but needs help with banking and major purchases 1
Cannot handle money independently 0

For each category, choose best description of person's highest level of functioning and rate (0 or 1). Summary score ranges from 0 (dependent) to 8 (independent).

Sources: M. P. Lawton and E. M. Brody, "Assessment of Older People: Self-Maintaining and Instrumental Activities of Daily Living," *The Gerontologist* 9, no. 3 (1969): 179–186; copyright © The Gerontological Society of America. Reproduced [Adapted] by permission of the publisher.

could mean just answering the phone. Inability to use a phone entirely is considered *dependence*. The other areas are just as nuanced—and just as important. They are shopping, food preparation, housekeeping, doing the laundry, taking transportation, medication management, and financial management.

What you probably realize in studying the list of IADLs is that each one requires a variety of physical and cognitive functions to carry out. For example, food preparation requires gross motor control to go from refrigerator to counter to stove and it requires fine motor control to cut, slice, or dice food. It demands good enough vision to read labels and measure the quantities of ingredients. Cooking necessitates a certain amount of safety awareness. Even heating food in the microwave entails realizing whether the container with the food is "microwave safe."

Understanding your family member's overall health state is more complicated than adding up measures of physical functioning, mental health, cognition and the number of diseases. All these components interact in sometimes subtle and sometimes obvious ways. That's why someone with mild dementia might be able to manage reasonably independently, just requiring some help with finances and other higher-level functions, but if she has macular degeneration (causing visual impairment) and Parkinson's disease (resulting in difficulty using the bathroom) in addition, then she might no longer be able to compensate for her weaknesses in some domains with strengths in others. Your family member's physician should assemble all the pieces for you so you can see the big picture. Your job is to make sure you understand each of the constituent parts listed in box 2.2 and that you *ask* about health state, recalling that the whole may be more than the sum of the parts.

Box 2.2

Components of the Health State

- Diseases

- Physical functioning

- Emotional factors

- Cognition

CHAPTER 3

Thinking like a Geriatrician

Geriatric Syndromes

If you're going to be in charge of your family member's health, or at least of his health care, you should probably take a page from the geriatrician's playbook. Geriatricians think differently from other kinds of doctors. We look at the whole person, not just a bunch of organs such as the heart, kidneys, and brain. As I mentioned earlier, this means paying attention to the overall health state, which is determined by physical function, cognition, and the emotional state as well as individual diseases. But what's unique about geriatricians is not just the holistic focus—other physicians, such as palliative care doctors, share that orientation—and it's not just the emphasis on function, although that is another crucial difference. It's also the focus on what are

called *geriatric syndromes*. These are groups of symptoms that aren't necessarily the result of a specific disease involving a single organ system. They typically arise from the interaction of several different systems. Often, they have little to do with the organ you may initially think is affected—incontinence may not be due to a bladder problem and acute confusion may be unrelated to a brain disease. I'm going to tell you a little about several of the most common geriatric syndromes: delirium, falls, incontinence, and polypharmacy (taking many medications). Dementia and depression, which are often considered geriatric syndromes, fit more neatly into traditional disease categorization and will be discussed in the chapters on the most common chronic diseases.

Delirium

If your relative has delirium, he has difficulty paying *attention*. You will find that you can't get him to focus. Moreover, this inattentiveness comes and goes over the course of a day: one minute, your family member is his usual self, the next minute his mind wanders. In fact, he is often quite sleepy and might doze off in the middle of a conversation. Paradoxically, some delirious people are unusually alert rather than sleepy. The technical term is that they have hyperactive rather than hypoactive delirium. While all of these symptoms wax and wane, the initial onset is *sudden* rather than gradual. The final problem, which explains why this syndrome is also referred to as an *acute confusional state*, is the inability to think straight, known as "disorganized thinking." You may find that your family member has trouble figuring out that he has to put his socks on before his shoes. He stares at the socks and shoes and doesn't know what to do with them—even though normally, he can dress himself.

That's the portrait of delirium—someone who fairly abruptly shows trouble thinking and paying attention, who may be unusually sleepy or uncharacteristically jumpy, but whose symptoms fluctuate over the day. It sounds straightforward, but it is often mistaken for dementia, especially by physicians who don't know the patient. Disorganized thinking, after all, is part of dementia as well as delirium. And if

the clinician doesn't evaluate the patient several times over the course of a few hours, she may miss the waxing and waning that is characteristic of dementia. But you, as the caregiver, know what your family member's baseline is; you will be aware of sudden changes; and you typically see your family member sufficiently frequently to pick up the variations in level of alertness. That means you are uniquely qualified to detect delirium early and potentially to stop it in its tracks.

The most common single cause of delirium is probably *medication*. Multiple different classes of medicines have a high propensity to precipitate delirium. One such class is called anticholinergic medications: this includes all sorts of drugs from tricyclic antidepressants to over-the-counter cold preparations. Antianxiety medications such as the benzodiazepines are another class of drugs that can result in delirium, particularly those that are very long-lasting, such as diazepam (brand name Valium). Pain medications, especially drugs such as morphine and oxycodone, form another group of medications that are big-time offenders. And the list continues.

Not only can medicines produce delirium, so can infection. Pneumonia can result in delirium as can a bladder infection. In fact, your family member might not have any other sign of an infection *other* than delirium: He might not develop a fever or a cough even though he has pneumonia, and he might not have pain on urinating even though he has a urinary tract infection.

Any of a variety of chemical imbalances, often referred to as metabolic abnormalities, can also trigger delirium. Dehydration is common in older people and severe dehydration typically causes blood chemistries such as the sodium level to be off-kilter. Unfortunately, older people often don't experience thirst, so the first sign of dehydration could be acute confusion. An abnormally high calcium (as occurs sometimes with bone metastases from cancer) or a very low calcium (as happens with certain glandular problems such as a malfunctioning parathyroid gland) can also result in delirium. While metastases to the bones typically cause pain, in fact rather severe pain, confusion from an elevated calcium may be the first manifestation of this problem.

The most effective treatment of delirium is treatment of the underlying cause or causes, whether by removing the offending medication, treating the precipitating infection with antibiotics, or correcting the triggering metabolic abnormality by giving plenty to drink. If you live with your family member, visit him regularly, or telephone frequently, you have a good chance of intervening promptly enough to make a difference.

Delirium is often extremely unpleasant for your relative. The disorganized thinking found in delirium may take the form of hallucinations or delusions—seeing or hearing things that aren't real or believing untruths—that can be frightening or alarming. True, your family member might have pleasant hallucinations: I remember one patient who was convinced there was a very sweet child in her room with her. Delusions may also be comforting: I had one patient who was convinced I was her favorite aunt. But more often, your relative with delirium will see demons or wild animals or think he is being poisoned. Delirium is also distressing for you as the caregiver to witness. Your good-natured, appreciative family member is abruptly transformed into someone who is paranoid, uncooperative, and confused. None of your strategies for soothing or reassuring him seem to work. He needs to be watched like a hawk since his judgment is impaired; he's so befuddled and sleepy that he's apt to spill hot tea on himself or fall when he gets up to go to the bathroom. Over and beyond how disturbing delirium is both for you and its victim, it's dangerous. Hospitalized patients with delirium are far more likely to die in the next year than their counterparts of the same age who don't develop delirium, even when every effort is made to adjust for differences in how sick they were. They also stay in the hospital longer and are more likely to need to go to a rehab facility after discharge.

Because delirium has such serious consequences, it is sometimes called a medical emergency. But you should realize that early detection and prompt intervention can make an enormous difference in the outcome of this disorder. Full-blown delirium in the hospital setting is extremely serious. That doesn't mean, however, that if you see signs of incipient delirium in the home setting you should rush to the nearest hospital emergency department with your family member. It does mean that you should know what delirium involves so you can be vigilant and report your concerns to your family member's doctor promptly. Together, you can decide whether an empiric approach makes sense or whether a comprehensive evaluation is appropriate. With an empiric approach, for example, you would stop a new medication, begin a course of antibiotics for a probable bladder infection, or vigorously treat constipation (severe constipation can cause delirium), depending on the circumstances. An extensive evaluation in the emergency department, by contrast, will include a physical examination and blood tests, and often a chest x-ray, computerized tomography (CT) scan, or magnetic resonance imaging (MRI) of the brain as well.

Usually doctors think of the role of caregivers as strictly preventive. Once delirium actually sets in, they figure, treatment is up to the medical team. I think about this situation a bit differently: I view you as *a crucial part of the medical team*. Standard treatment, apart from determining and then eliminating whatever caused the delirium, entails use of powerful antipsychotic medications such as haloperidol (brand name Haldol) or its second-generation variants such as quetiapine (brand name Seroquel). It focuses on trying to keep your relative safe while the delirium gradually abates, which sometimes includes physical restraints—jargon for tying him to the bed or chair. Antipsychotic drugs have side effects; in particular, they can be sedating, they can cause dizziness, and they may lead to

falls. Tying down your family member, leaving aside the question of whether it is an effective strategy, violates his dignity. Your family member may be floridly delirious, he may think he's on another planet, but he may nonetheless perceive restraints as a monumental infringement on his freedom. There is another, far more humane way to treat delirium.

Instead of starting with chemical and physical restraints—psychotropic drugs are just restraints in the form of a pill—try the human touch first. In progressive hospitals, the staff will utilize a "sitter," an aide to stay with your relative. Even better than a hired assistant is a known and beloved caregiver—you. And rather than taking the environment as a given, modify your family member's surroundings. If he keeps getting out of bed and you're worried he will fall—falling is the next geriatric syndrome we will get to shortly—put the mattress on the floor. It's a good deal harder to hurt yourself when you're only six inches from the floor. Ideally, keep your family member at home, where the surroundings are familiar, rather than admitting him to the hospital, where everything is unfamiliar and potentially frightening. You may think that since you don't know as much as the nurses and doctors, surely your family member would be better off in a medical facility. Maybe. But, if you are able to handle the medical complexities, you should consider taking care of your family member at home. Your familiar presence and knowledge of your family member contribute to the treatment. (For more about the evaluation of delirium, see chapter 38, "Confusion.")

Causes of Delirium

D Drugs (and alcohol)
Opioids
Antianxiety drugs (benzodiazepines)
Antipsychotics
Antidepressants
Antihistamines

E Electrolytes
Low sodium
Acute kidney injury
High calcium
Low blood sugar

L Lack of drugs
Pain
Withdrawal from drugs or alcohol
Recent dose reductions

I Infection

R Reduced sensory input
Lack of sight—no glasses, visual impairment due to stroke
Lack of hearing—no hearing aids, noisy environment

I Intracranial pathology
Bleeding in the brain (subdural hematoma)
Brain tumor
Confusion after seizures
Brain infection (encephalitis)

U Urinary or fecal retention
Constipation (can lead to urinary retention and urinary infection)
Pain/distress from constipation/retention

M Medical
Heart attack
Liver failure
Kidney failure

Falls

By the time they reach eighty, many people are anxious about falling. They know, and you as a caregiver know, that a bad fall can denote the beginning of the end. Falling isn't exclusively an orthopedic issue, though it's usually the orthopedist who is called if a fracture results; nor is it a just a neurologic issue, though many people who have fallen get a CT scan of the brain, either looking for the cause or the result of the fall. And it's not strictly a cardiac issue, though a heartbeat that's either very fast or very slow can result in fainting or falling. Falls are a classic geriatric syndrome: They are very common in older adults, they typically result from the interaction of multiple underlying factors, and they often have a major impact on quality of life.

Making sure your relative doesn't unintentionally hit ground (that's what falling is) requires the coordination of a whole host of systems. It involves balance and judgment. It requires muscle strength. It's useful to have good vision and intact sensation in his feet, as well as what is called proprioception—awareness of where his feet are. These are all the internal factors that prevent falling. There are also external factors that make a difference such as good lighting and proper footwear.

A single fall can wreak havoc; it is also the best predictor of subsequent falls. Moreover, once your family member has had a bad fall, he may be so frightened of having another one that the fear gets in the way of going out and doing things he enjoys. The resulting social isolation causes other problems such as depression. So, what can you do to prevent falls?

The most obvious things you can do are the kind of interventions that an occupational therapist would recommend during a "home safety evaluation," something that you might in fact want to request. This approach looks at factors outside your family member (exogenous factors) that contribute to the risk of falling: the classic example is throw rugs. My mother used to like putting scatter rugs in various places in her home to protect her carpet or even the bare wood floor. After I had explained to her several times how hazardous these were—they slide around and they're easy to trip on—and she politely ignored me, I finally went around her apartment scooping up all the rugs and took them to the basement and hid them. A related issue is clutter. People tend to accumulate stuff in their homes. Not surprisingly, older people have more stuff than younger people since they've had longer to acquire things. Unfortunately, having lots of knickknacks or end tables or stacks of newspapers means a greater opportunity to bump into something on the way from, say, the living room sofa to the front door.

One suggestion for a useful intervention that might not be met with much resistance from your family member is obtaining better lighting. Aging eyes may need as much as ten times greater illumination than youthful eyes for reading or other activities. Although your family member might not let you buy more lamps for him, or won't turn them on if you do, he probably won't protest if you replace all the bulbs with higher wattage variants. You will want to install railings along staircases and grab bars in the bathroom so your family member has something reliable to hold onto.

A few more measures you should consider don't involve modifying the outside world but rather affect the way your family member relates to his environment. Number one on the list is proper footwear. The importance of footwear is vastly underrated. Wearing socks without shoes is a bad idea especially on slippery surfaces such as bathrooms and kitchens. And a major culprit in falling, especially in women, turns out to be shoes that don't fit well or have high heels. A good pair of well-cushioned shoes can go a long way to preventing falls. If your relative considers sturdy, Oxford-style shoes esthetically unappealing, you can point out that running shoes seem to be all the rage. If shoelaces are problematic because your relative does not have the dexterity to tie them, Velcro straps may be a satisfactory alternative.

In addition to good shoes, think about assistive devices such as a cane or walker. Your family member may resist the idea, complaining that it makes him feel old. He probably worries that using a device will draw attention to his deficits. You may have noticed that in assisted living facilities, not to mention nursing homes, most of the residents use a cane or a walker. That's partly because institutions have a high proportion of people with mobility problems, but it's also because device use is socially acceptable. It's the norm. Everyone does it. Suddenly, the stigma vanishes. If your family member lives in an independent setting and has balance problems, you probably want to try to persuade him to swallow his pride. The alternative may be a hip fracture.

Along with thinking about the ways that the external environment poses risks, you should be alert to a variety of health conditions—internal factors—that can predispose to falling. Impaired vision can cause falls, at least indirectly by resulting in your family member missing a step or miscalculating distance. In many cases, vision can be improved with new glasses or by cataract surgery. I am generally skeptical of surgical intervention in frail, old people, but cataract surgery is a glaring exception. Almost no one is too old or too debilitated for cataract surgery. Of course, your relative should have a long enough life expectancy to make even a minor procedure worthwhile and if he is nearly blind from some other problem such as macular degeneration then cataract surgery may have nothing to offer. You should also realize that virtually everyone who lives long enough will get cataracts. The age of onset is highly variable—I have friends in their sixties who have already had cataract surgery in both eyes, while my ninety-two-year-old mother has had one cataract removed, her other eye is perfectly fine. Just as I'm not enthusiastic about procedures in older people, similarly I'm reluctant to see a frail, elderly person go to multiple specialists. Eye doctors are an exception. Whatever else you do, make sure your family member has a good eye exam.

Another health issue that plays a role in falls is osteoporosis or thinning of the bones. Strictly speaking, this doesn't cause falls, but it may result in breaking a bone if your family member does fall. There are sophisticated ways to measure bone density or the thickness of various bones, tests that your relative's doctor may wish to order, and there are potentially beneficial but possibly toxic medications that she may prescribe in select circumstances. What you can do is make sure that your family member gets adequate vitamin D, which is essential for bone health. Opinions about just what amount is recommended have changed over time but most authorities currently suggest eight hundred units of vitamin D—for some reason, vitamin D is measured in units rather than milligrams. It's also worth pointing out that this goes for men as well as women. While women get a head start on men in developing osteoporosis—bone density typically begins to decline after menopause—men don't escape the scourge. About one-quarter of hip fractures occur in men and hip fractures are generally associated with osteoporosis.

I don't want to suggest that medications are the source of all evil—medications can be both life-saving and quality-of-life-enhancing—but they are also fraught with risk. In particular, they are a leading cause of falls, so beware. Any medication that affects cognition or is sedating, whether deliberately or as a side effect, can result in a fall. That makes antianxiety drugs and antidepressants major offenders. Other medications may contribute to falls because they are associated with dizziness: a number of drugs for high blood pressure or to treat angina are notorious for causing dizziness. What's especially tricky is that although you have to be especially vigilant about monitoring for side effects when your family member starts a new medication, you can't let down your guard just because he's gone a month without any problems. Diuretics, for example, one of the mainstays of treatment for high blood pressure as well as for congestive heart failure, may be well-tolerated—until your family member goes out in

the hot sun and gets a little dehydrated. Neither the lack of fluids nor the medicines alone would have gotten him into trouble, but the combination is a fall waiting to happen.

Last but not least, certain disorders such as Parkinson's disease specifically affect gait and balance. If your family member is falling a lot, his physician should evaluate him for evidence of Parkinson's or some other neurological disorder—a stroke, for example, can cause weakness on one side of the body, leading to falls. But if he has been diagnosed with Parkinson's and is receiving treatment, you should watch for worsening of his walking. Such changes may mean he needs an adjustment in the dose of his medicine (both too much and too little medication, paradoxically, can cause problems) or that he would benefit from a different drug entirely. Sometimes the changes are subtle, so only his caregiver will notice. Reporting what you observe can prevent a hip or wrist fracture.

One more word about preventing falls. There's now reasonably good data indicating that Tai Chi can help preserve balance and prevent falls. Some studies have found the fall rate to decrease by nearly 50 percent. I don't expect you to teach your family member Tai Chi yourself, but you could put in a good word for the class at the neighborhood senior center.

Causes of Falls

- **Impaired Vision:** Cataracts and glaucoma alter depth perception, visual acuity, peripheral vision, and susceptibility to glare.

Solution: Add color and contrast to identify objects, such as grab bars and handrails.

- **Home Hazards:** Most homes have falling hazards.

  Solution: Add grab bars in the bathroom, install proper railings on both sides of stairways, improve the lighting, remove loose rugs, and fix uneven or cracked sidewalks.

- **Medication:** Many drugs (for example, sedatives, antidepressants) reduce mental alertness, affect balance and gait, and cause a fall in systolic blood pressure when going from sitting to standing. Mixing certain medications increases these effects, causing falls.

Solution: Have a home care professional carefully monitor medications and look for interactions.

- **Weakness, Poor Balance:** Weakness and lack of mobility lead to many falls.

  Solution: Exercise regularly to boost strength and muscle tone.

- **Chronic Conditions:** Parkinson's, heart disease, and other conditions increase the risk of falling.

  Solution: Enlist specially trained caregivers to ensure that patients follow their treatment plans, assist them to doctor appointments, and recognize red flags.

Incontinence

Incontinence is another major geriatric syndrome. It sounds as though it's just a symptom, presumably a symptom of some larger condition, much as a runny nose is either a symptom of a cold or of an allergy. But like other geriatric syndromes, it's common in old people, rare in young or middle-aged people, and is often caused by several different factors, making it "multifactorial." And as all caregivers know, if your family member has incontinence it looms large in his life, affecting his care needs, his quality of life, and even where he lives.

As with most other geriatric syndromes, incontinence comes in several varieties. Incontinence can be due to urge, stress, or overflow; it might be due to a combination of factors; or it could be related to difficulty getting to the bathroom. Probably the most common form is *urge incontinence*. That's where your family member has a sudden sensation of needing to go—and then immediately loses his urine before he has time to make it to the bathroom. The most familiar type is *stress incontinence*, in which your relative loses his urine when he coughs or strains. This problem is especially common in women, whose muscles may have been weakened by childbirth, but it is found in men as well. In *overflow incontinence*, there's trouble emptying the bladder, so it just gets fuller and fuller, like a balloon filled with water, until the pressure in the bag is so great that it overcomes the resistance at the bladder outlet and urine dribbles out. This type of incontinence is particularly common in men, who often develop an enlarged prostate gland that prevents the bladder from emptying. *Functional incontinence* is the technical name for a problem that has little to do with urinating and everything to do with mobility: if your relative can't get to the bathroom in time, whether because of paralysis (perhaps resulting from a stroke), physical restraints (perhaps instituted because of delirium), or because he moves slowly, and if he can't access a bedpan, eventually he will have no choice but to urinate in the chair or bed. Finally, there's *mixed incontinence*, which just means it's not exclusively one type or another but rather a bit of two or more kinds of incontinence.

Your role as a caregiver isn't to diagnose incontinence. But it is, first and foremost, to make sure the problem is brought to the attention of your family member's physician. Doctors have an annoying habit of not asking about continence and patients are often too embarrassed to report it. Doctors don't ask because they are often ill-equipped to make a diagnosis themselves: even gynecologists and urologists may have only a rudimentary familiarity with the diagnosis and treatment of this principally geriatric problem, and primary care doctors even less. This is one situation where your family member is best off with a geriatrician—at least to see in consultation. Your role in the evaluation of incontinence, other than bringing up the topic, is to help clarify the history. Various tests may help the doctor determine what kind of incontinence your family member has, but the single, most crucial piece of information is the *history*, the explanation of when the problem occurs. Ideally, your family member will provide the history. Sometimes, his physician will request that he keep a log to document whenever the problem occurs and to spell out what was going on at the time. But often telling the story suffices.

Once the physician has a good handle on what type of incontinence your family member is experiencing and initiates treatment, you may have a role in implementing the treatment plan. For example, one strategy for treating urge incontinence is regular "toileting." This means going to the bathroom approximately every two hours. If your relative has urge incontinence, he has voluntary control over voiding but also suffers from involuntary spasms that force urine out at unwanted moments, so a regimen of frequent bladder emptying may help by preventing the urine from accumulating.

Personal hygiene is a major issue if your family member is incontinent. You may be in the best position to institute a system of bathing and laundry that helps keep your relative comfortable and odor-free. You will need to figure out together whether that system should involve a third party. Providing personal care is a whole different ball game from making doctor's appointments or going shopping for groceries. You want to help your family member retain his dignity—without yourself contributing to a diminished sense of self. This may mean it would be better to hire a home health aide to help with toileting and bathing than to undertake these tasks yourself. A neutral third party whose job description includes these responsibilities may make a lot of sense—if you can afford to do it and if you find the right person. Gender often plays a significant role here. It's rare for a man to feel comfortable helping his mother shower; a woman may similarly feel conflicted about bathing her father. But men helping men and women helping women are not necessarily conflict-free. I can't tell you what the right answer is, just that you need to talk about this openly with your relative.

Causes of Incontinence

Mnemonic: DIAPERS

Delirium
Infection of the bladder or urethra
Atrophic vaginitis
Pharmaceuticals, including alcohol, caffeine and artificial sweeteners
Excess excretion
Restricted mobility
Stool impaction

Polypharmacy (Lots of Medications)

Some people include "polypharmacy" when they list geriatric syndromes. It's not quite in the same category as incontinence or falls, but it is a problem that arises frequently in older people—and one that the discipline of geriatrics pays particular attention to. Polypharmacy is problematic for a number of reasons. Lots of drugs may mean high cost—taking nine or ten different prescription drugs can be a financial hardship. You don't want your family member choosing between taking his medications and eating lunch or turning up the thermostat. A complicated drug regimen may be difficult for him to follow. I once had a patient with Parkinson's disease who was told by her neurologist to take a pill every two hours. That approach was, in principle, superior to using long-acting medicines, but it was virtually impossible for her to follow. All medications carry the risk of side effects so the more medications your relative takes, the greater the risk of one or more side effects. Finally, drugs sometimes interact with one another, so if your family member takes lots of medicines, odds are one or another will cause some problem with a different one.

Medication management, whether your family member takes one medicine or ten, is probably going to be a key issue for you. It is for the vast majority of family caregivers—nearly 80 percent of people who say they provide some kind of medical or nursing function for their family member report they deal with medications. And the more medicines your family member is on, the greater your responsibility. Medications are pivotal to your family member's health and well-being: the right medicines can significantly improve his lot and the wrong medicines can cause disaster. You may think that I'm biased because I'm a medical doctor and arguably most of what medical doctors do is to prescribe drugs. But any bias aside, medications are *objectively* invaluable to older people. They can cure problems such as pneumonia; they can make up for a deficient hormone, as with diabetes or an underactive thyroid gland; they can help people breathe if they have asthma or emphysema; they can remove unwanted and dangerous extra fluid in people with heart failure—the list goes on and on. As a result, medicines can keep your relative out of the hospital; they are recognized as so important—and sometimes so expensive—that they are now covered by Medicare (if you purchase a Medicare Part D plan).

What do you need to know about medication? I remember reading a study of care in rest homes years ago, in which the author was shocked to discover that the nursing assistants who dispensed medications didn't know a thing about them. I thought at the time, but do patients know about the pills they take? Do families know? The right inference, I think, is that *someone* intimately involved in the administration of medications needs to know what they're being given for, what the side effects are, and how to look for signs of over- or underdosing. Patients who have the necessary wherewithal can keep track of their own medicines.

Anyone who has a caregiver, whether paid or unpaid, whether a family member or someone else, should expect that someone to be knowledgeable in the same way.

The reality is that not only is polypharmacy a geriatric syndrome, but polypharmacy can be the cause of most other geriatric syndromes. Certain medications, including some antihistamines and some antidepressants, can cause delirium; sedating medication such as antianxiety drugs can cause falls; and diuretics (called "fluid pills" because they result in the excretion of fluid) can cause incontinence. That's the wonderful world of geriatrics—everything is related to everything else, and caregivers are the jugglers-in-chief.

Since medications are so very important, I'm going to suggest that you learn a little bit of geriatric pharmacology. Not a whole lot of technical material, but enough to make it easier to understand and remember crucial bits of information relating to each of the medicines your family member takes. For a drug to work, it has to get into your relative's system. Most medications for home use are taken by mouth (there are some notable exceptions, such as those that come in a patch and are absorbed through the skin). For oral medicines to have any chance of doing what they're supposed to do, they have to be swallowed and make it down to the stomach. That turns out to be no small matter if your relative has dementia or Parkinson's disease or a stroke—these disorders all result in trouble swallowing. Sometimes a liquid will go down when a pill won't. Sometimes the pill can be ground up and taken in applesauce the way you give pills to a young child. Once your family member successfully swallows the medication, it will usually reach the stomach without difficulty—unless your family member has "gastric outlet obstruction" (a blockage from an ulcer or tumor) or even very severe "gastroparesis" (inability of the stomach to push food into the intestine, often associated with severe diabetes). From the stomach, medicine has to be absorbed into the bloodstream and distributed to wherever it's supposed to go. Absorption is seldom a problem in old age, though again there are some exceptions: when you read on the pill bottle that a medicine shouldn't be taken with food, that generally means that it won't be absorbed properly if it is.

Once the drug has reached the bloodstream the potential problems begin. Drugs often bind to proteins in the bloodstream—they lock onto receptors on the surface of albumin, the major protein found in the blood, like a key into a lock—and it's only the "free drug," the drug that is left over after all the protein binding sites are filled up, that is effective in treating whatever condition it's been prescribed to treat. What this means is that if your family member is profoundly malnourished and has a very low amount of albumin in his blood, the binding sites will be used up very quickly. Translation: A lower than usual dose of medication will be enough to do the job, and the standard dose of medication can cause side effects.

Getting the drug to where it needs to go can be problematic for another reason: some parts of the body such as the brain have a special barrier to keep out substances that don't belong. The brain may keep a drug out even though the medication has to reach the brain to work—if, for example, it is being used to treat cancer that has spread to the brain or to treat an infection involving the central nervous system. As a result, the medicine either won't work or has to be given in extremely high doses to ensure that at least some of it gets past the "blood-brain barrier."

The distribution of drugs, that is what happens to them once they reach the bloodstream, is also affected by whether the drug is "lipophilic" (literally, fat-loving) or "hydrophilic" (water-loving). Lipophilic drugs will be absorbed by fat, which functions as a kind of slow-release system. Over time, as the level in the blood falls, the drug will make its way from the fat into the blood. The net effect is that lipophilic drugs such as diazepam (brand name Valium) can hang around for a very, very long time.

The last piece of pharmacology for you to know relates to the metabolism and excretion of drugs. The reason that medications have to be taken at regular intervals is that they are constantly being destroyed and eliminated from the body. There are two main places where this happens: the liver and the kidneys. This is useful to know because as your relative ages, he will probably develop some degree of kidney malfunction; even in "normal" aging, the kidney function is diminished. The result is that the dose of medication needs to be reduced, otherwise toxicity (side effects) is very likely. Knowing whether your family member has renal impairment, and if so whether it's mild, moderate, or severe, will help you be alert to the need for dosage modification of many drugs. You also need to understand that some medicines are broken down, "metabolized," by the liver. In those cases, assuming the metabolized version of the drug is harmless, the presence or absence of kidney problems is unimportant. However, what does matter is whether the liver is working normally. Liver function is typically preserved in older people— unlike kidney function—except with certain conditions such as cirrhosis of the liver or multiple liver metastases from cancer. Needless to say, there is more to geriatric pharmacology than what I've mentioned, but I think this basic understanding will stand you in good stead.

Odds are that your family member will have one or more of the geriatric syndromes I reviewed in this chapter (box 3.1) and is at risk of developing others. You will find that familiarizing yourself with the major geriatric syndromes—falls, incontinence, delirium, and polypharmacy, as well as depression and dementia, which I discuss later on (see chapter 29, "Alzheimer's Disease and Other Dementias," and chapter 31, "Depression")—is a good investment. You don't need an RN or MD degree to serve as an effective partner with your family member's physician, but you will greatly benefit from knowing the lay of the land. You will be better at your job, and you'll find it a good deal easier, emotionally and intellectually, if you develop a modicum of geriatric expertise.

Box 3.1

Geriatric Syndromes

- Delirium
- Falls
- Incontinence
- Polypharmacy
- Dementia
- Depression

CHAPTER 4

Determining Your Family Member's Health State

I have emphasized that, as a caregiver, you need to understand your family member's overall health state, what I call the big picture. I said that older people can be characterized as *"robust, frail, has dementia, or is dying."* I also suggested that *physical functioning, cognitive functioning,* and *emotional functioning* all come together with diseases or with medical conditions—some of which may be geriatric syndromes—to determine the overall health state.

Now that we've talked about the various types of functioning and geriatric syndromes, and assuming you already have a good sense of what diseases your family member has, it's time to put all the pieces together. Your family member's doctor should be the one to determine if she's robust, frail, has dementia, or is dying. But once you are familiar with all the ingredients of the health state you will be in a better position to understand just *why* your family member meets the criteria for her particular overall state. And just in case your family member's physician is

not forthcoming with the big picture, you are now equipped to formulate your own sense of your family member's general condition—and then seek confirmation from her physician.

So how do we arrive at a sense of your relative's underlying health state from information about her diseases (what they are and how severe they are), her physical functioning, her emotional functioning, and her cognition? There's no neat little point system that lets you assign a point for this and a point for that, add them all up, and arrive at a conclusion. Health status cannot be computed like the Katz Activities of Daily Living (ADL) scale or the Global Depression Scale (see chapter 2, "Ingredients of the Underlying Health State," for more on these scales), though there is something called the Charlson Comorbidity Index (comorbidities are just all the diseases that coexist in one person) that attempts to measure prognosis based solely on disease states.

The Charlson Comorbidity Index was originally designed in the 1980s as a way of quantifying how sick hospitalized patients are and how likely they are to die in the next year. Patients are given points for each disease: the riskier the disease, the greater the number of points. The current version, which has been used to predict ten-year mortality, has fifteen categories. It assigns six points for metastatic cancer, one point for heart failure, and four points for age over eighty, among other measures.

What I recommend instead is an approach that is less technical and less precise but that I think gets to the heart of the matter. I suggest reasoning backwards from each of the various possible states and, in each case, asking, does this capture who my family member is? Let's start with the extremes.

Dying

Ask yourself, does my family member have a life-threatening illness? Typically, this would be the advanced phase of a chronic condition such as cancer, heart failure, or a neurologic problem such as dementia or Parkinson's disease, but it could also be a sudden, fulminating infection or a major accident. If the answer is no, she's probably not dying—even if she is, say, ninety-five years old. If the answer is yes, then ask yourself, is my family member extremely limited in what she can do for herself? If not, if she's still reasonably independent, it's much less likely that she's going to die in the next few months than if she has reached a point where she needs most everything done for her. If, however, she has both a life-threatening disease *and* has

become very dependent, then you have to wonder how close she is to the end. Some people can continue in this state for a year or more, but however much time they have left, they are typically on the final leg of life's journey. This approach may sound vague, but it turns out that one of the most reliable ways that physicians have to predict who is nearing the end of life is to ask themselves the "surprise question": Would you be surprised if this patient died within the next year?

If they answer that they wouldn't be surprised, then even if the person lives, she is most likely approaching the end.

If you're pretty sure your family member can't be considered to be dying, ask yourself if she's got dementia.

Dementia

You can begin by asking yourself if your family member carries a diagnosis such as Alzheimer's disease, vascular dementia, or Lewy body dementia. If she does have one of these disorders or if you're already pretty confident she has dementia, ask if the cognitive impairment is severe enough to get in the way of everyday activities. Does your family member need help with more complicated tasks such as grocery shopping and food preparation and paying bills? If those are her only limitations, she may have dementia but it isn't very severe. Or does she need help with personal hygiene and getting to the bathroom? If she unambiguously has problems with say, memory, language, and judgment, and she also needs assistance in these very fundamental activities, her underlying health state is dementia. She could, of course, have very advanced dementia and be close to the end of life, but then you would have already figured out she had moved into the arena of the dying. And if she has dementia, but it's so mild that she needs only very modest assistance with matters such as handling her finances, then for purposes of this classification you may want to characterize her as robust—although straddling the fuzzy border with dementia.

If you are not sure whether your family member has dementia but you are worried that she might, you should request formal testing by her physician. I addressed briefly how physicians evaluate cognition earlier (see chapter 3, "Thinking like a Geriatrician: Geriatric Syndromes") and will discuss treatment of dementia later (see chapter 29, "Alzheimer's Disease and Other Dementias"). But if you want to have a quick and easy way of figuring out if your relative should undergo further testing for dementia, you can use the Mini-Cog (figure 4.1). This involves two tasks. First, give your relative three common words to remember, and a few minutes later ask her to repeat those words. Next, ask her to draw the face of a clock showing all twelve numbers and reading ten after eleven. That's all! There's a five-point score: one point for each word recalled correctly and two points for a satisfactory clock. A score of less than three means your family member should undergo more extensive testing. I'm always amazed at what can go wrong with the clock drawing. Sometimes people start with a circle that's much too small and simply don't have room to put in all the numbers. Another common error is to put the one and two in more or less the right places and then march off in a fairly straight line, writing three, four, five, etc., outside the clock.

Mini-Cog©

Instructions for Administration & Scoring

ID: _____ Date: _____

Step 1: Three Word Registration

Look directly at person and say, "Please listen carefully. I am going to say three words that I want you to repeat back to me now and try to remember. The words are [select a list of words from the versions below]. Please say them for me now." If the person is unable to repeat the words after three attempts, move on to Step 2 (clock drawing).

The following and other word lists have been used in one or more clinical studies.[1-3] For repeated administrations, use of an alternative word list is recommended.

Version 1	Version 2	Version 3	Version 4	Version 5	Version 6
Banana	Leader	Village	River	Captain	Daughter
Sunrise	Season	Kitchen	Nation	Garden	Heaven
Chair	Table	Baby	Finger	Picture	Mountain

Step 2: Clock Drawing

Say: "Next, I want you to draw a clock for me. First, put in all of the numbers where they go." When that is completed, say: "Now, set the hands to 10 past 11."

Use preprinted circle (see next page) for this exercise. Repeat instructions as needed as this is not a memory test. Move to Step 3 if the clock is not complete within three minutes.

Step 3: Three Word Recall

Ask the person to recall the three words you stated in Step 1. Say: "What were the three words I asked you to remember?" Record the word list version number and the person's answers below.

Word List Version: _____ Person's Answers: _____ _____ _____

Scoring

Word Recall: _____ (0-3 points)	1 point for each word spontaneously recalled without cueing.
Clock Draw: _____ (0 or 2 points)	Normal clock = 2 points. A normal clock has all numbers placed in the correct sequence and approximately correct position (e.g., 12, 3, 6 and 9 are in anchor positions) with no missing or duplicate numbers. Hands are pointing to the 11 and 2 (11:10). Hand length is not scored. Inability or refusal to draw a clock (abnormal) = 0 points.
Total Score: _____ (0-5 points)	Total score = Word Recall score + Clock Draw score. A cut point of <3 on the Mini-Cog™ has been validated for dementia screening, but many individuals with clinically meaningful cognitive impairment will score higher. When greater sensitivity is desired, a cut point of <4 is recommended as it may indicate a need for further evaluation of cognitive status.

Figure 4.1. Mini-Cog

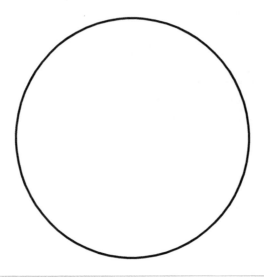

Clock Drawing

ID:_____ Date:_____

References

1. Borson S, Scanlan JM, Chen PJ et al. The Mini-Cog as a screen for dementia: Validation in a population based sample. J Am Geriatr Soc 2003;51:1451–1454.

2. Borson S, Scanlan JM, Watanabe J et al. Improving identification of cognitive impairment in primary care. Int J Geriatr Psychiatry 2006;21: 349–355.

3. Lessig M, Scanlan J et al. Time that tells: Critical clock-drawing errors for dementia screening. Int Psychogeriatr. 2008 June; 20(3): 459–470.

4. Tsoi K, Chan J et al. Cognitive tests to detect dementia: A systematic review and meta-analysis. JAMA Intern Med. 2015; E1-E9.

5. McCarten J, Anderson P et al. Screening for cognitive impairment in an elderly veteran population: Acceptability and results using different versions of the Mini-Cog. J Am Geriatr Soc 2011; 59: 309-213.

6. McCarten J, Anderson P et al. Finding dementia in primary care: The results of a clinical demonstration project. J Am Geriatr Soc 2012; 60: 210-217.

7. Scanlan J & Borson S. The Mini-Cog: Receiver operating characteristics with the expert and naive raters. Int J Geriatr Psychiatry 2001; 16: 216-222.

Figure 4.1. Mini-Cog

Frailty

Next, we come to frailty. Begin by asking if your family member has a single disease that affects many areas of functioning, typically a neurologic condition such as multiple sclerosis, Parkinson's disease, or stroke. This one disease may result in her having trouble walking, thinking, and urinating, to list a common triad. If your family member has a condition like this, consider how severe the impairments are—does she need a great deal of help in more than one arena? If so, then odds are your family member is frail.

If your family member does not have just one disease with widespread effects, then ask if she has multiple conditions—a common constellation is diabetes, arthritis, high blood pressure, and coronary artery disease, though the number of permutations is nearly infinite. In that case, you need to think about whether the combination makes her vulnerable to yet other problems. Has she landed in the hospital after a run-of-the-mill flu turned into something a good deal more serious? Did she go to the hospital or ambulatory surgery center for what was supposed to be a simple procedure and end up with complications? With confusion? The last time she was hospitalized, did she have to go to rehab afterward because she was in no shape to go directly home? If the answer is yes, your relative may well be frail.

Another approach to figuring out if your family member is frail is to count up the number of medications she is on. Taking nine or more different prescription drugs doesn't by itself prove your family member is frail, but it raises a red flag, especially if each medicine must be taken several times a day so the total number of pills could be thirty or more. Using that many medications predisposes someone to all kinds of side effects and interactions. Adding one more pill to the mix—as is likely in the event of a new, acute medical problem—can all the more easily tip your family member over the edge. And that sort of precarious balance between feeling well and feeling sick, between being independent and becoming dependent, is exactly what frailty is all about.

Frailty is tricky to define, but a number of tools can help screen for frailty. One of the simplest is the "Frail Questionnaire," which consists of just five questions and has the convenient acronym "FRAIL" (table 4.1).

The most extensively studied index of frailty is based on the work of Dr. Linda Fried, a physician who sees frailty as related to advanced cardiovascular disease. She looks for weight loss, a sense of chronic fatigue (or, as she calls it, exhaustion), avoidance of all exertion (or low energy expenditure), slowness, and weakness as measured by poor grip strength. The presence of three or more of these factors is associated with an increased risk of falls, increased disability, hospitalization, or death.

Table 4.1

"FRAIL" Questionnaire Screening Tool

3 or greater = frailty; 1 or 2 = pre-frail

_____ **F**atigue: Are you fatigued?

_____ **R**esistance: Can you walk up one flight of stairs?

_____ **A**erobic: Can you walk one block?

_____ **I**llness: Do you have more than five illnesses?

_____ **L**oss of weight: Have you lost more than 5 percent of your weight in the past 6 months?

Source: Adapted from table 3 in M. Singh, R. Stewart, and H. White, "Importance of Frailty in Patients with Cardiovascular Disease," *European Heart Journal*, 35, no. 26 (July 7, 2014): 1726–1731, https://doi.org/10.1093/eurheartj/ehu197.

What's important for you to realize is that frailty is not the same as disability, which is a physical or mental impairment that substantially limits one or more major activities of daily living. Nor is it the same as "multimorbidity," which is the presence of several chronic diseases. The essence of frailty is the loss of "homeostasis," the critical ability of the human organism to right itself, to compensate for any imbalance or disruption. Homeostasis is what is responsible for our going to the bathroom less often if we are dehydrated—our brains and our kidneys work together to try to keep us from collapsing. Homeostasis is the reason our body temperature doesn't rise when we go out on a very hot day or fall if we go outside on a very cold day—we sweat (in the first instance) or constrict the blood vessels to our hands and feet (in the second) to compensate for our environment. If your family member is frail, she will have great difficulty adjusting to these sorts of disruptions. As a result, she might start out with a simple flu, then end up with pneumonia, which puts a stress on her heart, perhaps causing a heart attack, which can lead to fluid backing up in the lungs, and so on. Because frail people tend to experience this kind of cascade of problems, they often end up hospitalized; and since even minor problems can snowball, those same seemingly minor problems often result in further loss of physical functioning. You can see why frailty is also associated with high rates of nursing home placement and of death.

Physicians aren't terribly good at identifying frailty and telling you and your family member that's what's going on. But without recognizing that frailty has set in, you won't be able to appreciate just how devastating a seemingly mild, acute illness or a new drug or moving to a new environment can be. You won't be able to decide wisely whether it makes more sense to try to treat your family member at home or in the hospital. Once you realize that even though no one of your family member's medical conditions is very severe, she is at high risk of developing problems from their combined impact, you will be on the way to grasping what frailty is all about.

Robustness

If your family member doesn't fit into any of the above categories—perhaps she has only a few health problems that are readily controlled with just a couple of medications—or whatever her difficulties, they don't translate into problems going about daily life—then she is probably robust. I'm not going to be spending much time talking about robust health, simply because most people who are robust don't need caregivers. You might be called upon to help for a brief period of time, say after an operation or during a bad bout of flu, but long-term caregiving is rarely an issue for the robust. The one exception that comes to mind is mental illness: a person with recurrent depression or chronic schizophrenia may well need caregiving. Such people don't fit neatly into my typology but are perhaps most productively considered to be frail since their chronic disease makes them vulnerable to all sorts of other problems.

Health State and Goals of Care

Let's say that you've figured it out: you know whether your family member is frail, has dementia, or is close to death. Now what? That knowledge will affect what treatments make sense for her. If she is frail, she is probably not in a good position to have a lung tumor removed surgically. If she has dementia, it may not be advisable to undergo chemotherapy for breast cancer, a treatment necessitating regular visits to the oncologist's office for intravenous treatments that produce side effects such as nausea and vomiting. If she is dying and breaks a hip, it may make more sense to stay home in bed rather than to have a hip replacement operation.

More fundamentally, understanding the big picture will enable your family member to engage with her physician and with you to discuss her *goals of care*. I touched on this at the beginning of this book when I spoke about the significance of determining the health state (see chapter 1, "Why Health State Matters"). There's a great deal of emphasis in medical practice today on honoring the preferences of individual patients: when faced with different possible approaches to treatment, each with its own pluses and minuses, the patient is supposed to decide which one she prefers. Often that involves a great deal of technical information, understanding exactly what each option involves. But what it should involve is a recognition that "preferences" are based on your relative's goals, on what she hopes medical care will accomplish. And those goals aren't just based on philosophical or religious beliefs; they are rooted in the person's situation, which includes her health state.

Once you and your family member have a reasonably good sense of her health state, you can discuss her most important objective of health care. Is it to live as long as possible, no matter what? Is it to remain physically and emotionally comfortable, even if that means forgoing potentially beneficial treatments? Or is it to be as independent and functional as possible, willing to tolerate some discomfort in exchange for the possibility of continuing to be able to walk and see, to think and hear? If your family member is able to say which of these three goals is most important, it's up to the physician to sketch out what kinds of treatment are most consistent with her goals when-

ever a problem develops. Naturally, most people want all three: they want to live longer *and* remain independent *and* be comfortable. Unfortunately, sometimes they cannot have it all, living longer, for example, may be at the cost of becoming more dependent. They have to *prioritize* their goals.

This kind of planning for the future based on the health state has to be done in conjunction with a physician. Ideally, your relative's physician will explain what her goals imply in terms of treatment. For instance, if your family member wants to focus on independence, intensive care unit (ICU) treatment may not make sense because a prolonged stay in the ICU leaves frail, older people debilitated and in need of greater assistance. If she wants to focus solely on comfort, admission to the hospital is seldom warranted, except if pain control of a condition such as cancer cannot be achieved at home.

Your family member's goals may well change as her condition evolves, so it's important to periodically review her health state (box 4.1). The process is sometimes difficult, but it makes choosing the right treatment in times of crisis far easier for her and for you (see chapter 49, "Planning for Future Medical Care").

Box 4.1

Older people may be robust, frail, have dementia, or be dying. Knowing in which category your family member belongs will help determine the goals of care and treatment choices.

PART II

Going to the Doctor

Your family member is going to encounter physicians at all the stops along his medical journey: the office (sometimes called "the clinic"), the hospital, and the skilled nursing facility. If he's exceptionally lucky, he will see the same physician in each location; more commonly, he will be cared for by a different person at each site. Often, he will have multiple doctors at each point in his travels through the health-care system—a generalist and several specialists, physicians such as cardiologists or neurologists. For most people, the majority of medical care is delivered in the outpatient setting, what I'm calling the office, and the lion's share of that care is provided by a primary care physician, who used to be called a general practitioner (GP), but is now usually either an internist (specialist in internal medicine) or a family physician (specialist in family medicine). The decisions made in the office and occasionally, if the primary care doctor or members of her team make house calls, at home, are the ones that you, as the family caregiver, are most apt to need to implement. You will find that partnering with your relative's physicians, wherever they practice, is a good strategy. Nowhere is it more important than in the office, so that's where we will begin.

CHAPTER 5

The Role of the Primary Care Physician

Chances are your family member already has a primary care physician, though sometimes primary care doctors retire, move away, or give up the practice of medicine. Or perhaps your family member just moved to the area, maybe to be near you, and you need to help him find a new doctor. Unfortunately, you may discover that your family member does indeed have a primary care doctor, but she is just not what is needed at this stage of life. I'm going to start with a few generic comments about what a primary care physician should ideally be like. It will be up to you to figure out if your family member's doctor fits the bill.

Accessibility

If your family member is going to be able to see his primary care doctor, that physician's office needs to be *accessible.* I mean literally—located where he can get to it. Many physicians practice in a doctor's office building that is adjacent to or attached to a hospital. That's very convenient for physicians who need to go back and forth between the office and the hospital and it means the office is in close proximity to all the x-rays and procedures you could possibly want, but it may be a place you have to drive to reach. If your relative does drive, or you drive him, once you get there you may be faced with one of those indoor parking garages that spiral endlessly and never seem to have enough spaces in which to park or room in which to maneuver, no matter how large they are. All in all, not necessarily the most convenient location for your family member to reach. Most offices these days are accessible in ways mandated by the Americans with Disabilities Act: they are located in an elevator building or can be reached via a ramp.

Once your family member is inside the office, he has to be able to make his way into the examining room and get onto the examining table. Geriatric-friendly offices are designed to accommodate wheelchairs and they have examining tables that can be lowered and raised electrically. Those aren't features you can take for granted: I've seen offices that are so small it's impossible to maneuver in them and examining tables that patients literally have to climb onto—or else they will be examined while sitting in a chair, which isn't a proper way to examine someone. Then there are the little things: do the chairs in the waiting room have arms? Your family member may not be able to rise out of his seat without a surface to push off from. Is there a specially designed scale that allows someone with a mobility disorder to be weighed? I remember weighing a pa-

tient on one of my first home visits as a young physician: I was so pleased with myself for recognizing the importance of measuring the patient's weight and for finding a standard bathroom scale in her house, but when she attempted to stand on the scale, with me right behind her as her spotter, we both ended up on the floor.

Accessibility also means availability. Is the physician in the office most days? Is there adequate coverage when she isn't? One of the services that "concierge" practices offer—those relatively new arrangements in which the patient pays a fee, often thousands of dollars a year, on top of Medicare premiums and co-payments, in exchange for certain extras—is 24/7 availability. Even concierge practices don't really provide around-the-clock coverage by the primary care physician; they have to rely on some kind of coverage system. But what you don't want is to be routinely directed to the emergency department of the nearest hospital if you happen to call outside regular business hours.

Ability to Communicate

The next job of the primary care physician, after simply being available and accessible, is to *communicate*. That requires the ability to listen as well as to explain medical matters clearly. A good communicator has to have empathy and be able to elicit your family member's concerns—not just symptoms and medical details such as when the pain started and

what makes it better or worse. Doctors learn to "take a history" in medical school; what they don't always learn is how to put a patient at ease so he will feel comfortable discussing his anxieties and fears. If your family member has difficulty hearing, the physician needs to compensate by speaking face-to-face to facilitate lip reading and by speaking slowly and clearly. Outfitting the office with a "pocket talker" (available through Williams Sound at www .williamssound.com) or similar device that amplifies hearing can help, too. And if your family member doesn't speak English, it's essential that the physician have interpreter services. That doesn't necessarily involve having someone on site to translate; there are also ways to reach a trained medical interpreter by telephone.

Communication is tremendously important, but so is *medical competence.* For geriatric patients that means familiarity not only with the usual topics in internal medicine, but also with geriatric syndromes. (For more about falling, delirium, incontinence, and polypharmacy see chapter 3, "Thinking like a Geriatrician: Geriatric Syndromes," for dementia and depression see chapter 29, "Alzheimer's Disease and Other De-

mentias," and chapter 31, "Depression.") One of the most important roles for a primary care physician is to be on the lookout for one or more geriatric syndromes and to be prepared to evaluate your relative if he has such a condition. I'm not saying the primary care physician needs to be a geriatrician, a physician who completed a one- or two-year fellowship in geriatric medicine. Many family physicians and general internists have all the requisite skills and knowledge to take care of your family member, but not all do. That's why you need to develop at least cursory familiarity with the geriatric syndromes yourself. If you are aware that falls, incontinence, and so forth are often important issues in older people, you can make sure your family member's doctor at least asks about them.

Capacity to Perform Geriatric Assessment

Another skill necessary for the primary physician, along with familiarity with geriatric syndromes, is the capacity to perform a *geriatric assessment.* It's one thing for the physician to ask about trouble walking or carrying out basic activities such as bathing or toileting; it's another to test your family member directly, to observe how he performs. The physician doesn't necessarily have to measure function herself, but she should have someone in her office, typically a nurse

practitioner or physician assistant, who does. And the physician doesn't have to ask about every geriatric syndrome or test each basic activity of daily living (ADL) at every visit. But at the time of the annual physical, evaluating these quintessentially geriatric concerns, and not just the heart and lungs, is critical. Ironically, many physicians are so accustomed to listening to the heart and lungs that they regard these actions as the core of the physical examination. In general, however, there is less to be learned by placing the stethoscope on the chest than there is, say, by taking off your relative's socks and shoes or asking him to get up from his seat and walk across the room.

Willingness to Partner with You

You may not have figured out yet how much you want to participate in your family member's medical appointments. That's something you have to decide for yourself, but if you are going to be involved in carrying out "doctor's orders"—whether it's making sure your family member takes his medications or changing dressings or administering tube feedings—you need to establish a relationship with the primary care physician. Once you start playing a role in making decisions about issues such as home versus hospital care and do-not-resuscitate (DNR) status (or, as I prefer to call it, DNAR, for do-not-attempt-resuscitation), or you are the one to figure out what services are needed at home, you are going to have to interact with the physician. Doctors aren't always used to involving families. In fact, we are trained to respect "individual autonomy," which is often taken to mean that the patient is to be treated in isolation, apart from family and community. In geriatrics, as in much of medicine and of life in general, that model doesn't work well. It's important for physicians to listen to their patients, to respect them as individuals, and to tailor treatment to their preferences, but it's also essential for physicians to recognize that patients are part of a family and a community. Acting as though your relative is independent of his surroundings is foolish and unrealistic, especially if he is an older person who depends on you, his caregiver. The physician needs to know if there is someone to check the blood sugar three times a day—if that's what she thinks should be done to monitor your relative's diabetes. The physician needs to know if your family member gets dizzy after he takes his blood pressure medicines—and you, the caregiver, may be the best person to report this problem.

Relationships are two-way streets. You have to be willing to go with your family member to at least selected medical appointments and you need to be ready to engage with the physician, but the physician has to be open to involving you as well. You will need your family member's permission to be privy to medical information about him; ideally, your family member will appoint you his health-care proxy so that you are legally empowered to make medical decisions on his behalf if he is unable to do so himself. But the physician has to be willing to listen to you, to speak with you, and when necessary to teach you how to administer treatment, if caregiving is going to work. Medical care for complex older adults is most effective when the physician partners with the family.

Participation in a Network

Speaking of partnerships, there are other clinicians who often work together with the primary care physician to provide comprehensive care. As I alluded to in conjunction with geriatric assessment, these professionals include nurse practitioners (NPs) and physician assistants (PAs). Your family member may be accustomed to interacting exclusively with a physician and be a bit leery of an arrangement involving a whole team of people but will usually come around after direct experience. For those of you who are not familiar with NPs and PAs, they typically bring a great deal to the practice (see chapter 6, "What to Expect from Nurse Practitioners and Physician Assistants"). They probably focused on the family unit during their training and are comfortable doing assessments of mobility and cognition. They may even have been on the "geriatrics track" when in school. A well-oiled medical group will make use of the special competence of these advanced practice clinicians, as they are also called, to complement the work of the physician: the NP or PA will diagnose the more straightforward medical problems, leaving the complex ones to the MD; the NP or PA will spend time teaching you and your family member how to manage a chronic condition such as diabetes. If there's an advanced practice clinician working with your relative's doctor, that person is another potential ally for you, another partner in care.

Beyond the other members of the medical team who work in the same office as your family member's physician are a host of other "providers" who are likely to play an important role. There is the "coverage group," the other physicians who are on call when your relative's regular physician is not available. These doctors should be people your family member feels comfortable with since, odds are, he will be interacting with them as well as with his primary care physician. There are the specialists, from the podiatrist who cuts your family member's toenails to the medical specialists (cardiologists, nephrologists, neurologists, and so forth) who address diseases of particular organ systems to the surgical specialists (ophthalmologists, orthopedists, etc.) who deal with problems that might require an operation to fix. These specialists form the network of which your family member's primary physician is a part (see chapter 8, "What to Expect from Medical Specialists"). That network can be defined by shared membership in a multi-specialty group practice (Kaiser Permanente, the Palo Alto Medical Clinic, and the Mayo Clinic are examples of very large multi-specialty group practices) or by participation in a hospital system (Hospital Corporation of America and Tenet Healthcare are examples of such systems).

Over and beyond coordinating care with individual physicians, your relative's primary care physician has to interact with a local hospital. There should be an acute care facility with which the primary physician has some sort of relationship and where she sends patients when they need hospital level care. She very likely has "privileges" at that hospital, which means she can see patients who have been admitted and write notes in the medical record, though she may or may not actually be in charge of their care. Even if the primary care physician doesn't set foot in the acute care hospital, it's her job to relay information about your family member to the physicians who are taking care of him while he's there and to find out about what happened during his stay. Ideally, she'll be involved during his hospitalization, if not in person, then at least virtually, so she can weigh in if she is concerned about the direction in which his treatment is going.

Finally, another role of the primary care physician is to arrange for "services" for your family member. These include the services of a visiting nurse for short-term, often post-hospital care; treatment by a physical therapist after an injury, stroke, or to help recover from generalized weakness; assistance from a home health aide, someone who can help with personal care; and other, less unequivocally medical needs such as Meals on Wheels (home delivered meals) or adult day health care (a day care program for adults).

This job description is long and detailed because you may want to carry around a mental checklist to make sure your family member's physician is fulfilling all these roles. If she's not, you may need to suggest supplementing her care, perhaps with a geriatric consultation. Or you may need to find a new doctor for your family member. The key points to look for in a primary care physician are summarized in box 5.1. You'd prefer not to disrupt a longstanding relationship if it's a good one, but sometimes what worked twenty years ago is no longer viable today.

Box 5.1

Primary care physicians should be

- Accessible
- Available
- Good communicators
- Knowledgeable about geriatric syndromes
- Willing to partner with caregivers

CHAPTER 6

What to Expect from Nurse Practitioners and Physician Assistants

You are almost undoubtedly familiar with the concept of a primary care physician (see chapter 5, "The Role of the Primary Care Physician"). You might also find yourself interacting with "advanced practice clinicians," including nurse practitioners (NPs) and physician assistants (PAs), sometimes also called "mid-level practitioners." I'd like to talk a bit more about what you can expect from these important members of the health-care team.

Training of NPs and PAs

First, a word about their training compared to that of a physician. Physicians begin with a bachelor's degree from a four-year college where they can major in whatever they like but need to take courses in biology, inorganic chemistry, organic chemistry, and physics to apply to medical school. They then spend four years in medical school, which classically consists of two years of classroom learning and two years spent doing "rotations" in the hospital (and occasionally in an office setting) to expose them to the practical aspects of treating patients. At the end of all that, they are technically physicians but cannot actually practice medicine until they have done a residency, a three- (or four- or five-) year training program that is a true practicum: they apply the more theoretical knowledge gained in school under supervision from a more experienced physician. A residency in internal medicine is three years in duration as is a residency in family medicine. Surgical residencies, by contrast, last five years. Specialty training—becoming a cardiologist or oncologist, if you are an internist, or a hand surgeon or a plastic surgeon if you went into surgery—requires a fellowship after residency.

After all those years of school and supplementary training, physicians want to put their knowledge and skills to work. Not surprisingly, many don't want to spend their time on routine medical problems such as bladder infections or the flu. They tend to like the challenge of difficult or unusual cases. For patients and their families, of course, a bladder infection or the flu may be anything but routine. It can turn their lives upside down, threatening the tenuous stability a frail elder might have achieved living alone at home. A relatively minor illness can trigger other conditions or evolve into something more serious. From your perspective as a caregiver, you might not always want or need a physician's level of sophistication.

The path to becoming an advanced practice clinician is considerably shorter. Like doctors, future PAs have to go to college and earn a bachelor's degree. They need to take a few courses in biology and chemistry as undergraduates. Then, usually after working in the medical field for a few years, they apply to a PA program at a full-service university or in a freestanding professional school. In either case, their course of study parallels a medical student's but it's highly compressed. Instead of two years of basic science and two years of

clinical rotations, they usually have a year of coursework, combining basic and applied biology, and a year of brief rotations. After graduation the newly minted PA is ready to be employed, though increasing numbers are doing a residency, again mirroring physician training. The net effect of all this is that PAs are equipped to do much of what physicians do—take a history, diagnose, and treat disease—provided the illness is relatively routine. PAs are perfectly adequate for diagnosing and treating many of the problems an older person develops, and in light of physicians' low level of interest in what they consider the more mundane medical problems, PAs may be better suited to the job.

The nurse practitioner pathway isn't just an abbreviated version of the medical track. Instead, it's firmly grounded in the nursing tradition. In fact, NPs are usually registered nurses before they study to become an NP. They typically major in nursing in college, graduating with a bachelor's degree in nursing. At some point, often after a number of years of work experience, they decide to get a master's degree in nursing and become a nurse practitioner. They also take classroom courses and then engage in supervised clinical practice. Their training tends to be holistic, focusing on the patient as part of a family and a community. While NPs can do many of the same things that MDs—or PAs—do, they often complement the work of a physician rather than replace it. They will be the ones who teach patients, along with family members, how to manage their diabetes. They will perform functional and psychosocial assessments. While an NP can diagnose and treat common ailments and some work very independently, the NP's particular strength is often in performing these complementary roles.

Role of NPs and PAs

What you should realize is that because of their training in working as part of an interdisciplinary team, their skills in coordinating care, and their interest in working with patients as part of a family, mid-levels, especially NPs, may play a crucial role in your relative's care. They often serve as the glue that allows older patients with multiple chronic conditions to get the kind of coordinated care that they need.

In theory, mid-levels can improve the primary care experience for older adults. But do they? Studies have found that when an NP "comanages" frail, geriatric patients with an internist, the patient is more likely to receive high-quality care than if the internist works solo. In addition to strong communication skills and a whole-person perspective, NPs may also know more than internists in certain domains—most have available to them a "geriatric nurse practitioner track" in their training programs. They may have formally studied how to assess gait, mobility, hearing, and vision, tasks that internists assume will be carried out by physical therapists, audiologists, or ophthalmologists. Moreover, with the shortage of primary care physicians, the use of nurse practitioners instead of physicians for the evaluation and treatment of the most common medi-

cal conditions can help solve medicine's manpower problem. By creatively divvying up primary care responsibilities, physicians and mid-levels can ensure that each has more time to devote to your family member.

We've been talking about the office setting but mid-levels are increasingly used in the hospital, where they take over the more routine medical work, and in the skilled nursing facility, where they may be the principal on-site practitioners. Don't bristle when the doctor doesn't show up at the bedside in the hospital or the rehab but a PA or NP arrives instead; you may find they are more willing than physicians to take the time to listen to your concerns or to explain what's going on. The division of labor between physicians and mid-levels in the rehab facility is often such that it's the advanced practice clinician who broaches such important subjects as whether you and your family member would want attempted cardiopulmonary resuscitation (CPR) in the event of a cardiac arrest—a procedure, incidentally, that's extremely unlikely to be effective in the rehabilitation setting, but more on that later. The advanced practice clinician may also be the one to talk about whether or not to hospitalize your family member rather than taking care of her in rehab or to raise the possibility that hospice would be a useful supplement to her medical care.

Mid-levels also sometimes provide medical care at home, where they can be invaluable. We'll talk more later about home visit programs, which are a rarity in the United States. But when medical care at home is available—and I'm talking about an approach that's more comprehensive than a visiting nurse who comes to the home a few times after a hospitalization, for example—it's often a PA or NP who travels from the office to do the evaluation. Like visiting nurses, they can report back to the primary care physician, but they can also function independently. For the frail, older person who has difficulty getting to and from the doctor's office but who isn't so sick as to need to go to a hospital emergency department, this arrangement is ideal. Advanced practice clinicians may be equipped to draw blood, perform an electrocardiogram (EKG), give an injection, and sometimes to start an IV and give fluids or intravenous medicines. In addition, they may have the skills to evaluate your family member in her home environment: Are the rooms light enough?

Are they so cluttered with furniture and riffraff that they're just asking for your family member to fall? What's in the refrigerator? Is your family member eating properly? Does the bathroom have grab bars?

The advanced practice clinician is a good ally for you, in whatever environment you find him or her. Many caregivers report that they bear the responsibility for carrying out a variety of medical or nursing procedures—from providing nutrition through a feeding tube that was surgically inserted into the stomach to operating a home dialysis machine—but never received adequate instruction in what to do. If you aren't a nurse, there's no good reason why you should know how to give an injection or put someone on a bedpan, let alone operate a sophisticated machine. A technician may have given you some basic information when your family member first went home with a feeding tube or on dialysis. A visiting nurse might have taught you a trick or two so you could troubleshoot when there was a problem. But your most sophisticated guide is likely to be an NP or PA (box 6.1).

Box 6.1

Roles of Nurse Practitioners and Physician Assistants

- Coordinating care
- Working with families
- Providing transitional care
- Assessing mobility
- Medical diagnosis and treatment

CHAPTER 7

What to Expect from Nurses, Social Workers, and Therapists

As a physician discussing how to deal with your family member's medical problems, I'm naturally most familiar with the physician angle. Some of what doctors do is often also performed by "mid-level practitioners," otherwise known as "advanced practice clinicians" or sometimes as "physician extenders" (see chapter 6, "What to Expect from Nurse Practitioners and Physician Assistants"). But there are numerous other people who can and often do contribute to the health and well-being of older people. According to government statistics, five million "allied health providers" work in over eighty professions in the United States. These include technicians—the person who actually takes the chest x-ray or draws blood—and therapists—individuals who treat illness but in a different way from the approach taken by physicians. I'm not going to talk about all the different categories but will focus on four professions that I find particularly important in caring for geriatric patients. The four disciplines are nursing, social work, physical therapy, and occupational therapy. You will no doubt encounter all of them in the course of caregiving but to take maximum advantage of their skills and talents, you should know a bit more about some of them.

Nurses

Let's start with *nurses*. You are probably most familiar with nurses, certainly from the hospital, definitely from the skilled nursing home—if you've ever set foot inside one—and quite possibly from the doctor's office. I'm not talking here about *nurse practitioners*, whom I discussed earlier. Rather, I'm referring to either licensed practical nurses (LPNs), who have typically completed a two-year community college program specializing in nursing, or registered nurses (RNs), who have usually gotten a bachelor's degree in nursing upon graduating from a four-year college program. Sometimes people don't decide they want to go into nursing until after they've graduated from either a two-year or four-year college, at which point they can enter a special program dedicated exclusively to training nurses.

What both future LPNs and RNs learn in school is to function autonomously as well as to work collaboratively with physicians. Their "scope of practice," the jargon used by licensing boards to describe what nurses can and cannot do, includes a very long list of procedures from giving injections to evaluating a patient who has fallen to assessing skin breakdown (pressure ulcers or, in common parlance, bedsores). In nursing homes, they are often on the front lines: together with nursing aides, they are the ones caring for some of the frailest and most vulnerable people on the planet. It's up to the nurse on duty in the rehabilitation center to decide when to call a physician and what to tell the physician when she calls. I've gotten calls such as, "Mrs. Smith fell on her way to the bathroom, but she's okay now. Her vital signs are fine and she has good range of motion in all her joints," or "Mrs. Jones got out of bed and fell; she's moaning in pain and her leg is externally rotated; I think we need to send her for x-rays." In practice, it may be up to the nurse on duty to determine whether to send a patient to the hospital.

In the office setting, the nurse typically serves as an assistant to the physician. She—it's still usually a she—may function as a kind of chaperone, simply standing in the room during a gynecologic exam. Or she may be the one who measures your relative's weight, blood pressure, heart rate, and temperature before the physician comes into the room to do an examination. In some practices, nurses are the teachers par excellence, helping patients and families with such important tasks as learning how to administer insulin shots and how to adjust their insulin dose in response to the results of finger stick monitoring. What I'd like to emphasize is something you might not be aware of, that nurses increasingly serve as gatekeepers to physicians or to various services that your relative may need. When you call because there's an urgent problem, say your family member is short of breath or has a fever, you are more likely to speak to the nurse directly than to the doctor. If you know the nurse and have a relationship with her, she's going to take you seriously when you say you are really worried because your family member seems very sick. She can make things happen, whether it's by relaying your concerns to the physician, advising you to bring your family member in right away, arranging a home visit, or suggesting that you call 911.

Sooner or later your family member is likely to need help from a visiting nurse, someone who works for a Visiting Nurse Association (VNA) in your area. A visiting nurse isn't going to be part of your family member's life for very long because Medicare will not pay for ongoing care (see chapter 48, "Paying for Health Care"), except in unusual circumstances such as the need for monthly B12 injections. She'll come a couple of times after your family member has been in the hospital or perhaps the skilled nursing facility. She, or perhaps a nurse employed by the hospital or your family member's doctor specifically for this purpose, may be providing *transitional care.* It turns out that the period right after your relative gets home from the hospital or rehab is an especially tricky time (see chapter 20, "Discharge Home"). After being in a supervised environment—your family member may have had to wait entirely too long for a nursing assistant to come and help him get to the bathroom, but there was always someone around, 24/7—for days or even weeks, suddenly he's back in his own home or perhaps yours. He's very relieved, but he may not remember exactly what medications he's supposed to take even though the nurse at the hospital gave him a chart that shows all his pills, what they're for, and how often they should be taken. So, one very useful task the nurse performs is *medication reconciliation.* That means looking at what medications your family member was taking before he went into the hospital and what he was discharged on and figuring out which ones he actually should take. Sometimes, he may have bottles for two different blood pressure medications or two antidepressants or two anti-ulcer medicines and he is expected to take one but not the other—or neither of them. The transitional care nurse can also make sure your family member has a follow-up appointment with his primary care physician and whomever else he should be seeing after he's settled in at home.

These three roles: liaison to the primary care physician, educator, and transition manager can be lifesavers for your family member. That's not to say that all the other things that nurses do are of less value, just that these three are functions you may not fully appreciate and should know about.

Social Workers

Another type of professional that you've probably run into somewhere along the line is a *social worker*. Social workers, like nurses, are quite heterogeneous. A few have a bachelor's degree in social work, obtained from a four-year, vocationally oriented college. The majority attended a four-year college and then went on to get a master's degree in social work (MSW) from an approved graduate school. There are school social workers, family social workers, palliative care social workers, and geriatric social workers (to name a few variants). From your perspective as a caregiver, two areas of expertise are likely to be very relevant: knowledge of community resources, on the one hand, and mental health services on the other. *Clinical social workers* provide psychotherapy and counseling. They often address depression, anxiety, and other emotional issues, functioning much like a psychiatrist—but without the ability to prescribe medications and based on narrower, more focused training. *Medical social workers* sometimes provide counseling and support to families, but they often spend much of their time connecting patients with appropriate resources—information about Medicare Part D programs (drug coverage), adult day health care, Meals on Wheels, and so forth. Both roles, sometimes embodied in the same person, can be vital to you and your family member.

If you're like most caregivers, you're going to experience moments of doubt, uncertainty about whether you are competent at caregiving and doubt about whether your shoulders are broad enough to take on this extra burden. You're going to feel all sorts of other emotions, too. First, there's guilt: Are you doing enough? Are you sufficiently compassionate? Or are you spending so much time on caregiving for your parent that you are neglecting your spouse or your own children? Then there's ambivalence: Do you want to do this? Do you just want to wipe your hands of all your responsibilities? Do you sometimes wish your family member were just, well, dead? And then, on top of guilt and ambivalence, there's anxiety: Did you forget to put out your family member's pills? Did you put that dressing on the way you were supposed to? You may well find that you're tired, maybe even exhausted. Your family member's physician, if she inquires about "caregiver burden," may recommend respite, perhaps arranging for your family member to stay at an assisted living facility for a week or two while you get away. That's a good suggestion and may be something you can act on once a year. But on an ongoing basis, what you may need is continuing support (see chapter 53, "Caregiver Support").

Some families can provide support to each other, if for example, you have several siblings with whom you share caregiving responsibilities. You might be able to laugh together or commiserate with one another. Unfortunately, siblings are as often a source of frustration as of sustenance—they live on the other side of the country, they're too busy, they're too scatterbrained; whatever the justification, they don't help out. An alternative is a support group which meets, say, once a month. Other caregivers can give you good ideas about how to solve various problems you might have encountered, or you might conclude you're actually doing fairly well, comparatively speaking (see chapter 53, "Caregiver Support"). For many people, the ideal source of support is a clinical social worker who's trained to listen and to advise.

What I find particularly appealing about clinical social workers for this role is that the best of them offer concrete suggestions *and* talk therapy. It's analogous to what I've experienced as a physician: if I can help someone very concretely by treating pneumonia or addressing physical pain, I have more credibility when I move on to sensitive issues such as advance care planning or preferences for end-of-life care. A good social worker will understand that there are multiple sources for your suffering, ranging from lack of resources to psychological stress. Addressing more than one of those sources can go a long way to helping you. Moreover, you may think you are facing a technical problem when, in fact, the social worker will correctly identify that the problem has more to do with your insecurity or your fears than your lack of ability. Alterna-

tively, you may think your problem has to do with a fundamental aspect of your relationship with your family member when there's an easy fix: if your father doesn't like you to get him dressed or bathed, it doesn't mean he doesn't trust you, just that he, like many other parents, finds it humiliating to receive personal care from his adult children. What is needed is a home health aide, not psychotherapy.

I suspect that what makes clinical social workers so effective, and so essential, is that they understand the importance of *relationships*. That means your relationship with your family member and your relationship with the others who are impacted by your caregiving, most commonly your spouse, and not infrequently your siblings and your children (see chapter 52, "Involving the Rest of the Family"). But it also means your relationship with the social worker. Having someone you trust go through the caregiving journey with you can make an enormous difference. Your relative's primary care physician may be able to refer you to a social worker; social workers are also regularly members of both geriatrics and palliative care teams, so they will form part of the evaluation if your relative has a geriatric or palliative care consultation. Social workers are also on the staff of hospitals, skilled nursing facilities, Visiting Nurse Associations, and hospices. Alternatively, you can find a social worker through the local Area Agency on Aging, a federally mandated program.

Physical Therapists and Occupational Therapists

A very different kind of health-care clinician is the therapist. I'm referring here to physical therapists and occupational therapists, not psychotherapists. We talked quite a bit about the importance of *function:* the ability of your family member to get around, whether he can use the bathroom, whether he can feed himself and, on a somewhat higher plane, whether he can prepare meals for himself or go shopping or balance his checkbook. The therapists I'm speaking of now are experts in precisely this sort of function.

Just to be clear, occupational therapists and physical therapists are both concerned with the fundamental activities necessary to get through the day. In the geriatric context, occupational therapists aren't concerned with your relative's job, with his employment; rather, they're concerned with whether your family member can use the stove or maneuver safely in the kitchen. There's another division between occupational and physical therapists that's roughly accurate: occupational therapists tend to focus on the hands and arms, while physical therapists tend to focus on the legs and feet. That division of labor sometimes breaks down, but after a hip fracture or total knee replacement, your family member is going to be referred to a physical therapist to work on getting back on his feet, and after a wrist fracture, he's probably

going to see an occupational therapist. Sometimes the two professions overlap in their competence: a home safety evaluation can be carried out either by a physical therapist or an occupational therapist, though the physical therapist may be more focused on whether your family member can maneuver in the home and the occupational therapist on whether he can perform various activities such as using the stove or running the washing machine.

Let me give you a few examples of ways in which therapists can be tremendously helpful to you and your family member. The first area is mobility. If your relative can't get around, he's going to be far less independent and far needier than if he can. Now "getting around," in the contemporary United States means traversing short distances, either by walking independently or with an assistive device, and traveling for miles, by car, bus, or train. A physical therapist can promote self-sufficiency in both cases. She can figure out what kind of assistive device, such as a walker or cane, is needed and teach your family member how to use it correctly.

I'm regularly impressed with how many older people use the cane on their "bad side" instead of on their "good side," as they are supposed to. Others have a cane that's too tall or too short or use a single-tipped cane instead of a tripod cane (for information on how to select the right sized cane and how to use one, see chapter 9, "What a Geriatric Assessment Is and When to Ask for One"). An evaluation by a physical therapist will avoid these pitfalls. Suppose your family member needs a walker for balance and safety. He'd like to go out with you, whether for pleasure or business, whether to a restaurant for lunch or to a medical appointment. But he has trouble getting into your car and you don't want to strain your back lifting him. A physical therapist may be able to teach you, and him, how to transfer to the car.

One of the greatest threats to mobility is falling. In the extreme case, someone with a broken leg is going to have very diminished mobility. In fact, someone with a broken wrist who depends on a walker for getting around may also have diminished mobility as it's hard to use a walker when your wrist is out of commission. Even without broken bones, just worrying about falling can prevent older people from going out. A physical therapist can often work with your family member to teach "safety awareness" and other strategies for avoiding falls. Ironically, while many older people feel secure at home and see the outside world as threatening, the place where they fall most often is in their own home. At home, they may have a false sense of security. A safety evaluation, undertaken by either a physical or occupational therapist, can point out a few critical risks. Some of these may be obvious to you, such as those scatter rugs that slip and slide on the wood floor, but your family member may be more willing to get rid of the

rugs if the occupational therapist tells him to than if you do. Some of the risks may be less obvious to you, such as the need for better lighting. Older eyes need far greater intensity light bulbs to see than younger eyes do, so illumination that appears satisfactory to you may in fact be inadequate for your family member (for more on falls, see chapter 3, "Thinking like a Geriatrician: Geriatric Syndromes").

The second major area where therapists can be useful, principally occupational therapists, is self-care. This gets to the activities of daily living (ADLs) and instrumental activities of daily living (IADLs)—what a person needs to be able to *do* in order to function independently (see chapter 2, "Ingredients of the Underlying Health State"). Some deficits are easier to compensate for than others: if your family member can't go to the supermarket to buy food, for instance, maybe he can learn to arrange for home delivery online. But if he can't wipe himself after he goes to the bathroom, he's going to need a full-time aide. An occupational therapist can reeducate your family member how to perform all sorts of tasks that he used to take for granted but that may have become very challenging. The occupational therapist can order a variety of gadgets, ranging from a large-button, amplified telephone (figure 7.1) to a jar opener designed for someone with arthritis in his hands. Again, some of these devices you can find advertised in AARP's magazine or other magazines featuring technology for seniors. Some are expensive. Others are more likely to be found in supply catalogs used by occupational therapists and some may even count as "durable medical equipment" and be covered by Medicare (for examples of other gadgets, see chapter 24, "Arthritis").

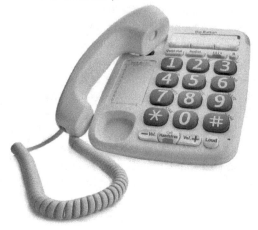

Figure 7.1. Large-button telephone

I haven't even mentioned the most common situation in which your family member is likely to benefit from the services of a physical or occupational therapist—after a traumatic injury or after a prolonged hospitalization resulting in deconditioning. In these situations, the physician will order therapy, either in the hospital, in the rehabilitation facility, or at home.

Nurses, social workers, occupational therapists, and physical therapists all have a critical role to play in your ongoing care of your family member (see box 7.1). Seeking them out and getting to know them once they have become involved in your relative's life can make a difference to you both.

Box 7.1

Roles of Nurses, Social Workers, Therapists

- Nurses: liaison to primary physician, educator, transition manager
- Social workers: counseling and support, arranging concrete services
- Physical and occupational therapists: safety awareness, improving daily function, recuperation after injury or illness

CHAPTER 8

What to Expect from Medical Specialists

Fewer than half of all visits to the doctor made by older patients are to their primary care physician—in contrast to the situation forty years ago, when nearly two-thirds of all outpatient visits were to the family physician. This specialty orientation is part of what makes American medicine as technologically sophisticated as it is, but it can be downright dangerous for frail older patients (figure 8.1).

Don't get me wrong—if your family member has acute appendicitis, she needs an operation and I'm not advocating that a general practitioner perform it on the kitchen table. She needs a surgeon, just as she will need an orthopedist if she falls and breaks her hip or an ophthalmologist if she develops cataracts. Oncologists (cancer specialists), nephrologists (kidney specialists), and cardiologists (heart specialists) sometimes have an important role to play in your family member's health care.

The problem with specialists is that they almost invariably take a narrow organ-specific or disease-specific view of your relative. They are concerned with her lungs or her liver, her heart or her kidneys, her cancer or her arthritis. They may know about all the latest treatments for "their" diseases, but that can be a problem if your relative has more than just that one disease. It's a rare older person, certainly not anyone who is likely to need a caregiver, who is perfectly healthy except for one well-defined medical problem. Even if your family member doesn't have five—or six or seven—other medical problems that have the potential to affect the disease the specialist is concerned about, or if she isn't on five or six or seven other medications that have the potential to interact with whatever new medicine the specialist prescribes, her overall health is essential to consider in deciding how to approach any medical problem.

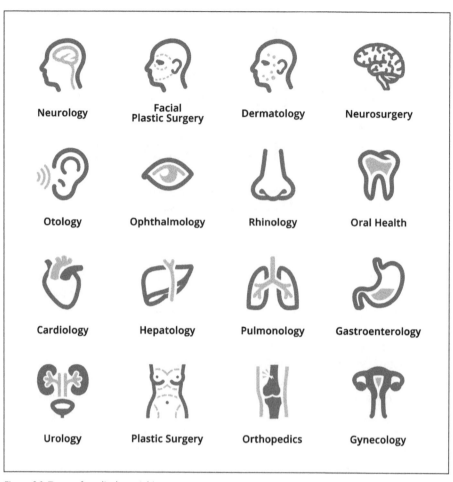

Figure 8.1. Types of medical specialties

Consequences of Taking a Narrow View

L et me give you a few examples. These are situations I've seen many times in clinical practice. Suppose your relative takes insulin injections for diabetes. Maintaining "tight control," keeping blood sugars within a fairly narrow range, is considered the gold standard in the treatment of diabetes because it offers the best chance of avoiding nasty complications such as neuropathy (pains, tingling, and numbness in the legs) and retinopathy (abnormalities of the retina, one of the parts of the eye critical for vision). But the time frame for development of those complications is *at least* five years. Moreover, the effect of excessively low blood sugar is that your family member will feel faint or even pass out, and the result of feeling faint or passing out may be falling—and breaking a bone. Which would she rather: run the risk of neuropathy in five years, when she might not be alive, or accept a substantial risk of a broken bone next week? If an endocrinologist sees your relative to evaluate her diabetes, he is apt to emphasize the importance of tight control; when a primary care physician sees her, he is more likely to emphasize moderately good control of the blood sugar and advocate doing everything possible to avoid falling.

Here's another example. Say your family member has Parkinson's disease, a neurological disorder that results in a tremor, generalized slowness, and a characteristic shuffling gait. The mainstay of treatment for Parkinson's disease is the drug L-dopa which replaces a brain chemical that is lacking in Parkinson's. One of the main side effects of L-dopa is a fall in blood pressure. That alone can cause problems if it leads to dizziness and falls. But suppose that, in addition to Parkinson's, your family member has congestive heart failure, one of the most common diseases in older people, and her cardiologist has her on a slew of medicines to control her heart disease—several of which lower blood pressure. It's entirely possible that if your family member *only* had Parkinson's, she could tolerate the L-dopa the neurologist prescribed, and

if she *only* had heart failure, she could tolerate the beta blocker her cardiologist prescribed. Unfortunately, she has both conditions and the only way she can be optimally treated, from the perspective of each specialist, is to undertreat the other disorder. Now some specialists appreciate this dilemma—but maybe only after there's been a bad outcome. Or they may simply be unaware of what other medicines their patient is taking. Electronic medical records are supposed to prevent this kind of poor coordination of care but some physicians don't use an electronic medical record. Some physicians find that their system is incompatible with the system used by other clinicians involved in their patient's care.

There's another more fundamental problem with specialty care. The treatments and medications used by doctors have typically only been tested in patients who have nothing else wrong with them other than the condition for which they are being treated. Heart failure drugs are tested in people who are healthy except for their heart failure, diabetes drugs are tested in people whose only medical problem is diabetes. What this means is that physicians don't know whether the patient with congestive heart failure *and* diabetes *and* glaucoma *and* osteoarthritis will respond to treatment as well as someone who has heart failure and *no other conditions*. In a similar vein, some of the procedures and drugs used in the diagnosis and treatment of disease have not been tested in any older people, even in older people who don't have multiple other chronic conditions. You shouldn't think this necessarily means that the treatment will be less beneficial or more harmful in your family member. Sometimes, the procedure may prove to be *more* effective—when powerful intravenous blood thinners were first used as "clot busters" in patients having a heart attack, the widespread assumption was that they were too dangerous to use in older people. It turned out that they were actually more effective in older people than in their younger counterparts, probably because the older people on average had more serious heart attacks and, therefore, stood to benefit more from dissolving the blood clot producing the problem. But at least as often, the treatment is less effective or riskier than in healthier people.

Is the Specialist Essential?

Specialists tend to be well-versed in the latest, most sophisticated technology. Because they want to help, they are eager to prescribe the newest, most powerful treatments for their patients. Unfortunately, they have no way of knowing whether your family member stands to benefit. If your relative goes to a specialist, it will be of paramount importance to discuss the risks of treatment along with what's known about its effectiveness in people like her. You will also want to address whether there's another approach to treatment that offers a reasonable shot at success but comes with fewer side effects.

In light of these concerns, my judgment—and this is an instance where I'm offering you my opinion, not fact—is that you think carefully about whether your family member really needs that visit to the specialist. Suppose she already goes to the primary care doctor on a regular basis as well as the podiatrist and the dentist. Maybe she's going to physical therapy to work on her mobility and to the audiologist to have her hearing aid checked. Just because she's gone to a neurologist, a cardiologist, and a nephrologist for years, does she have to keep going? Or can she follow up only if there is a specific issue for them to address, an issue about which her primary physician would like guidance? I've seen patients faithfully go to see their kidney doctor— even after they've decided unequivocally that they will not go on dialysis if their kidney function deteriorates further, after they are already following a special "renal diet," and after they already have a list of medications to avoid because their kidneys are not working optimally. I've seen patients religiously visit their cardiologist, who orders an echocardiogram every year to check how much worse their heart failure has gotten, even though there is nothing he will do with the information. These all too common occurrences lead me to suggest that in your interactions with *all* physicians, if the doctor proposes a test, whether an electrocardiogram (EKG) or an echocardiogram or something more invasive such as an angiogram, you should always ask, how will the results change what we do? If the answer is, let's see what it shows and then we can discuss it further, that's not good enough. Unnecessary testing—and a recent survey of physicians found that they thought nearly 30 percent of all medical tests are superfluous—is costly, both to society as a whole in terms of the cost of medical care and to your family member in terms of the risk of side effects.

Coordinating Medical Care

If your family member sees more than one physician—I'm assuming that she has a primary care physician, so any others in her life are likely to be specialists—you should be sure they communicate with each other. You might think you could take this for granted, and in the best of all worlds, you would be able to take it for granted. But we live in a fragmented, complex health-care system and you shouldn't assume that the specialist will send the primary care physician a report, or that the primary care physician has sent the specialist a summary of your family member's active medical problems, medical history, and a list of her current medications. And as I indicated before, electronic medical records can help overcome communication problems, but the physicians have to copy each other on the notes they write or the other party won't know there's a note to read. The safest course of action is to remind the specialist to please send a report to the primary care physician. It's up to the specialist to figure out if that means flagging a note in the electronic record, sending an email to the primary

care doctor alerting him that there's a new note about your family member, or doing things the old-fashioned way by dictating a letter and sending it through the mail.

As a general rule of thumb, you will want *most* of your relative's medical care to be provided by her primary care physician (see chapter 5, "The Role of the Primary Care Physician"). Bear in mind a few noteworthy exceptions in addition to the examples of a broken hip or a cataract I mentioned earlier. If you have already concluded that your relative needs a procedure, for example injection of a painful joint with steroids, and the primary care physician does not provide the service, she will need to see a specialist, in this case a rheumatologist. If your family member has a rare disease, for instance Multiple Systems Atrophy (a neurologic condition that can mimic Parkinson's disease), she will benefit from specialist care, in this example a neurologist. Certain diseases are treated exclusively by specialists: cancer, if it is going to be treated with chemotherapy, necessitates the involvement of an oncologist.

Geriatricians, Generalist Specialists

Finally, you might want your family member to see a geriatrician. Most geriatricians are technically specialists; primary care geriatricians, although they exist, are relative rarities. It's just too labor-intensive for most physicians to consider an exclusively geriatric, primary care practice. I had a good friend who went into solo practice caring exclusively for older patients and she just couldn't make it work financially, an experience shared by many who try similar models. The net effect is that, if your family member sees a geriatrician at all, she will probably see a geriatrician in consultation. Geriatricians know about functional status and geriatric syndromes, they are leery of long lists of medications, and they are aware of the potential perils of diagnostic tests and procedures. But geriatric consultants, unlike some other specialists, know that implementation of their recommendations will likely fall to the primary care doctor so they understand that their effectiveness depends on good communication (for more on geriatric assessment, see chapter 9, "What a Geriatric Assessment Is and When to Ask for One").

The specialists your relative has seen before can continue to play a role in her care, as can new specialists with expertise in whatever new medical problems develop (box 8.1). But like rich desserts, they should be taken in moderation.

Box 8.1

> Specialist physicians are important for
>
> - Surgical procedures
>
> - Rare diseases
>
> - Consultation with primary care physicians
>
> Remember to ask:
>
> - How will the results of this test change what we do?
>
> - Is there another alternative with fewer risks?

CHAPTER 9

What a Geriatric Assessment Is and When to Ask for One

Geriatricians don't have a procedure, unlike cardiologists, who perform cardiac catheterizations or gastroenterologists who do colonoscopies. Even relatively low-tech specialists such as endocrinologists sometimes do procedures; for example, they may biopsy the thyroid gland if it is enlarged or contains a lump. This involves inserting a needle into the gland just below the Adam's apple and taking out a snippet for a pathologist to examine under the microscope. But the closest geriatricians come to having a procedure, a special test for which they can actually bill Medicare, is the comprehensive geriatric assessment, sometimes abbreviated CGA.

There is surprisingly little agreement on just what this kind of assessment consists of, except that it is multidisciplinary (preferably interdisciplinary—more later on the distinction) and includes several aspects of life that are important to the health and well-being of older people, and that are not routinely part of a standard annual physical examination. The part that is similar to a conventional exam is the medical piece, which entails a review of diseases and diagnoses, but even that differs from the norm by paying attention to geriatric syndromes. Those syndromes, as I mentioned earlier, are falling, delirium, incontinence, and polypharmacy as well as depression and dementia (see chapter 3, "Thinking like a Geriatrician: Geriatric Syndromes," chapter 29, "Alzheimer's Disease and Other Dementias," and chapter 31, "Depression"). Because these disorders make up an important part of the evaluation, the physician's examination will of necessity include a gait exam, mental status exam, and a review of the medications your relative is taking. Beyond the physician's contribution, there is usually a psychosocial assessment that is often conducted by a social worker and a functional assessment that is typically performed by a nurse or nurse practitioner. The CGA requires a team, although the precise members of the team vary somewhat in different settings. Usually there are affiliated team members who can be called upon as needed to add other components to the assessment. In some cases, a physical therapist is needed to more fully address mobility or a psychiatrist to determine if depression is present. The entire process commonly takes several hours and may even be spread over two visits, especially if ancillary exams or tests are necessary.

Outpatient CGA is a particular form of geriatric consultation. It is usually requested by the primary care physician, but sometimes by the patient or family and, rarely, by a specialist. An oncologist or cardiologist trying to determine if a particular patient is able to tolerate the rigors of some form of treatment might, for example, request a geriatric consultation to help guide the decision. That consultation is best carried out by a team since it isn't focused on a narrowly defined question such as "Why is this patient incontinent and how can he be treated?" or "Does this patient have dementia?"

The Interdisciplinary Team

Let me say a little more about teams in general and CGA teams in particular. A team in medicine means a group of people who function as an integrated unit. Like sports teams, they are most effective when the team members interact and complement each other rather than each working quasi-independently. But medicine is historically a very individualistic pursuit: physicians aren't accustomed to working with others so much as they are to working alongside others or ordering others around. Sometimes they substitute for each other, as when a physician goes on vacation and hands over her patients to a "covering physician," or when an intern in the hospital finally goes home after a twenty-four-hour shift and passes the baton to another intern. These ways of functioning are all very different from the truly interdisciplinary team model.

A genuinely interdisciplinary approach entails a division of labor—the social worker evaluates the emotional stresses in your relative's life and asks about family dynamics; the nurse actually tests activities of daily living (ADLs) and asks both the patient and caregiver about independent activities of daily living (IADLs); the physician takes a history and performs a physical examination, focusing on geriatric syndromes—and then all the pieces are integrated, sometimes via a joint discussion, sometimes by the physician, who assembles the parts. The idea is that the physician can't possibly understand why your family member is so limited in his instrumental activities of daily living, say, unless she realizes he has dementia. The doctor can't appreciate why your relative comes across as cognitively impaired even though he performs well on his mental status exam until she appreciates how depressed he is. And the physician might unnecessarily embark on an extensive evaluation of your relative's constipation if she didn't find over-the-counter antihistamines for his allergies in one of the bottles of medication you brought along. In short, a geriatrician might perform some elements of a comprehensive assessment at the time of a routine visit, but the best interdisciplinary consultations involve multiple participants, each with her own expertise, that are woven together to form a coherent whole.

Inpatient Comprehensive Geriatric Assessment

Comprehensive geriatric assessments can also take place in the inpatient setting. The Veterans Administration (VA) pioneered the approach and has developed special Geriatric Evaluation and Management (GEM) units for this purpose. Some community hospitals have adopted the model as well. Patients are typically admitted for an acute problem—a flare of congestive heart failure or a urinary tract infection, for instance—and once they are medically stable, they are transferred to the GEM unit for further diagnosis and treatment. Physicians at the VA have found that selected patients do better in the GEM environment than on a conventional medical floor.

Who benefits from a geriatric assessment? It's important to state up front that it's not necessary—or useful— for everyone. CGA makes most sense when it is targeted, reserved for the oldest and frailest people, who are the most complicated to understand and treat effectively. That's the group that the American Geriatrics Society says should have a CGA. It's most helpful if your relative is seeing many different specialists and has an internist as a primary care physician who is not particularly knowledgeable in the diagnosis and management of geriatric syndromes. CGA can be useful if your family member is considering a major life change such as a move to a nursing home and you or your family member are not sure whether this is the right step. The purpose of the CGA in this case is not to determine whether it's the right decision or not, which is at least in part a decision that reflects personal preferences; rather, it's to try to optimize your relative's health and functioning. After various medications have been eliminated from his regimen, drugs that were causing confusion or unsteadiness, his incontinence has come under better control, and he has several gadgets to facilitate bathing, dressing, and eating, the urgent need to go to a nursing home may dissipate. Perhaps just as often, your family member will still have needs that are so extensive and so constant as to require nursing home level care—but at least you will have peace of mind, knowing you did everything you could to improve his situation.

How can you arrange for an outpatient comprehensive geriatric assessment? They aren't universally available.

Ideally, your family member's primary care physician will know or figure out how to obtain a CGA and make the referral. That approach also increases the likelihood that the recommendations stemming from the evaluation will be followed. As I mentioned in discussing the recommendations from a geriatric consultation, one of the best ways to assure that the consultation will prove useless is to ignore the suggestions it produces. In general, primary care physicians are much more apt to be receptive to advice they have solicited than to recommendations they didn't ask for in the first place.

Alternatives to Comprehensive Geriatric Assessment

Because CGA isn't always an option, there are a few alternatives you should know about that more or less serve the same purpose. First, there is geriatric consultation, which I talked about before, typically provided by a geriatrician rather than a whole team. The geriatrician is equipped to perform some of the parts of the assessment and can refer your family member to practitioners of other disciplines such as physical therapy, nutrition, or social work as needed. You might end up with multiple separate visits instead of the one-time, one-stop-shopping approach of a CGA, and you won't benefit from the integration of the various recommendations unless you return to the consulting geriatrician for yet another visit. Second, in the hospital setting, there are several hundred, specialized, geriatric inpatient units called Acute Care for the Elderly (ACE) units scattered across the country. Unlike the VA's GEM units, the ACE units take care of the patient from admission to discharge. They aren't a type of "step-down unit" for ongoing care after the acute problem is under control; they are simply an alternative to a standard medical floor. I'll talk more about ACE units when we discuss hospitalization (see chapter 14, "Acute Care for the Elderly Units"). Suffice it to say here that their focus is improving the hospital stay rather than looking comprehensively at health and well-being. Part of their mission is good discharge planning and, if they're going to be as sure as they can be that your family member will get the requisite care after leaving the hospital, they have to pay attention to things such as mobility, cognition, and social supports—some of the linchpins of a comprehensive geriatric assessment. The limitation of this quasi-CGA is that it is performed while your family member is acutely ill and the findings may not be generalizable to some later point in time when, with good luck and good care, your family member will be doing better. Of course, any CGA is of limited validity, bound in time to the moment when it is conducted, but an in-hospital assessment is carried out at a particularly vulnerable point in your relative's life.

Similarly, your family member can get some semblance of a comprehensive assessment if he happens to be in a skilled nursing or rehabilitation facility, recovering after a hospitalization for an acute problem. Just as I will have more to say about ACE units when we talk about hospital care, so, too, I'll have more to say about rehab-style geriatric assessment when we discuss those facilities (see chapter 19, "Hospital-Lite— Another Role for Rehab"). I'll point out now that, by law, rehabs are required to complete a comprehensive evaluation of their residents at the time of admission and this assessment is supposed to serve as the basis for their entire plan of care. To facilitate such an evaluation, the Centers for Medicare and Medicaid Services require that nursing facilities complete the Minimum Data Set (MDS), a long and complex survey of the resident's physical, cognitive, emotional, and psychosocial status—exactly what a CGA does.

Earlier, we spoke about your family member's underlying health state and I explained that his ability to function in daily life, his psychological state of mind, and his cognition are all ingredients of his overall health state, along with the more traditional medical diagnoses. A CGA is another way to systematically determine health state or, if you already know whether your relative is robust, frail, has dementia, or is dying, it's a way to understand his current condition more precisely. Just as a conventional annual exam can both uncover new diagnoses and determine the severity of each already known diagnosis, just as a physical exam is used as the basis for developing a new plan or revising the old plan for managing established diseases, a CGA is a way to address all the major components of your family member's health.

A comprehensive geriatric assessment can be a valuable supplement to routine medical care for your family member (box 9.1). It's a way to try to adjust the treatment of his diseases and improve his daily functioning so as to maximize his quality of life.

Box 9.1

Comprehensive Geriatric Assessment focuses on

- Physical function
- Medical problems
- Cognition
- Psychological issues
- Interdisciplinary assessment

PART III

Going to the Hospital

E ach year, your family member has at least a one-in-five chance of being hospitalized. If she's over age eighty-five and needs help with her daily activities, her risk of hospitalization is closer to one-in-two. And if she does go to the hospital, her sojourn will typically disrupt her life significantly. The modern hospital is a palace of technology with the potential to cure her of all sorts of ills, but it can also leave her weaker and needier than ever. Being prepared for the experience, knowing something about choosing which hospital to go to, what to expect when you're there, and how to deal with the staff can vastly enhance your relative's stay.

CHAPTER 10

The Perils of Hospitalization

I promised that I would let you know when I'm giving you my opinion rather than either facts or an approach to thinking about a problem. I'm going to begin the section on hospital care by telling you that I have a strong preference for keeping frail elders out of hospitals altogether. I realize this is not always possible and that it may not be the course that you and your family member choose. Just so you understand my perspective and are in a better position to make sense of the remaining chapters about hospitals, I'm going to start with an explanation of why I'm so leery of them.

It's important to recognize that anyone who is hospitalized these days is likely to be really sick. If your family member is very ill, she's probably going to have tests and procedures, and these tests and procedures are associated with complications. Many of the complications have nothing to do with the hospital itself; they are related to your family member's illness and its treatment. For example, your family member might develop a rash from the antibiotic she is taking for pneumonia, whether she takes the antibiotics at home or in the hospital. Or she might go into kidney failure from the dye that is injected during a computerized tomography (CT) scan, an x-ray taken to evaluate abdominal pain, regardless of whether the CT scan is ordered by her primary care physician at the time of an office visit or by the hospital physician during an inpatient stay. But other complications are related to the process of hospitalization itself. Your family member might wake up during the night and have to go to the bathroom but because she is in an unfamiliar place, she might trip and fall as she tries to make her way in the dark. Alternatively, she may have trouble sleeping since she's in an uncomfortable bed away from home. The physician may prescribe a sleeping pill to help but this may lead to a new problem: confusion caused by the sleeping pill.

Even problems that appear to be related to the disease for which your family member was admitted or its treatment might actually arise from an interaction between the treatment and the hospital environment. That antibiotic-induced rash might be due to an antibiotic to which your family member was known to be allergic—except the crucial information was buried in her office chart and inaccessible to the hospital staff. While the kidney failure triggered by a CT scan was the result of a fairly common reaction to dye, your family member might only have gotten the CT scan because it was so convenient to obtain in the hospital. For her to have a CT scan as an outpatient, her doctor would have to order it, you'd have to schedule it, and then your relative would have to travel to either a hospital x-ray suite or a freestanding radiology clinic to have the procedure done—quite possibly on an empty stomach, predisposing her to dizziness and falls. When getting a test is such an ordeal, the physician might think twice about ordering it. In the hospital, all that's needed is the click of a mouse and the test is ordered. If any special preparation is required, the nurse will make sure it is taken care of and when it's time for the test, an orderly will show up with a stretcher and transport your family member to the right place.

The Dangers of Multiple Tests

Hospitals are potentially perilous because the standard of care in the hospital is often inimical to the best interests of frail older people. When your family member is admitted, she will receive a standard battery of tests. Sometimes this is even dignified with a special name, the "admissions order set," and it customarily includes multiple blood tests (a blood count, chemistries such as electrolytes, glucose, and measures of kidney function), a urine test, a chest x-ray, and an electrocardiogram (EKG). It's a basic law of statistics that if your relative has enough tests, at least one of them will give false positive results, come back abnormal just by chance, even though nothing is actually wrong with her. But in the hospital, if a test result is off, the physician will almost invariably order other tests to try to get to the bottom of the "problem," even though the real problem is with the interpretation of the test. It's not that the technician made an error or that the radiologist read the film incorrectly; rather, it's that no test is perfect. A perfect test would always come back positive in the setting of disease and negative in the absence of disease. A very good test is only rarely positive in the absence of disease. But even if a test is inaccurate only 5 percent of the time, that means, roughly speaking, 5 percent of all tests performed will lead to false positive test results. If she has twenty tests—and hospitalized patients are subject to far more than twenty tests—at least one of them is apt to come out falsely positive. The follow-up test or treatment, whatever that might be, could be quite unpleasant for your family member, not to mention that it will make her anxious because she believes something is wrong with her.

I've seen many hospitalized patients treated for a "urinary tract infection" because the urinalysis they had on admission showed some bacteria—even though the majority of older women and many older men *always* have bacteria in their urine. This finding alone is of no consequence unless it is associated with symptoms such as burning on urination or the urge to go to the bathroom frequently. Other false positive test results can cause even more trouble: I remember one case of a woman in her eighties whose physician considered doing a spinal tap to look for evidence of advanced syphilis after a blood test came back positive for syphilis, although the patient had no symptoms of disease and had been sexually inactive for thirty years—and even though positive test results were far more commonly false positives than true positives.

A Cascade of Complications

Sometimes it's not just one problem that results from hospitalization, it's a whole cascade of problems. A seemingly minor occurrence triggers another difficulty that leads to yet a third issue. That seemingly innocuous urinary tract infection, for instance, results in an order for an antibiotic. But the antibiotic, in addition to killing off the bacteria in the urine that weren't causing any trouble, also kills off bacteria in the intestines that were actually serving an important function. Without the normal bacteria to check their growth, a dangerous organism called *clostridium difficile* can get out of hand, causing severe diarrhea. Now your family member, who never even had a bladder infection to start with, has a rip-roaring case of diarrhea and ends up dehydrated and dizzy. This time when she wakes up at night to go to the bathroom, she's sure to fall. If she's really unlucky, she might break her hip. Events have spiraled out of control. It happens all the time in hospitals.

If you list the main complications that are directly or indirectly associated with hospitalization, you find delirium, falls, polypharmacy, and functional decline head the list. If this sounds a lot like the leading geriatric syndromes, it is. *Delirium*, or acute confusion, is precipitated by a whole host of interventions that are common in the hospital, quite apart from the condition that led to your family member being admitted (see chapter 38, "Confusion"). Heading the list are medications. A hospitalization is almost invariably associated with the introduction of several new medicines, with a good chance that at least one will cause confusion. Then there are environmental factors, especially in places such as the intensive care unit (ICU) which disrupts the sleep/wake cycle with alarms, perpetual illumination, and constant activity. The phenomenon is so common that it has been called "ICU psychosis," which is just another name for delirium that develops in the ICU.

Falling is another hazard of hospitalization, even though "injurious falls," or falls that cause a significant injury, now result in Medicare penalizing the hospital with a lower rate of reimbursement. As I mentioned before, falling may be caused by medications or simply by stumbling in an unfamiliar environment. In addition, many hospitalized patients are kept at bedrest, either as part of their treatment or because of concern that they *might* fall if they get up unassisted; the result of prolonged bedrest, however, is what I call "Jell-O legs" which also predisposes someone to falling.

Polypharmacy is the norm in the hospital. Some of the new medications may cause delirium or falls, but they can cause other problems as well. They may, for example, cause constipation and while that doesn't sound like a major issue, severe constipation, in addition to being very uncomfortable, can trigger other symptoms ranging from confusion to difficulty urinating. Medications may cause a rash, which again doesn't sound so bad, but rashes are

itchy, and itching will lead to the doctor prescribing an antihistamine, and antihistamines tend to be sedating and to cause constipation—and suddenly your relative is undergoing another cascade of complications. Medications can also interact with other medications and the more pills your family member is taking, the more likely she is to have one of these "drug-drug interactions." These can be serious: for example, with blood-thinning medications, certain drugs can elevate the level, causing bleeding; with anti-epileptic medication, some drugs can depress drug levels, resulting in seizures.

All in all, an estimated one in three older patients is worse off in terms of her ability to function on her own at the time of discharge than before admission. That's one reason that so many elders end up going to rehab before they go home—not to receive ongoing treatment for their acute problem but to recover from the hospitalization. We'll talk later about various strategies for avoiding or ameliorating these iatrogenic (doctor-induced) complications of hospitalization. But the most effective way to prevent them is to avoid the hospital altogether, which is precisely why I began by saying that my bias is that hospitals, while remarkable and sometimes lifesaving institutions, should be avoided by those who are frail whenever possible.

When Hospitalization Is Essential

"Whenever possible" doesn't mean always. Sometimes only the hospital can provide the treatment your family member needs. If she has fallen and broken her hip and wishes to regain her mobility, she will need an operation. If her knee or hip has degenerated to the point where she has a great deal of pain and trouble walking, she would benefit from joint replacement surgery. And if she has an inflamed appendix, it will need to be removed if she is to survive. But it's not just surgical problems that necessitate hospitalization. Certain medical conditions, such as a bleeding ulcer, a condition that is best treated with intravenous medications and blood transfusions, also warrant hospital care. Various procedures including insertion of a stent to prop open an artery and restore blood flow, whether to the leg, the heart, or some other body part, can only be done in a hospital—although interestingly, the standard of care is evolving and more and more procedures are safely carried out in "ambulatory surgery centers," freestanding facilities that are effectively mini-hospitals in an outpatient environment.

For those conditions that could, theoretically, be treated outside the hospital, there may nonetheless be compelling reasons for preferring the hospital. Hospitals offer incredible benefits—along with risks. Perhaps most importantly, they provide 24/7 nursing care. While your family member might complain that the nurse doesn't come as quickly as she'd like after she presses the "call button," she will come eventually. The ratio of nurses to patients may not be as high as you'd like but it's higher than in a skilled nursing facility, another potential treatment site. That means that whether your family member has to pass her urine, is having pain, or has developed shortness of breath, a qualified professional is available to respond to her needs. Hospitals also generally have good access to physicians, either on site or on call, in contrast to the skilled nursing facility, that at best has a physician who can be reached by telephone, and the home, where no physician may be available until the next day. In addition, the hospital offers one-stop shopping: an on-site pharmacy and fully equipped radiology suite, along with technicians for drawing blood and a lab for analyzing the blood that's been drawn. These features make the experience far more convenient for patients than if they remained at home and had to travel to disparate locations for various diagnostic procedures and treatments. It's this ready availability that is both advantageous and hazardous to your family member.

I'll talk more about home versus hospital care later on but at this juncture, I just want you to be aware of the principal risks and some of the benefits of hospital care (box 10.1). Armed with this knowledge, you'll be better positioned to try to avoid some of the potential complications if your family member does go to the hospital.

Box 10.1

Perils of Hospitalization

- Falls
- Confusion
- Polypharmacy
- Functional decline
- Unnecessary tests

CHAPTER 11

Choosing a Hospital

I f you call an ambulance in the event of an emergency, the paramedics will take your family member to the nearest hospital. If the situation isn't quite so dire, the choice of hospital will likely be dictated by where his physician has "privileges" (i.e., where she can visit or care for patients) or what facility she is associated with. If you live in a rural area, you might effectively have no choice—you'd have to travel an unreasonable distance to reach any hospital other than the local community institution. But sometimes, for example, if your family member needs an elective procedure such as a total hip replacement or surgery to remove her gallbladder, and if you live in an urban area, you will have the opportunity to consider the options.

The Rankings

I f you have choices and want to evaluate them, you have several places to turn, each of which offers its own version of a report card for hospitals. Medicare provides a way of learning about hospital quality with its Hospital Compare website (figure 11.1). As of February 2019, 3,724 hospitals across the country reported sufficient data for Medicare to rate them. Medicare gave each hospital between one and five stars, with the majority of hospitals earning two, three, or four stars; only 7.9 percent of evaluable hospitals were awarded five stars and 7.6 percent got one star. The ratings are based on a survey of recently discharged patients reporting on their subjective experiences as well as six objective measures. The subjective measures include such areas as how well patients thought physicians and nurses communicated, how satisfied they were with the noise level and cleanliness at the hospital, and how well the hospital prepared them for discharge. The objective measures include the mortality rate, the safety of care, the effectiveness of care, the readmission rate, the timeliness of care, and the efficient use of medical imaging.

Another very different approach to assessing hospital quality is offered by the not-for-profit Leapfrog Group (see figure 11.2). This organization is in the business of trying to improve quality by reporting on safety. Medicare uses the Michelin Guide five-star rating system; Leapfrog opts for letter grades from A to E. It assigns a grade to each of several domains such as hospital-acquired infections, surgical problems, preventive practices, and staff characteristics (that one is vague but refers to whether certified intensive care unit [ICU] physicians are on the staff and whether staff regularly receives special safety

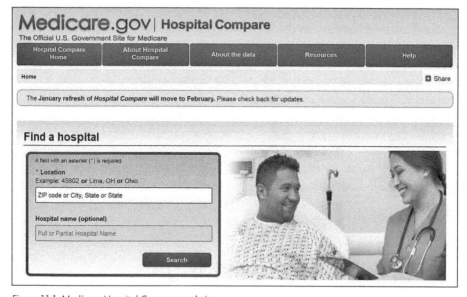

Figure 11.1. Medicare Hospital Compare website

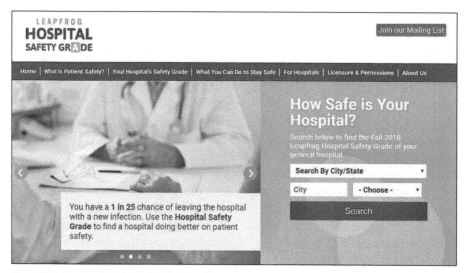

Figure 11.2. Leapfrog Hospital Safety Grade website

training). In some instances, it's desirable to have a high score (for example, widespread use of precaution gowns or fire drills that are designed to prevent problems) and in others, the lower the better (fewer cases of nasty infections with bacteria such as MRSA and *clostridium difficile*, two organisms that can wreak havoc in hospitals).

U.S. News and World Report also issues its list of "best hospitals" each year. This ranking of sixteen hospital specialties, from oncology to geriatrics, is based on physician opinion. Various experts are asked to name up to five hospitals they consider the best for difficult cases in their specialty. Hospitals are very eager to win this recognition: in the Boston area, hospitals put banners over their doorways and pay for ads on street corners touting, for example, that they are #5 in cardiology or #4 in cancer care.

The problem with all these sources is that their methodology varies; they each present one perspective. Medicare heavily weights the consumer's experience—important, but not a measure of medical competence or sophistication. Leapfrog presents the safety record—also important, but not the only thing that matters when your family member is hospitalized. *U.S. News* tells you about reputation, which may reflect some aspect of performance, though it's not entirely clear which one. As a result, the same hospital can get rave reviews on one appraisal and mediocre reports on another. One community hospital in my neighborhood, for example, got four stars from Hospital Compare and an "A" from Leapfrog but has no nationally ranked specialties according to *U.S. News and World Report*. A major teaching hospital nearby was awarded only three stars by Hospital Compare and a "B" by Leapfrog, but it boasts eleven, nationally ranked specialty services.

What Type of Hospital?

This brings me to another consideration: the *type* of hospital to choose for your family member. The various kinds of hospitals present different pluses and minuses for complex patients. I am only going to talk about hospitals that care for acute medical problems, not about psychiatric hospitals or long-term care hospitals. The American Hospital Association categorizes hospitals as *community hospi-* *tals* and *federal government hospitals*. Community hospitals, in turn, can be investor-owned (for-profit); they can be private, not-for-profit; or they can be owned and operated by a city or region. Federal hospitals are almost exclusively Veterans Administration hospitals. In this schema, a tertiary care megahospital, a hospital that is a magnet for referrals from all over the state and sometimes the entire country or even the world, and that has eight hundred or a thousand beds, is lumped together with a moderate-sized or small, local hospital that mainly provides care for "bread and butter" conditions such as pneumonia or heart failure. The experience for your family member is likely to be very different in these two environments.

Because hospitals are almost by definition unfamiliar, stressful, and anxiety-producing institutions, your family member is apt to find a smaller, less technologically intensive site of care more comfortable and less intimidating—what most laypeople refer to as their neighborhood or community hospital. If your family member is more comfortable and less intimidated, he is probably less likely to incur one of the many risks I talked about earlier, such as falls or confusion. He may also be more likely to have his own primary care physician serving as the "attending physician," or physician in charge of his care, rather than having a hospitalist or hospital employee responsible for his treatment. More on hospitalists later—they have much to recommend them, but a hospitalist is not your family member's regular physician, someone with whom he already has a relationship and who has ready access to his outpatient medical records (see chapter 12, "Working with a Hospitalist"). Community hospitals may not have the latest and greatest technology, though they are almost all quite sophisticated and have computerized tomography (CT) scanners, magnetic resonance imaging (MRI) machines, and the ability to perform cardiac echocardiograms. For most medical prob-

lems, they have ample technological sophistication and if they don't have something, they won't use it, which for frail patients is often an advantage, not a disadvantage—unless your family member has a rare disease or exceptionally complicated problem. If you know he has an unusual condition or a problem that nobody's been able to diagnose despite multiple attempts, he may be better off in a larger, more academically oriented hospital.

Suppose your family member does have an unusual disease, say a rare type of cancer or rare neurological syndrome, then you need to figure out how aggressive your family member wants treatment to be. That, in turn, reflects his principal goal of care. Does he want to live as long as possible, no matter what the consequences are for his daily functioning or his comfort? Does he want the doctors to focus exclusively on his comfort? Or is he somewhere in between—where most, but certainly not all, people are—he'd like to live as long as possible, but not if it means major losses in his already limited ability to carry out his daily activities. If his goal is to have as much time as he can, period, then he's probably better off getting treated in a tertiary care hospital, a major teaching hospital. If his goal is to be kept comfortable, then odds are he'll do better in a local community hospital. And if he's in the in-between group, it's hard to say for sure. The choice may depend on just how frail he is, how many tests and procedures he is able to tolerate. Or it may depend on whether he already has an established relationship with a specialist who is affiliated with one or the other institution.

Hospital Ownership:
For-Profit or Not-for-Profit

Another dimension along which hospitals differ is ownership—is the hospital you are considering a for-profit or a not-for-profit institution? This is an area where I have a bias: all things being equal, I trust not-for-profit hospitals with their volunteer boards more than I trust for-profit institutions that seek to make money and are accountable to shareholders. Studies confirm that on average, not-for-profits have a better track record for quality. That said, *all* hospitals are worried about their bottom line; they *all* try to make a profit, although the not-for-profits plow it back into the hospital whereas the owners of for-profits can pocket what was earned. *All* hospital CEOs are leery of money-losing units within their hospital—and geriatric units, psychiatry units, and palliative care units, which may be extremely beneficial for your family member, are almost always money losers. The not-for-profits, however, have a mandate to provide certain kinds of services to their patients even if they are not lucrative. This is another domain where you might not have a choice: in certain parts of the country, virtually all the hospitals are for-profit and in other states none of them are.

Another consideration is whether the institution is a teaching hospital or not. Teaching hospitals are where medical students get hands-on experience with patients; they are often where

freshly minted doctors spend upward of a year acquiring the supervised training they need to become physicians who can work independently. The teaching environment has its pluses and minuses for your family member. On the one hand, he will receive a good deal of medical attention. Rather than once daily rounds by the attending physician, with the bulk of care being provided by nurses, perhaps supplemented by a physician assistant or nurse practitioner, he will have a whole team of physicians. At the bottom of the pyramid is the intern (also called a first-year resident), a physician in her first year after graduating from medical school. The next layer is the junior (or second-year) resident, a physician who has completed an internship, and so on until you reach the attending physician, at the pinnacle of the pyramid, the senior physician in charge of your family member. The advantage of all these layers is that your relative will have fresh young minds thinking about him, considering all the alternative approaches to treatment and discussing with each other how to proceed. The drawback is that interns and residents are learners; they don't have the confidence that comes from experience, confidence that allows them to eliminate certain diagnostic possibilities from consideration and to focus in on the most likely explanation for your relative's symptoms. The net effect: they cast a wide net, which translates into more tests and procedures for your family member, an approach that may not be in his best interest. This is not just a theoretical concern—we know that teaching hospitals spend more money per patient than their nonteaching counterparts, a reality that is reflected in higher Medicare reimbursement to these facilities. But more isn't necessarily better for your family member when it comes to x-rays, blood tests, biopsies, and other interventions.

Hospital Systems

In today's world, the hospital industry has been marked by *consolidation*, by mergers, acquisitions, and the formation of entire hospital "systems." While all this buying and selling, wheeling and dealing, or marriage and divorce may seem unimportant to you as a caregiver, it matters in thinking about what hospital your family member should go to. All your careful preparation that leads to your family member seeking care in a small community hospital rather than a downtown tertiary teaching hospital may go by the wayside if the small hospital decides unilaterally to transfer your relative to its sister institution in town. The key operative word here is "unilaterally"; clearly, you should have input into any such decision. But increasingly, the way that hospital networks or systems operate is that patients are moved from one site to another, ostensibly to improve care, sometimes for the duration of their hospitalization and sometimes just for a day, to avail themselves of a procedure that is only available in the larger institution. Ideally, this fluidity offers patients the advantages of both types of hospitals. In reality, for complex, vulnerable patients, it may result in the worst of both worlds: They went to the small, local hospital in order to avoid the perils of say, a cardiac catheterization, and they ended up with the very test they didn't want *and* the disruption of traveling back and forth to another institution. Moreover, since they are often shipped back to their hospital of origin shortly after the procedure is carried out, the follow-up is going to be provided by physicians other than those who performed the exam—and it's during the follow-up period that your family member is most likely to run into complications.

How Useful Is That Procedure?

The bottom line is that you need to be extremely vigilant. It's not easy to say no to physicians, especially when they are arguing that a move or a test is in the patient's best interest; you don't want to feel as though you are depriving your family member of a beneficial, perhaps even lifesaving intervention. But that's the critical question: just how likely is the procedure to be beneficial *and at what cost?* Often, physicians see only the pluses and none of the minuses. If the endoscopy or the angiogram or whatever it is that's being proposed is extremely likely to be useful and almost certainly won't be harmful, that's terrific. Far more often, that positron emissions tomography (PET) scan or biopsy has a modest chance of proving useful and a considerable risk of causing harm. The specialist or the resident physician who is recommending the intervention may not know your relative well enough or have sufficient experience herself to engage in the delicate balancing act required to care for complicated patients like your family member.

A good bet may be to rely on your primary care physician to advise you about the choice of hospital (box 11.1). And better yet, in many situations, you will be able to keep your family member out of the hospital altogether.

Box 11.1

Choosing a Hospital

- Hospital rankings are one measure of quality
- Not-for-profit hospitals tend to perform better than for-profit hospitals in quality
- Local community hospitals may be better for common conditions
- Teaching hospitals (academic institutions) are advantageous for rare diseases

CHAPTER 12

Working with a Hospitalist

Hospitalists are the new kids on the block. Traditionally, your relative's primary care physician—or the specialist referring her to the hospital—continued to provide care once she was hospitalized. In the American hospital of the 1990s, a new breed of physician began to appear who worked exclusively in the hospital and took over responsibility for your family member only once she was admitted. The motivation for creating this new specialty was a desire to improve *efficiency*: hospitalists are physically on site, unlike your relative's primary care physician who has to make time in his office schedule to go to the hospital to see her. Only rarely do primary care physicians visit the hospital more than once a day, arguably to the detriment of patients such as your family member, who are often unstable with a rapidly changing course.

The new model, which spread rapidly across the United States, penetrating large hospitals first but extending into all types of hospital over time, makes a great deal of sense—in principle. For primary care physicians, who spend most of their day in the office, it is less disruptive; for your relative, it

means greater access to a physician; and for nursing staff, it allows easier, more direct communication with the physician in charge (instead of telephoning the doctor's office and hoping to be put through or leaving a message and receiving a return call from a frazzled doctor between patients, the nurse can page the hospitalist, who might appear in person minutes later). But while studies of the new model confirm increases in efficiency—patients tend to have shorter hospital stays—there has been no measurable improvement in the quality of care.

The absence of an increase in quality doesn't, of course, mean that quality is worse. But the evaluations do not separate out different types of patients—old versus young, complex versus straightforward, frail versus robust, patients with dementia versus the cognitively intact. Quite possibly, hospitalists are particularly advantageous for your family member because, being specialists in hospital care, they are well-acquainted with the hazards of hospitalization. Perhaps they know all about the risk of falls, delirium, polypharmacy, and functional decline in hospitalized elders. Maybe they are better attuned to these potential problems than are physicians whose practice is primarily located in the outpatient setting. Or perhaps the relative expertise of the hospitalist and the primary care physician varies depending on their particular degree of geriatric sophistication: at one extreme, the hospitalist may be naïve about geriatric syndromes, while the primary physician is well-versed in them; at the other extreme, the hospitalist is the sophisticated one and the outpatient doctor is the rube. Whatever the situation, the hospitalist is new to you and your family member, and he is someone you will need to get to know and work with. In particular, you will need to work with the hospitalist—sometimes with several different ones over the course of a single hospital stay—to convince him of the importance of your *engagement* in his patient's care, to inform him of her *baseline state*, and to be sure he understands and abides by any *advance care plan* you and your family member have developed.

Patient Engagement in Medical Care

The prevailing norm in American medicine is for patients to participate in decision-making about their care. But the paradigm assumes that each patient is autonomous and acts alone, not that she is a member of a family or has a caregiver, or for that matter lives in a community. The reality is that family members and caregivers, as well as the surrounding neighborhood or social network, often constrain individual decision-making. If your relative cannot see well but is supposed to self-administer insulin injections, someone else will need to pre-fill the syringes or be available to give the medication—or else another form of treatment will have to be substituted. If your family member has poor memory and is expected to take a pill five times a day, a system will need to be put in place to make that possible, either using preset smartphone reminders, telephone calls, or a caregiver who makes sure she takes her medications. But physicians may not appreciate these limitations on your relative's *executional autonomy*, the help she needs in carrying out a plan, even if she is able to participate in formulating the plan in the first place. Unless your family member has dementia, and sometimes fairly advanced dementia, the hospitalist physician may assume she is the only person with whom he has to interact, whether to obtain informed consent for a procedure or to discuss treatment options.

If you provide a significant amount of caregiving and participate extensively in your relative's day-to-day medical care, you will need to explain your role to the hospitalist. You will also need to obtain your family member's permission to allow the hospitalist to contact you by telephone or invite you to participate in planning discussions in the hospital. Without such explicit authorization, physicians are not supposed to talk about clinical matters with you, in the interest of protecting your family member's privacy and autonomy, as mandated by the Health Insurance Portability and Accountability Act (HIPAA). Communicating with the hospital staff prior to discharge is also very important to assure continuity of care. In most states, CARE (Caregiver, Advise, Record, Enable) legislation requires hospital personnel to record the name of their patients' caregivers and provide discharge information.

You clearly don't want your interactions with the hospital staff, whether the hospitalist or anybody else, to be confrontational. You don't want to find yourself in the position of being furious that you arrived at the hospital, only to find your family member was off having some procedure that you would never have wanted performed, if only you had known it was under consideration. You don't want to discover your relative has just received three doses of a medication that, in the past, has made her floridly delirious, but nobody checked with you first, even though the drug in question is one that many frail elders do not tolerate. Assuming your family member

is amenable to your active participation in her care, the best strategy is to introduce yourself to the hospitalist early on, making clear that you can be tremendously helpful to *him* (and, of course, to your family member) through your involvement, by assuring compliance with his instructions or supporting joint decisions about treatment or reiterating what he said about what to expect.

If you visit your family member in the evenings and the hospitalist comes by in the early morning or late afternoon, you might want to rearrange your visiting schedule or set up a regular way to communicate new developments. Most hospitals have a secure email system for transmitting confidential information or you can agree on a time to touch base by phone. If you don't come up with some kind of system, you may find that the hospitalist doesn't communicate with you at all—except in the event of an emergency—or that he interacts with whomever he does find at your family member's bedside, even if that's her ex-husband or a prying neighbor, rather than you, the person who has her health-care proxy and is her caregiver. On the other hand, if you do establish open lines of communication, you will have a better grasp of what's going on in the hospital and be in a better position to provide the requisite care once your family member goes home.

Clarifying the Baseline State

One of the major adverse events your relative is at risk of experiencing in the hospital is delirium, or an acute confusional state (for more about delirium, see chapter 38, "Confusion"). For physicians to recognize and correctly diagnose delirium, it's extremely helpful to appreciate that your family member is not at her baseline. All too often, the nurses and doctors involved in your relative's care first meet her during her hospital stay and don't realize that she isn't normally confused. She might even develop hallucinations or delusions that are likewise chalked up to dementia, whether or not she actually has dementia. Even if she does carry the diagnosis of dementia, the staff might not know that she doesn't usually experience hallucinations or delusions. One of the biggest favors you can do for your family member and for the hospitalist is to let the staff know what your family member is usually like.

In addition to describing her baseline mental status, you will want to say a bit about how much she can do for herself at home. If she's had a new stroke, it's imperative to know what she was like before the stroke to determine the goals of rehabilitation. If she couldn't walk without an assistive device before, or she couldn't dress herself or take a shower independently, then it would be foolhardy to expect she will do so after the stroke. On the other hand, if she lives in a house with stairs and used to be able to go up and down

on her own, then putting her at bedrest in the hospital for seven days and then sending her home without determining if she is still going to be able to cope with steps is also a mistake.

You may also be the best source of information about her usual medications. Even if both the hospital and your family member's primary care physician use electronic medical records, and even if the two records are compatible, and even if the hospitalist has access to the outpatient records (all big ifs), medication lists are notoriously inaccurate and out of date. Sometimes physicians add new drugs to the list but forget to remove old ones. The correct dose may likewise be uncertain. Sometimes specialists add to or modify the medication list but those changes don't make it onto what is supposedly the master list. If you keep your own records of your family member's medications, both past and present, you might also be the best source for determining if a proposed medication, while not a drug your family member is currently taking, was something she took in the past. Perhaps it was discontinued because it didn't work. Maybe she developed an adverse reaction, whether a rash, nausea, diarrhea, or confusion.

Knowledge of your relative's home situation will also help the hospitalist figure out whether she can safely return home after the acute episode has subsided or whether, for example, she might need a rehab stay. As the hospitalization appears to be drawing to a close—perhaps the intravenous medication and the continuous cardiac monitoring are no longer necessary and have been discontinued—you may want to clarify with the hospitalist how close to her baseline your family member now is in terms of her level of function-ing. Without a basis for comparison, the physician has no way of knowing just how much the patient has recovered. You may be surprised, too. If you re-quest that your family member get out of bed, dress, and walk around, you may discover how much weaker or shakier she is than she was at home.

Advance Care Planning

If I talk a great deal about advance care planning and establishing goals of care, it's because I think that these discussions have the potential to significantly affect what tests and treatments your family member has (see chapter 49, "Planning for Future Medical Care"). If your relative has an out-of-hospital do-not-resuscitate (DNR) order that she and her physician signed, you should give a copy to the hospitalist. Ditto if she has completed a Physician Orders for Life-Sustaining Treatment (POLST) form or the variants used in other states—MOST (Medical Orders for Scope of Treatment) in West Virginia, MOLST (Medical Orders for Life-Sustaining Treatment) in Massa-chusetts, and so forth. These are actual medical orders, enshrined in law by the states that honor them, so, in principle, they should be accepted as valid by any health-care institution. The reality is that hospitals usually accept as bind-ing only medical orders written into their medical record system by their staff physicians. These are *intervention-specific* directives: the DNR order says,

in effect, if my heart stops beating and I'm not breathing, do not attempt to revive me with cardiopulmonary re-suscitation (CPR). The POLST specifies for a whole raft of potential medical interventions, starting with CPR and intubation and moving on to artificial nutrition and hydration, dialysis, and other treatment modalities commonly used in very sick people: "I want to have the treatment" if my physician recom-mends it for my condition, or "I don't want the treatment," or "I'm not sure." While it's a good idea to communicate these sorts of preferences to the hos-pitalist if you and your family member have already discussed them, you should also talk to the hospitalist more generally about *goals of care*.

Remember that the default assump-tion in the hospital is that your family member wants all available treatment to extend life or correct a medical problem, regardless of how risky or how uncertain the benefit. Letting the hospitalist know if your family member favors a different approach is essential to assure she receives care that makes sense for her. You might, for example, inform the hospitalist that your family member is at a point in her life when her main concern is to be kept comfortable. If what your family member values above all is maintaining her current level of function—her present ability to walk or talk or think or hear—that information is crucial to communicate. Often, hospital-based physicians, like physicians generally, assume that either a patient wants "everything" or "nothing"; they interpret "nothing" to mean morphine and oxygen. You are going to have to make clear if your family member falls between these two extremes. It will then be up to you (ideally in concert with your relative) and the hospitalist to determine which of the various treatment possibilities is most likely to be consistent with your family member's overriding goal.

Goals of care have the potential to shape all kinds of decisions that are made in the hospital. Would your family member be better off in the intensive care unit (ICU) or on a medical or surgical floor? Which makes more sense, the standard of care or a variant strategy? Consider first the question of the ICU. An ICU, by definition, offers more intensive nursing care, more intensive monitoring, and ready access to a whole array of technology that is used exclusively in the ICU setting (most hospitals, for example, do not provide ventilator care or continuous peritoneal dialysis outside selected units). On the other hand, the constant bustle in the ICU makes it conducive to triggering delirium. Delirium is so commonly associated with the ICU that it's been called "ICU psychosis." Frail older pa-

tients who spend long periods of time in the ICU have a poor prognosis if they are able to leave the hospital at all, both in terms of survival and in terms of their quality of life, for several months after discharge.

Now let's think about whether the "standard" approach is necessarily the best one for your family member. I'm thinking about several serious medical problems that are customarily addressed surgically, such as an inflamed gallbladder (cholecystitis) or an ischemic bowel (the intestinal analog of a heart attack, in which tissue dies from lack of adequate blood supply). The presumption in both cases is that your family member will have the best chance of surviving if she has an operation. But for someone with multiple other medical problems, in addition to the acute problem, someone who at baseline leads a fairly tenuous existence, surgery is especially risky. Not only do such patients have a higher-than-average risk of dying, but they also run a considerable risk of suffering from a cascade of complications and further decline in their ability to function if they do survive. Your family member may not be satisfied with an entirely hands-off approach, either. She may be willing to receive antibiotics (in the case of a gallbladder problem) or intravenous fluids with no food by mouth for a few days (in the case of ischemic bowel). These are forms of what I call "intermediate care," intermediate between maximally aggressive treatment and care focused exclusively on comfort. Physicians are often uncomfortable offering what they consider a second-rate treatment—but it may be just the thing for your family member if her primary goal of care is to maintain her previous level of functioning. I don't expect you to know just what intermediate options might exist in your family member's situation. But if you help the hospitalist understand the goal of care on which you and your relative have agreed, the hospitalist can strategize about a solution.

To work successfully with a hospitalist, you need—above all—to establish a relationship (box 12.1). In the outpatient setting, you can gradually establish a relationship with your relative's physician. In the hospital, everything is accelerated. You will have to learn quickly to trust each other, but if you succeed, it will pay off amply.

Box 12.1

Working with a Hospitalist

- Establish an open line of communication
- Clarify your relative's baseline state, both level of physical functioning and cognition
- Provide information about the goals of care, including a Physician Orders for Life-Sustaining Treatment (POLST) or a do-not-resuscitate (DNR) form when available

CHAPTER 13

The Technological Imperative

Technology can be lifesaving and it can dramatically improve your relative's quality of life. Sometimes high-tech treatments are even more effective in older people than in their younger counterparts: it turns out that clot-busting drugs, medications that are used to stop a heart attack in its tracks, are particularly worthwhile in older people. The paradox—at least it seems to be a paradox, because powerful drugs are also more likely to cause side effects when used in the elderly—arises because older people have more at stake. If your family member has a heart attack it will tend, on average, to be more massive and more devastating than if he were younger, so he may have more to lose if he *doesn't* get clot-busting drugs. But it's essential to be very selective about what technological interventions your family member will have. The crucial questions about any test or procedure are always: How much of a difference will it make, what harm might it cause, and what are the alternatives?

Risks of Low-Tech Procedures

Even seemingly harmless technology carries risk in susceptible, hospitalized patients. Take the lowly intravenous catheter (IV). Leaving a catheter in your relative's vein, whether to give medication, fluids, or "just in case," means having something mechanical inside him, what doctors call "a foreign body." This specific device is a conduit between his deepest recesses—the bloodstream—and the outside world. It's a great way for bacteria, which are generally ruthlessly excluded from the blood vessels, to make their way inside, giving them unfettered access to every organ in the body as the blood courses through the veins to the heart and from the heart back into the circulation. Physicians and nurses try to prevent bacteria from taking advantage of this doorway to the body's inner sanctum by using "sterile technique" when inserting the catheter in the first place and when using it to administer a drug or other substance. But despite their efforts, catheter-associated infections remain a problem, especially when the catheter is of a special variety that is threaded all the way into one of the big veins close to the heart.

The IV catheter can cause other problems for your family member as well: it can irritate the vein where it's lodged, producing a local "phlebitis," or inflammation of the vein, which is painful. And sometimes the IV catheter creates its mischief indirectly: for example, your relative may be "restrained," or tied down, to prevent him from pulling out the catheter. Restraints in the form of a strap, belt, or what are essentially soft handcuffs are an affront to personal dignity. In addition, they can trigger a whole cascade of problems: for instance, if your relative's hands are tied down, he won't be able to get up and walk so he will stay in bed, becoming weaker and more debilitated.

What's important to remember is that not everyone who is in the hospital needs an intravenous catheter. I remember many years ago reading reflections by a British physician on visiting an American hospital emergency department. One of the first things he noticed was that all the patients had an IV. Before they had been evaluated by anyone, long before they were seen by a physician, they had an IV placed. When the British doctor asked why, he was told that if they were sick enough to be in the emergency department, they just might need emergency medication; hence, the IV. In English emergency departments, at least at that time, patients only had an IV inserted if a physician had determined that they would receive something important through it.

Now think about another simple medical device, the Foley catheter. This is a tube that goes into the bladder and is left there for the purpose of collecting and measuring the urine as it is produced. It's generally easy to insert and once it's in, the tube is connected to a bag that hangs over the edge of the bed or the side of a chair. The only maintenance required is to empty the bag when it fills and to periodically change the catheter. But this innocuous bit of technology, like the IV, can cause no end of mayhem. It is also a foreign body and it connects a normally sterile part of the body, the bladder, with the external world. It is intended to transport fluid from the inside to the outside, but there's no reason it can't also provide safe passage to organisms seeking to invade the body's inner recesses. As a result, the most common complication of an "indwelling Foley catheter," that is a catheter inserted into the bladder and left there for days at a time, is a bladder infection.

Like the IV, the Foley catheter can also produce complications indirectly. If your relative has a Foley catheter, he probably won't need to be restrained to prevent him from pulling out the catheter—the tube is safely out of sight, with the bag looped over the side rails of the hospital bed—but the tube itself serves as a de facto restraint. It's difficult for your family member to maneuver with a tube hanging out of his bladder. Add to that an IV pole and perhaps EKG leads and your relative is effectively immobilized, with all its associated risks.

Risks of High-Tech Procedures

If these everyday basic devices are fraught with risk, more complex devices are correspondingly more dangerous. Many of these risks will be reviewed with you when the physician seeks informed consent for a procedure—although the litany of bad-things-that-could-happen is often presented in much the way that television ads for medications list the major possible side effects: sotto voce. In the case of the television commercial, the incantation of adverse consequences often coincides with visual images of happy couples cavorting in the fields (in the case of Viagra ads, timed to correspond to the narrator's comment that "if you have an erection lasting longer than four hours, call your doctor"). You and your family member may both be so distraught by the news that there might be a tumor lurking in the abdomen that you don't fully process the comment, say, that the dye used in the computerized tomography (CT) scan that is planned can result in kidney failure. An intensive care unit (ICU) room with both high- and low-tech equipment is depicted in figure 13.1.

Other risks of technology will go unmentioned because physicians are unaware of them or don't appreciate their importance. Chief among these is "functional decline," the phenomenon I keep coming back to, in which basic self-care capability deteriorates in response to factors such as bedrest, sedating medications, and hospital food. Physicians typically do a good job of telling you about the major risks of tests or procedures such as death, bleeding into the brain, or sustaining a stroke. But if your family member has advanced illness or multiple conditions affecting his daily life, he may be less worried about catastrophic complications than about the more modest problems. Those seemingly minor problems have the potential to make him so dependent that he can no longer live at home or to cause his quality of life to plummet.

I want to make sure you understand the drive to use technology in the hospital because you may be the only counterweight to this powerful force. The issue isn't just that physicians can't possibly tell you about all possible side effects of a proposed treatment and that they may not realize what effect the intervention might have on your family member, although these are concerns. The issue is that *from the physician's point of view*, the potential benefits of technology likely outweigh its risks.

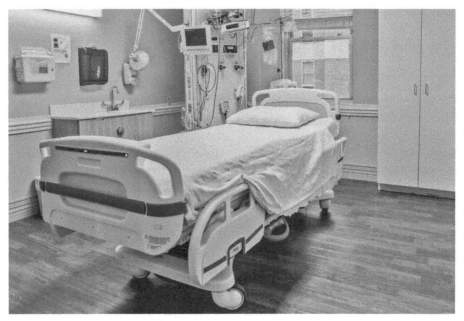

Figure 13.1. Technology in an intensive care unit room

What Is the Cost of Certainty and Is It Worth It?

We learn in medical school, and it's hammered in during residency, that certainty is of paramount importance. A well-known and well-respected oncologist summarized this perspective nicely when he told a patient, "There's no point worrying about what the treatment involves until we know for sure what the diagnosis is." But with people who have an advanced illness or are frail or are near the end of life, the real question, in my view, should be "Is there any possible diagnosis for which we have a treatment that you would find acceptable?" Occasionally, you or your family member may simply want to know what's going on for purposes of prognosis. Even if there is no treatable disease that your relative might have or no disease treatable in a way that your family member could tolerate, you might still want to know what to expect over time. You might also want some sense of how much time your family member has left. More often, patients and families are satisfied if they know that all treatable diseases have been eliminated from consideration. Living with uncertainty may not always be easy for you, but it's very disconcerting for physicians. We want *answers*, even if we don't have any good *solutions*.

Not knowing the truth is intellectually unsatisfying. Physicians are detectives; we like to track down diseases, to find patterns in seemingly disparate symptoms, to create clarity where there was darkness. And as long as we have no diagnosis, there's going to be lingering doubt, worry that we might have missed something treatable. But if the physician goes through the rigorous process of enumerating all the potential causes of your family member's problem, carefully articulating what would be required to diagnose each one and thoughtfully determining whether the treatment in each case would be feasible, there's no reason for anxiety. You will need to agree that it's acceptable to dispense with the diagnosis under these conditions. If you or your family member complains, if you don't understand why the physician isn't pursuing the "answer," then the physician is likely to fall back onto what's effectively the easier path—ordering the test.

You should realize that doing whatever needs to be done to "find the answer" isn't always worth the effort. I deliberately say "effort," because sometimes the attempts at getting a good biopsy sample to look at under the microscope fail. And I say "effort" because it may require a major effort by your family member to go through whatever diagnostic tests are proposed. That's even before they have a chance to cause mischief in the form of an adverse reaction, whether to anesthesia, dye, or the procedure itself. That's before the results come back, triggering still more tests. The bottom line for you is to *ask the physician* what difference the answer, if you get one, will make in treating your family member. If the only possible explanations for your family member's condition are two untreatable, fatal diseases, maybe you don't need to know which it is. If there's a possible explanation that's easily treatable such as a stomach ulcer, and another possibility that's poorly treatable and invariably fatal, such as stomach cancer, you might decide that the prudent approach is to empirically treat for an ulcer and hope for the best. Don't let the doctor put you off by saying, "We'll cross that bridge when we get to it." The real issue is whether you want your family member to try to cross the bridge. What if it's a rickety bridge and he might fall in the river below? What if the land on the other side is inhospitable?

Sometimes—and this is one of the major arguments made for pursuing a diagnosis—it's helpful to know the truth, even if it doesn't guide treatment. Knowledge might make a difference in planning for the future, in whether you decide to go on that trip to visit the children and grandchildren sooner rather than later, in figuring out whether or not your family member should move into assisted living or a nursing home. The same reasoning leads some young people to be tested to see if they are going to come down later in life with a progressive, ultimately fatal neurologic condition such as Huntington's chorea. In that example, fewer than 15 percent of at-risk individuals (anyone who has a parent with Huntington's disease has a 50 percent chance of being affected since it is an autosomal dominant condition) choose to get tested. They prefer uncertainty to living with what might be very disturbing information. They also recognize that all tests have false positives and false negatives: that is, some of the people who are told they won't get the disease actually will get it (or, in the case of your family member, he will be told that he doesn't have whatever devastating condition he was being tested for, when actually he does), and others who are told they will develop the disease in fact will not—or else will die of something else before the condition has a chance to develop. False reassurance or an incorrect diagnosis may be worse than not knowing at all. What this implies is that even when it's cheap and easy to get "an answer," you may prefer not to know.

If it's expensive and difficult to find out the truth, that adds another layer of complexity to decision-making. But just because the technique for making a diagnosis isn't expensive and burdensome doesn't mean you should forge ahead blindly. This situation is particularly tricky because the physician may blithely order tests without your appreciating the potential consequences. More and more noninvasive or minimally invasive tests have been designed in recent years which is a wonderful development, but unless there is a comparably noninvasive treatment for whatever condition is diagnosed, these tests are not without peril.

Technology may be your friend, but it may also be your enemy (box 13.1). Remember that physicians are almost always aware of the most severe risks associated with a particular procedure but may not recognize how devastating other, less dramatic problems may be for your frail relative. Don't make any assumptions—just ask!

Box 13.1

Technology in Frail Elders

- Even low-tech procedures carry risk
- High-tech procedures carry even greater risk
- Decline in the ability to do everyday activities is one of the major risks of technology
- Ask: What will it take to make a diagnosis and what difference will it make?

CHAPTER 14

Acute Care for the Elderly Units

Across the country, about two hundred hospitals have an ACE (Acute Care for the Elderly) unit. These are special inpatient units or designated areas of the hospital that are tailor-made for vulnerable older patients. If your family member is a high-risk patient but is not over age sixty-five or if your hospital is not one of the select few, you won't be able to take advantage of these facilities. I thought it would be worth telling you a little about the virtues of the ACE model to encourage you to lobby for your family member to be admitted to the ACE unit if your hospital has one, to advocate for your hospital to develop one if it doesn't have one, or to try to ensure that your family member receives some of the benefits of an ACE unit even if she is not actually in one.

The idea of the ACE unit originated with the recognition that hospitals often produce all those problems I discussed earlier such as delirium, polypharmacy, and falling (see chapter 10, "The Perils of Hospitalization"). Frail older people frequently leave the hospital more disabled than when they came in. The net result is that the potential benefits of hospitalization are often overshadowed, if not outweighed altogether, by the problems they create. The initial response to this situation was to try to improve the hospital environment. That turned out to be extremely difficult: it's a complex system with many parts and affected by lots of players including physicians, nurses, administrators, insurers, regulators, and even the companies that supply devices and medications. Instead of trying to redesign the entire institution, a few geriatricians wondered if they could carve out a small part of the hospital for geriatric patients and do things differently in that section of the institution.

The Design of the ACE Unit

University Hospitals of Cleveland was the first private institution to develop what it dubbed an ACE unit. Building on the earlier success of the Geriatric Evaluation and Management units created by the Veterans Administration and the concept of comprehensive geriatric assessment, the new unit was designed to focus on acutely ill older people throughout their hospitalization. The Cleveland model and all the ACE programs that followed had four distinctive features: a unique environment, a focus on function, a strong discharge planning program, and a strategy to avoid iatrogenic complications.

Every ACE unit is a little different from every other unit in the *way* it implements the model. A typical ACE unit versus a conventional hospital room are depicted in figures 14.1 and 14.2. Modifications of the environment, for instance, almost always include the use of raised toilet seats but might also involve a dining room where patients can eat with family members. The units generally have handrails along the walls for your family member—or her visitors—to grab onto as they walk, but some also boast rooms for family conferences and a small gym to facilitate physical therapy on site. Every ACE unit tries to deliver "patient-centered care," treatment that is specifically tailored to the needs of your relative, and all of them use an interdisciplinary team to design the plan of care and to visit the patient at least once a day to monitor progress and revise the plan. While the core geriatric team usually consists of a physician, nurse, and social worker, it might also include a pharmacist or physical therapist. Some hospitals ask a staff geriatrician to oversee the care alongside the usual attending physician; others substitute a geriatric physician for the internist, much the same way intensive care units (ICUs) often employ an "intensivist" for their patients; still others expect that hospitalists will retool to become quasi-specialists in geriatric care.

The staff members of ACE units are acutely aware that your family member is at risk of deteriorating in her ability to function independently while hospitalized. They routinely insist that your relative get out of bed early in her stay—sometimes sooner than you may think is reasonable. They make use of physical therapists and gym equipment, whether on the unit or elsewhere in the facility. They try to prevent delirium with strategies to help your family member sleep at night that include hot chocolate and backrubs rather than sleeping pills. This approach was actually specifically tested in a study a number of years ago and proved to be at least as effective and far less toxic than medication. It is common practice to review your relative's medications regularly to make sure she is not taking a drug that's on the Beers List, a list of "potentially inappropriate drugs for the

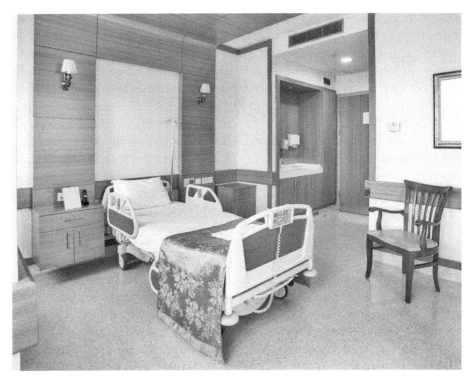

Figure 14.1. Acute Care for the Elderly unit room

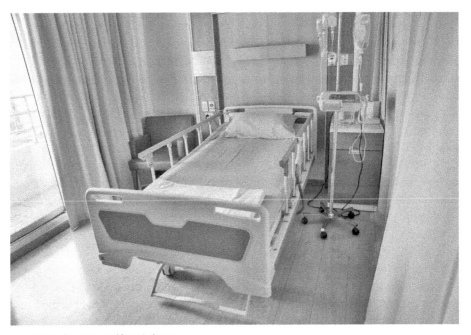

Figure 14.2. Conventional hospital room

elderly." At the same time, the medical orders for your family member are checked, sometimes by a pharmacist, to keep the total number of drugs to a minimum and to think about what she will take after discharge. Which brings us to the final common feature of ACE units—a focus on discharge starting on day one. Instead of waiting until your relative is medically ready to go home and discovering that discharge is impossible because you cannot provide the extensive care she now requires, or finding out that she needs a hospital bed or a ramp to get into the house, a nurse or social worker assesses the home situation early on and makes preliminary post-hospitalization plans.

Every study that's been carried out of ACE units, and there are several, including a few randomized controlled trials, the "gold standard" of testing in medicine, has shown that they are helpful. At the very least, they improve patient and family satisfaction. Because they tend to shorten length of stay, they either save money or cost no more than standard care. In some settings, function improves compared to usual care. They are no panacea—if your family member is admitted to an ACE unit, she might still develop delirium and functional decline; she is still likely to be put on new medications, sometimes more than is ideal, and she might still fall. She would probably be better off at home, if at all feasible (see chapter 10, "The Perils of Hospitalization"). But the hospital-associated adversity associated with ACE units occurs, on average, less often than in the rest of the hospital.

I should mention that some hospitals call their ACE units by another name but they are similar. The Veterans Administration system, for example, which pioneered the idea of a special area of the hospital devoted to geriatric care, continues to call their units "Geriatric Evaluation and Management units." GEM units or GEMUs are a little different from the contemporary ACE model in that they are typically not geared to managing acute medical problems: patients must first go to some other part of the hospital and be stabilized; only then can they be transferred to the GEM. It's analogous to the patient in a private hospital who starts out in the ICU, where a level of care is available that cannot be provided on a regular medical floor, and is subsequently transferred to the ACE unit. It's similar to the situation in a non-VA hospital in which there is a list of "eligibility criteria" for admission to the ACE unit—not only do patients have to be over age sixty-five and have some degree of baseline functional impairment, but they typically have to have a *medical* rather than a *surgical* problem and to require care that doesn't entail a type of monitoring the ACE cannot offer.

Because hospital administrators are often loath to dedicate fixed resources to a special geriatric unit, especially a unit that is not self-supporting (though they often do result in lower overall costs for the hospital), some hospitals have developed what I call ACE-lite. They take some of the concepts enshrined in the ACE unit, such as the use of a geriatrician or early discharge planning and bring them to older patients, whatever part of the hospital they may find themselves in. The key to this approach is to "geriatricize" hospitalists so they request the individual services that, together, comprise the essence of ACE care. A geriatric hospitalist could, for example, order a physical therapy consult on your relative just for the purpose of "mobilizing" her as soon as possible—for getting her out of bed and walking. A geriatric hospitalist could request a consult with a social worker to look into the home situation and begin thinking about what resources your family member will need after discharge. Based on this assessment, you and the hospital can begin to make the necessary arrangements, whether ordering equipment or submitting the paper work to apply for Medicaid. A geriatric hospitalist could request the assistance of a pharmacist or, if he has had appropriate training, review the medications daily himself to make sure they are as safe and age-friendly as possible.

Why invoke hospitalists for this role? Why can't any and all attending physicians do exactly the same thing? In the best of all worlds, they would. I think that every physician who takes care of older patients in the hospital setting should know about the hazards of hospitalization, about geriatric pharmacology, and about fall and delirium prevention. Maybe one day we will achieve that goal, but in the meantime hospitalists, who are generally employed by the hospital and are subject to hospital rules and regulations, are good candidates to acquire at least hospital-specific geriatric wisdom.

Another variant of ACE-lite is the HELP program (Hospital Elder Life Program). This approach specifically targets delirium and functional decline

and, like the other ACE variants, makes use of geriatric-oriented physicians and nurses. HELP, unlike conventional ACE programs, is not located in a separate part of the hospital so it doesn't involve any modifications to the building's physical structure. Nor does HELP typically draw on pharmacists or discharge planners. What's unique about HELP is its use of volunteers. The volunteers are trained to help get your family member walking instead of depending exclusively on physical therapists for a task that may not require professional expertise. They spend time with your family member playing Scrabble or card games or reading aloud in the hope that ongoing mental stimulation will help stave off delirium. Volunteers can also help with other practical issues such as assisting at meal time: in many hospitals, the utensils arrive from the kitchen tightly sealed in plastic, beverages are inside containers that are nearly impossible to open, and the meal tray itself is deposited on a bedside table that may be totally out of reach for your family member.

Finally, some hospitals feature other specialized units that they call "geriatric." A geriatric psychiatry unit, for example, is a discrete program devoted to older people with mental illness. Geriatric Intensive Care units that are specifically geared to the older population also exist, though they are even rarer than ACE units. And sometimes the proportion of patients in conventional ICUs who are over age seventy-five is so large that these standard units come to regard themselves as geriatric. A number of years ago, I proposed the creation of geriatric hospitals—full-service hospitals that are entirely geared to the needs of patients like your family member and that integrate rehabilitation services so that she would not have to travel from the hospital to a skilled nursing facility (SNF) after discharge. Nobody has taken me up on the idea, but it reminds me to point out that what we do have are SNFs. In many ways, SNFs are effectively low-tech, geriatric hospitals. They offer 24/7 nursing care as well as simple diagnostic and therapeutic technology including x-rays, IV medication, and nebulizer treatments (special breathing treatment for asthma). In addition, they provide physical therapy, social work services, and medical care in the form of a physician, sometimes working in concert with a nurse practitioner or physician assistant. But they routinely use an interdisciplinary team approach to care and they are mandated by law to engage in some form of geriatric assessment (see chapter 19, "Hospital-Lite—Another Role for Rehab").

The bottom line is that, if your family member ends up in the hospital, one of these special units—or a related version—can help make her stay safer, more comfortable, and more effective than it might otherwise be.

Box 14.1

Characteristics of Acute Care for the Elderly Units

- Interdisciplinary team care
- Early discharge planning
- Awareness of geriatric syndromes
- Focus on function

Advantages of Acute Care for the Elderly Units

- Shortened length of stay
- Increased patient and family satisfaction
- Decreased risk of falls, delirium, and other complications of hospitalization

CHAPTER 15

Hospital-Based Palliative Care

M ost people either think that palliative care is exclusively for the dying or else they have no clear idea of just what palliative care is, but they figure it is irrelevant to them and their family member. The truth is that palliative care *isn't* just for the dying and it *is* appropriate for many frail older people, so don't be shocked if the physicians in the hospital request a palliative care consult for your relative. People who have several chronic diseases in addition to functional impairment can benefit from palliative care, just as people with a single, advanced illness can. So, what exactly is palliative care and how does it fit in with other treatment?

Palliative Care Provides an Added Layer of Support

A few years ago, the Center for the Advancement of Palliative Care (CAPC) in New York City learned from a survey of the general public that patients with serious illness and their families are very enthusiastic about having "an added layer of support." That's exactly what palliative care offers. True, it's intended for people with serious illness, but that doesn't mean the illness is necessarily in its most advanced stage. Palliative care is sometimes confused with hospice, a program for people who really are in the final stage of life and who generally have opted for a comfort-oriented approach to care. Hospice is one type of palliative care, but the palliative umbrella covers much more.

If you associate palliative care with cancer patients, you are right that it is widely used in oncology, but it's by no means just for people with cancer. Plenty of people with congestive heart failure or dementia make use of palliative care, as do a small but increasing number of people with conditions such as Parkinson's disease and kidney failure. Palliative care is an interdisciplinary team approach to care (that should sound familiar after our discussion of Acute Care for Elders [ACE] units and geriatric consultation) that focuses on symptom management, psychosocial support, and improved communication for patients and families. Your family member may well need some or all of these strategies while in the hospital.

According to the National Coalition for Hospice and Palliative Care (https://www.nationalcoalitionhpc.org/wp-content/uploads/2018/10/NCHPC-NCPGuidelines_4thED_web_FINAL.pdf), palliative care is

- Appropriate at any stage in a serious illness, and it is beneficial when provided along with treatments of curative or life-prolonging intent.

- Provided over time to patients based on their needs and not their prognosis.

- Offered in all care settings and by various organizations, such as physician practices, health systems, cancer centers, dialysis units, home health agencies, hospices, and long-term care providers.

- Focused on what is most important to the patient, family, and caregiver(s), assessing their goals and preferences and determining how best to achieve them.

- Interdisciplinary to attend to the holistic care needs of the patient and their identified family and caregivers.

Availability of Palliative Care

Hospital-based palliative care consultation is now available in the majority of American hospitals. Hospital administrators have discovered that palliative care services are good for business—they shorten hospital stays, save money for the institution, and increase patient and family satisfaction, all without causing other problems. Requesting a consult is an option to consider if your family member is having symptoms that aren't well-controlled, such as pain or delirium, or if you aren't convinced that the course the doctors are pursuing is consistent with his goals of care. You may well find an ally on the palliative care team to help you navigate the confusing and sometimes impenetrable hospital hierarchy.

That said, it's important to recognize that geriatrics and palliative care are not interchangeable; they are distinct specialties, each with its own strengths. Palliative care isn't as focused on function as is geriatrics and tends to devote more attention to pain than to falls. Many palliative care clinicians are only gradually becoming as conversant with dementia as they are with cancer. If you're lucky, the physician member of the palliative care team will be "double boarded" in both geriatrics and palliative care; that is, she will have done fellowships in the two specialties and be equally comfortable with both. Increasing numbers of clinicians, as well as articles and books, are dedicated to "geriatric palliative care."

You should also know that, just as there are ACE units, which are specialized geriatric inpatient areas of the hospital, so, too, there are inpatient palliative care units. Not very many, but there might be one in the hospital your family member goes to. Each hospital with such a unit has its own admissions criteria, though in general these facilities are restricted to patients who are close to the end of life and have an acute problem, such as delirium or pain, that is overwhelming the capacity of the regular hospital staff. Odds are that transfer to such a unit won't make sense for your family member unless he is dying or has a very short life expectancy.

Another fact worth knowing is that some palliative care teams that help care for patients in the hospital will also provide care for them at home. If your family member does have a palliative care consultation while in the hospital and if you find it helpful, then you may want to inquire about what will happen after discharge. If you or your family member click with a member of the palliative care team, that's important, sometimes as important as whatever assistance that person provided in the arena of symptom management or advance care planning. Don't just say goodbye and thank you when your family member leaves the hospital; see how the relationship can continue. Even if your relative doesn't survive the hospitalization, the palliative care team may continue to help you by offering bereavement counseling.

When Is Palliative Care Consultation Useful?

So, let's get back to describing hospital-based palliative care consultation. What kinds of problems might warrant calling in the palliative care team? I spent ten years seeing patients in palliative care consultation and probably the most common reason for calling me was to have a conversation with the patient and the family about their goals. Typically, the physician felt that one or the other—patient or family—did not fully grasp the clinical situation and, as a result, was asking for treatment that was very burdensome and unlikely to be beneficial. Usually, the hospital staff had already tried to discuss what was going on but without much success. In other cases, the physician knew that a conversation about the patient's goals was needed but didn't feel comfortable initiating it. In some instances, the family members disagreed about how much treatment was too much and how much was too little. The attending physician requested the help of the palliative care team to mediate among the various factions. And occasionally, although not very often, the patient or family requested a meeting to talk about the big picture, about where things were headed, and wanted someone with special expertise in communication to help out. My role was to help patients formulate and prioritize their goals of care after I communicated with whatever specialists were involved to make sure I fully understood the clinical situation.

A related situation that often triggers a palliative care consultation is the need to make a specific medical decision. Should your family member try second-line chemotherapy after he relapsed with first-line treatment? Should he start dialysis? Perhaps the oncologist or the kidney specialist has reviewed the options with you and your family member and summarized their pros and cons, but you are still struggling. Your sneaking suspicion is that the specialist is biased or maybe even has a vested interest in your making a particular choice. You'd like to discuss the possibilities with someone who is able to look at the issues from your perspective and from your relative's point of view, who can listen to what matters to both of you and help you figure out which path is most consistent with your interests. Moreover, bringing in the palliative care team rather than just a single person facilitates addressing the social and economic aspects of decision-making as well as the strictly medical component. The team will make sure certain important questions are addressed (as an example): Who's going to take your family member to dialysis three times a week, if that's the approach he opts for? Who's going to take care of him if he doesn't go to dialysis and decides instead to let his kidney disease take its natural course and he begins to become weaker or more confused? If implementing the plan of care requires moving into an assisted living facility, how will your family member pay for that? Can he afford it? What about if he stays home and needs a home health aide for four hours every day? How much will Medicare cover and what will he have to pay out of pocket?

Another problem that commonly precipitates a palliative care consult request is pain that persists despite the usual medications and other maneuvers. This situation frequently arises in cancer patients, but could also be an issue for your family member if he has a painful acute problem—say a hip fracture or recent surgery or a skin ulcer—and cannot tolerate the medicines that were prescribed to alleviate his suffering. It's worth pointing out that while consultants are usually asked to address some aspect of whatever problem led to the hospitalization, sometimes they are called on to look into an unsolved mystery, an issue that the primary care doctor had never dealt with satisfactorily. For example, suppose your family member had major mobility problems at home because of painful, debilitating peripheral neuropathy (nerve pain). He's been tried on morphine and its cousins but invariably became either confused or profoundly constipated, so he's been going without any medication. As a result, he hardly ever leaves his second story apartment: walking is just too painful and he lives in a walk-up. A palliative care consultant might be able to suggest a different regimen such as an anticonvulsant or a non-opioid pain medicine. A geriatric-oriented, palliative care consultant, or perhaps the physical therapy member of the palliative care team, might advocate an exercise regime or installing a chairlift to enable your relative to go up and down the stairs.

Just as some hospitals have ACE-lite, a way to obtain some but not all of the features of an Acute Care for Elders unit, some hospitals similarly have palliative care–lite (see chapter 19, "Hospital-Lite—Another Role for Rehab"). If your family member is on a specialized hospital floor, say the cancer wing or the orthopedics department, chances are there is a social worker attached to that unit who has expertise in the issues that commonly arise with treatment of their specialty's problems. For example, the social worker on an oncology floor might know the ins and outs of how to obtain coverage for new, and extremely expensive, targeted medications. She probably has dealt with this matter before and knows how to contact the drug manufacturer to request medica-

tion for "compassionate use" or how to apply for a "patient drug assistance program." Compassionate use means treatment for a serious illness with a new, unapproved drug if no other treatment is available. A patient drug assistance program enables patients to receive medications at a substantial discount if the drug is not covered by their prescription drug plan (or they don't have such a plan) and payment of the retail price will cause a significant financial hardship. Similarly, the orthopedics unit probably has its own dedicated physical therapist(s) who are likely to be knowledgeable about what gadgets could be useful at home or which rehab facility is best suited to addressing your relative's needs after discharge.

If you feel overwhelmed by your family member's needs, by how complicated his care is, odds are the reason is that his care *is* complicated. His problems are often best addressed by a team, not just a single person. While much of the treatment provided in a hospital is physician-centric—directed and delivered by doctors—the hospital can also provide interdisciplinary care. Ideally, the interdisciplinary team is already operational and just needs to be activated for your family member, as on an ACE unit or when a geriatric or palliative care consultation has been requested. But sometimes you will need to prod the attending physician to mobilize the individual components of what, together, makes up team care.

Box 15.1

Roles of Hospital-Based Palliative Care

- Managing symptoms
- Eliciting and prioritizing goals of care
- Translating goals into treatment
- Helping make difficult medical decisions

PART IV

Going to the Rehabilitation Facility

I f you're not already familiar with the drill, you will be soon: first, your family member goes to the hospital, then she goes for rehabilitation (or rehab), and only then is she pronounced ready to go home. Rehabilitation is the middle ground between being sick and being well. What's remarkable about what I'm calling rehab, by which I mean post-acute or subacute care provided in a skilled nursing facility, is that it didn't exist fifty years ago. It didn't exist, practically speaking, in 1981, when I was finishing my residency in internal medicine. In those days, if you were sick enough to go to the hospital, you stayed there until you were well enough to go home. If you had completed a one-week course of intravenous antibiotics and were now taking pills for your pneumonia, but you were still too wobbly to make it to the bathroom on your own, you remained in the hospital until you had your strength back. The only kind of post-acute care that I recall was a hospital for inpatient rehabilitation, where you could get intensive treatment for a condition such as a stroke. Today, one-fifth of people on fee-for-service Medicare who are hospitalized are discharged to a skilled nursing facility, or SNF (pronounced "sniff"). For the oldest old (people over eighty or eighty-five) and those who had trouble carrying out their daily activities independently even before their hospitalization, the rate of SNF use is even higher.

All told, 1.7 million people who were enrolled in fee-for-service Medicare in 2015 had at least one SNF stay. Since 30 percent of the Medicare population are enrolled in a Medicare Advantage plan (a comprehensive, private alternative to fee-for-service Medicare), the true number is a little more than 2.4 million. Because Medicare pays a lump sum to Medicare Advantage plans for each patient they care for, it doesn't bother to collect statistics on each of the services those individuals use, such as a SNF or acute care hospital. In short, if you and your family member haven't yet been inside a SNF, you probably will be sooner rather than later.

Because the term SNF is also used to apply to facilities that provide long-term, nursing home care—in fact, the same buildings often offer both short-term and long-term care under the same roof—and because people receiving subacute care are usually recovering from an acute illness, I will refer to short-term care as "rehab." Part IV of *The Caregiver's Encyclopedia* is all about life in the rehab.

CHAPTER 16

Choosing a Rehab Facility

Maybe your family member has been to a rehab for post-hospital care several times before and there's a particular place she is happy with, or maybe there's only one option in the area. Alternatively, you may be dealing with the question for the first time: your family member is in the hospital and, out of the blue, you get a call from someone telling you she's the case manager and your family member will be ready for discharge to rehab in a couple of days. When you are given a few names of candidate institutions that you are encouraged to check out, you realize you have no idea how to choose.

Ratings

Where do you begin? Selecting a rehab presents many of the same challenges and opportunities as choosing a hospital, though you may have several options and at least a little bit of time to do some research. You can begin with the ratings. The main source is the government website, Nursing Home Compare. Like its hospital analog, Hospital Compare, this is a tool developed by the Centers for Medicare and Medicaid Services (CMS), the agency that creates the regulations for rehabs, collects data on their performance, and is the principal source of payment. In 2017, Medicare spent $28.4 billion on rehab care for fee-for-service Medicare enrollees alone. Like all report cards, Nursing Home Compare has its limitations, but it's a good place to start.

Keep in mind that the overwhelming majority of skilled nursing facilities provide both short-term care (what I'm calling "rehab") *and* long-term, residential nursing home care. They are "dually certified," which means they can accept both Medicare (for short-term patients) and Medicaid (for long-term residents). Nursing Home Compare (figure 16.1) evaluates both components of a facility's care even though the two parts are typically physically distinct—the rehab unit might consist of ten beds or it might have sixty beds, but those beds are grouped together, sometimes on a separate floor. In fact, the star rating assigned by CMS, the composite score that attempts to give you the big picture, is based on its assessment of the short-stay and long-stay parts of the facility combined. That assessment, in turn, relies on the staffing level (the number of nurses per resident or patient), the facility's performance on recent health inspections, and a variety of measures of the quality of care—called quality indicators—some of which are applicable to the short-stay part and some to the long-stay part of the facility. This rating system allows you to separate the unusually high performers (those with five stars) from the abysmal performers (those with one star). Even if the facility's principal problems are centered in its long-term care arm, you should be leery of the overall management if the rating is poor, as the administration will affect both components of the institution. But what you mainly want to focus on are the quality measures that are collected for short-stay patients.

In 2019, CMS expanded the list of factors it uses to rate the quality of care for short-stay patients from seven to thirteen. They can be grouped into measures that look at *physical functioning*, measures that look at *prevention*, measures dealing with *acute medical care*, and a variety of measures of *overall effectiveness*. The physical function

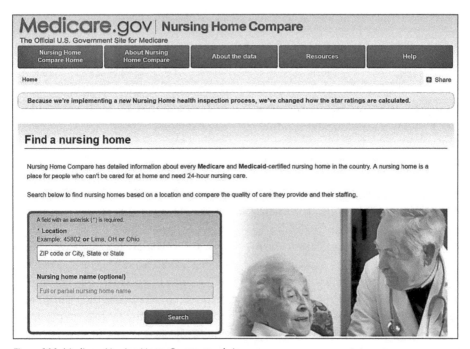

Figure 16.1. Medicare Nursing Home Compare website

measures include the percent of patients whose ability to move around improved and the percent whose function was assessed as part of a treatment plan. The measures addressing prevention include the percent of residents who both needed and received a flu shot or a pneumonia shot (the only indicators where a high rate indicates good quality and a low rate suggests poor quality), the percent with a new or worsening pressure ulcer, and the percent who experienced one or more major falls. Measures of acute medical care focus on the percent of patients prescribed an antipsychotic medication for the first time and the proportion who reported moderate or severe pain. The measures of overall effectiveness include the percent of residents with an emergency room visit, the percent discharged to their home, the percent rehospitalized during a rehab stay, and the percent rehospitalized in the thirty days after discharge from a rehab. These are composite measures that assess the effectiveness of care by looking at various outcomes that optimal care should have either promoted (such as discharge home) or prevented (such as readmission to the hospital). Finally, CMS throws in a *financial* measure: the average Medicare spending per beneficiary.

The rationale for each quality indicator differs. Consider, for example, the pain indicator. Your relative might be at rehab to recover from an operation, perhaps from knee replacement surgery or open heart surgery. Not surprisingly, she will experience postoperative pain. But if she is going to participate in physical therapy,

she needs to have good pain control. Rehabs have a history of doing a bad job at treating pain—hence the quality measure. Ditto for the proportion of patients who develop a new or worsening pressure ulcer (the technical term for a bedsore) while in rehab. Good preventive techniques, including use of a special low-pressure mattress and the practice of turning bed-ridden patients regularly, should prevent this problem. Likewise, the prescription of a new antipsychotic medication is a reasonable quality indicator. Such drugs have traditionally been overused in nursing facilities. They may be instituted because your family member is agitated or confused due to her underlying dementia, even though there is no good evidence that they are effective in this setting.

These are all reasonable indicators of quality. After all, you don't want your family member to be in pain, you certainly don't want her to develop a pressure ulcer, and you probably don't want her to be started on an antipsychotic medication. All things being equal, you'd prefer that she not be sent to the hospital emergency department and be rehospitalized, and your overall goal is most likely to get her back home. But these measures are not adjusted for the severity of illness of the individuals admitted. Now you might say that it's just as bad for someone who is very sick to get a pressure ulcer as it is for someone who is in better shape. But suppose the very sick person already had one pressure ulcer because she is extremely thin, malnourished, and immobile. Preventing that individual from getting a second area of skin breakdown is a good deal harder than keeping the perfectly intact skin of another patient from getting an ulcer in the first place. Moreover, a facility that doesn't fare well on the CMS quality indicators might nonetheless be a good fit for your family member if she's very ill and debilitated if it has experience and expertise in managing her sort of problems. A second limitation of quality indicators in general is that they encourage facilities to "teach to the test," they provide incentives to rehabs to focus on the particular issues on which they are going to be graded. Of at least equal importance to you and your relative may be the problems that the facility ignores or handles poorly, such as depression or incontinence.

Rating systems are a good place to start, but you should also pay attention to word of mouth. If your family member has a friend or neighbor whose opinion she respects and if that person has spent time at a particular rehab and had either a very good or a very bad experience, her impression is worth taking into consideration. Of course, it's entirely possible that the friend's situation was very different from your relative's and that generalizing from her experience is perilous, but what happened to her is, at the very least, a valuable piece of data.

What to Look for When You Visit a Rehab

The third and final step is to visit the potential rehabs. Usually, the case manager, or whoever is in charge of discharge planning at the hospital, will let you know about two or three options. These are facilities to which the hospital has sent patients before and with which they presumably have had a good experience. Sometimes the facilities are part of a "preferred network," a group of rehabs that have established lines of communication with the acute care hospital, a system that has the potential to promote better coordination of care for your family member. The case manager can call up the various candidate institutions and find out if they have a bed available; she can also have your family member "screened" by those facilities to see if she is eligible for admission, given her problems and her needs. For example, your relative might need a private room if she has a certain type of highly contagious infection—but the facility may have no private rooms available. Or she might need a certain kind of treatment such as total parenteral nutrition, a highly concentrated solution given intravenously, that the facility may not be equipped to provide. If you're going to visit, and typically you will only have a couple of days in which to do so, you probably want a few tips to guide your investigation.

When you arrive at the rehab, the first thing just about any visitor will do is use the sniff test. Literally, this means noticing if the place is permeated by an odor of urine—not a good sign. More generally, it means getting a general sense of the place. Is it clean? Is there a lot of hustle and bustle, indicating ongoing nursing and rehabilitative care? Do the nurses look stressed out or do they seem energetic? Are the aides sullen and hostile or warm and enthusiastic? You should beware of judging a place by the amenities, what's been dubbed the "chandelier effect." Some of the best rehabs don't look terribly attractive. Remember your family member isn't going to move in here; the idea is for her to spend at most a few weeks. An elegant lounge with a piano (particularly if no one ever plays it) is a good deal less important than a physical therapy room well-stocked with equipment.

You may also want to inquire whether the facility is for-profit or not-for-profit. Quality doesn't track perfectly with ownership status, but on average, not-for-profit rehabs are more likely to do a good job than their for-profit counterparts. Put differently, the rotten eggs are apt to be for-profit and the truly outstanding facilities are almost always not-for-profit.

Finally, you should look into the arrangements for medical care. The specific regulations vary from state to state, but in general the bare minimum is that a physician evaluate your family member within a relatively short period of time after admission and then see her again periodically. In many rehabs, the only professional staff on site all the time are nurses, either registered nurses (RNs) or licensed practical nurses (LPNs). The medical director makes rounds once a week. Period. In other rehabs, the physician is complemented by a physician assistant (PA) or nurse practitioner (NP) who is on site far more often. In one model, the PA or NP spends eight hours a day at the facility and is in regular contact with the supervising physician. A handful of facilities have their own medical staff who care for all the patients and who make rounds daily. Think about what your family member is likely to need. If she's just had knee replacement surgery, what's most important to her is the physical therapist, but if she's had a protracted hospitalization, suffering many medical complications after an initial admission for pneumonia or a bladder infection, more extensive medical care may be essential for her to get better. Even if the hospital course was relatively uneventful or if the reason for her initial admission was fairly straightforward, you will probably want a bit more than the minimum required by law.

You did it. You checked out the options using Nursing Home Compare, you asked around for recommendations from people you trust, and you visited a few places, making sure they were close enough to your home so that you can get there conveniently. If you and your family member live in different locations, it's more important that you be able to visit than that your relative live nearby since by definition, she's not going to be going back and forth from home to the facility. You made sure the facility passed the sniff test and that it has enough on-site medical care for your family member to be evaluated at the rehab rather than in the hospital every time she develops a problem. Now your relative is ready for discharge from the hospital and for the next challenge to begin.

Box 16.1

To choose a rehab facility, consider

- Past experience
- Word of mouth
- Ratings such as performance on inspections, patient/staff ratio, quality indicators
- Visiting the facility
- System of medical care

CHAPTER 17

How Rehab Runs

It's moving day: your family member is being picked up by ambulance or chair car (Medicare won't pay for transportation by a full-service ambulance unless it's clearly medically justified) and brought to the place where he's going to stay for the next few days or weeks. Maybe you drive over to meet him there; more likely, you'll come over later to see how he's settling in.

The first thing you notice about the rehab when you arrive is how quiet it is. I'm going to refer to "rehab," rather than "skilled nursing facility" or the abbreviation "SNF," to distinguish it from a nursing home that provides long-term care. From Medicare's perspective, however, it is called a skilled nursing facility, as is its long-stay counterpart, and with good reason: the place is structured and organized for and by nurses. If you come in the evening, you may have the eerie sensation that nobody's around. The physical and occupational therapists have gone home and you are not going to encounter any x-ray technicians or phlebotomists because there aren't any on the staff. During evening hours, there's a skeleton crew—fewer nurses, fewer nursing assistants, probably no unit secretary to greet you when you arrive on your family member's floor, and no physicians. But you will find a couple of critically important people, the individuals who run the rehab. Getting to know them will be invaluable for you, for your family member, and for the staff members.

The Professionals Who Run the Rehab

You need to understand that nurses run the show at rehab. If the physician (more often than not a man) is king in the hospital, the nurse (more often than not a woman) is queen in the nursing facility. That was certainly true of long-stay nursing homes, but when they morphed into short-term, post-acute facilities, it remained the dominant reality. Even in facilities with a nurse practitioner on staff or a physician who visits patients regularly, the nurse generally controls which patients they will see. In the acute care hospital, by contrast, physicians see all their patients every day. It's a well-kept secret that nurses have far more autonomy in the rehab setting than in many other practice sites. Much of the time they are on their own, taking care of people who only hours or days earlier were sick enough to be in the hospital, sometimes in the intensive care unit, perhaps in the operating room. They evaluate patients and they decide when to call for help. When they do call for help—it's often literally a phone call—the physician isn't likely to drop everything and drive over to assess the patient, so they talk on the telephone. The nurse serves as the physician's eyes and ears; the best ones have a fairly good idea of what the problem is and feel free to suggest to the doctor what tests should be ordered or medications prescribed. Ideally, the nurse will have read the hospital discharge summary and can let the physician know that your family member had a very similar problem when he was in the hospital, that they gave him such and such treatment, and he got better. Ideally, you will get to know the nursing staff, preferably on both the evening and day shifts, as they are your most critical allies.

The rehab team includes several other individuals you should get to know. One is the physical therapist. In many cases, the main reason your family member is in the rehab is to receive physical therapy, to literally get back on his feet. Perhaps your family member can tell the physical therapist exactly what he was able to do before he became acutely ill and required hos-

pitalization, how many steps he needs to climb to get to his bedroom, how far he has to walk to get to the elevator in the apartment building where he lives, and what assistive devices he used. But maybe he needs you to provide the details.

Another professional you might be less familiar with but who often plays an important role in rehab is the occupational therapist (OT). In the context of your family member, what the OT has to offer is working with your relative to ensure he can do all the things necessary to make it at home. In some instances, she will teach him new tricks or new skills and, in other situations, she will insist that your family member have additional help at home to compensate for his lack of proficiency. For example, can your family member wash his face and brush his teeth safely and competently—without falling down? Can he do an adequate cleaning job on some of the less accessible bodily regions? What about dressing? And if he's able to manage sweat pants and polo shirts, but can't handle button-downs, does he have the right sort of clothes at home? What about household tasks? Can he use the stove properly, without hurting himself or risking burning the house down? Many rehabs have a model kitchen on the premises so that patients can work with the OT to hone their skills.

Depending on the circumstances, you might want to track down the rehab social worker. I mention this because rehabs all have a social worker on their staff, but in many facilities, she is overburdened with responsibilities and has too many patients to attend to, so if there's something important your family member needs, you may have to be the squeaky wheel. You might know, for example, that your family member is running out of money and will need to apply for Medicaid soon, which is something the social worker can assist with. You might be wondering about adult day health care, a program for older people that provides socialization and supervision during the day while allowing the participants to continue living at home. That's something else the social worker can help you arrange. Or you might not have a clear idea of what your family member needs but have a strong sense that things aren't going very well at home. You'd like someone to talk to about your concerns and the rehab social worker may fit the bill.

Last but not least are the medical professionals—the nurse practitioner or physician assistant, if there is one, and the physician. You want to make sure they know you are interested and available. It's desirable to match names to faces. You certainly want to be sure they know what medications your family member was taking at home before the hospitalization, not just at the time of discharge. You want to transmit any advance care plan your family member may have, whether a living will; an out-of-hospital do-not-resuscitate (DNR) order; or a Physician Orders for Life-Sustaining Treatment (POLST) form. If you are the officially designated health-care surrogate, you should be certain the facility has a copy of the proxy designation in the medical record.

How the Rehab Staff Functions

The rehab professional staff, along with the nursing assistant who helps with personal care, will play a crucial role in your family member's life for whatever period of time he is at rehab. Indirectly, they have the potential to affect his life for a long time after that. Getting to know them individually and establishing a relationship is a good idea, but you also need to understand how they work together as a team.

Care at the rehab center is based on the concept of interdisciplinary team work. The goal of the rehab is to help your family member achieve maximal functioning, given the constraints of his disease (see figure 17.1). Optimal functioning, in turn, has a physical, an emotional, and a medical component.

The goal of hospital care, by contrast, is usually to diagnose and treat a particular disease; accordingly, the tests that the doctor orders and the treatments she prescribes are whatever is recommended for his symptoms. Hospitals often pay lip service to team work, but their structure tends to be hierarchical, with physicians on top, giving orders to everyone else.

The basic way that the rehab's interdisciplinary team functions is through a *care plan*. The care plan is the lifeblood of the rehab. It spells out the facility's *goals* for your family member and how the staff members propose *implementing* those goals. You might, for example, hear something like this at a care planning meeting: "Mr. S. had a stroke that left him weak on the right side and with difficulty speaking. We are going to focus on getting him therapy to help him return to his prior living situation or, if that proves impossible, to come up with an alternative arrangement. Along the way, we will monitor his blood pressure and the blood thinner the doctors started in the hospital to try to prevent another stroke." The goal, in short, is to enable your family member to function well enough to go home and the strategy for implementing that goal is physical therapy, occupational therapy, and medical management.

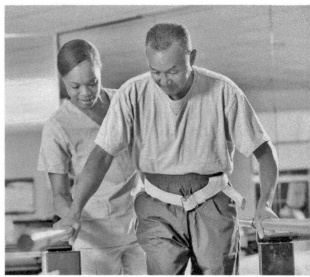

Figure 17.1. Rehabilitation focuses on function

In the hospital, by contrast, the attending physician (or, in teaching facilities, the medical or surgical resident, with the attending physician's blessing) performs an assessment and comes up with a plan, which she writes up in the medical record. The plan specifies what tests will be ordered, what medications given, what procedures carried out, based on the most likely explanation for your relative's problem. If you speak with his physician, you are likely to be given a brief summary of the plan, something of the form, "We need to get to the bottom of Mr. S's bleeding, so he's going to have an upper endoscopy and, if that doesn't give us the answer, a lower endoscopy. In the meantime,

we're not letting him eat anything; we are just giving him fluids by vein. We also have him on a strong anti-ulcer medication since he most likely has an ulcer or a severe irritation of the lining of the stomach." Or maybe, "Mr. S. broke his hip in a couple of places—it's a pretty bad break, so we can't just pin it back together. We're recommending putting in an artificial hip. It's routine surgery, but because of his history of heart problems, we've asked the cardiologist to come by and clear him before we take him to the operating room." The course of action is disease-driven, with the individual needs and preferences of the particular patient modulating the strategy slightly.

All rehabs are required to have a planning process: within seven days of admission, according to Medicare guidelines, the facility must develop a "comprehensive care plan," designed, at a minimum, by the attending physician, a registered nurse involved in the resident's care, a nurse's aide responsible for the resident's care, and someone from the dietary staff. Your family member will be invited to participate in the care planning meeting. And if he agrees, you can attend as well. In fact, Medicare feels so strongly about patient and family involvement that it requires facilities to justify why patients and families *don't* attend care planning meetings.

The care plan will guide what happens to your relative while he is at rehab. It specifies what treatments he will have, such as intravenous medications or physical therapy. It says how often he will have various services, such as physical or occupational therapy: Every day? Three times a week? The plan details what special equipment the facility will provide for him, such as a walker or an air mattress intended to prevent pressure ulcers. It indicates what kind of diet he is to receive, such as high protein, or puréed, or low salt. And it lays out just what it is that the

rehab stay is intended to accomplish, which effectively determines the endpoint for the admission. Care plans can be revised as time progresses; sometimes new strategies turn out to be necessary, sometimes new problems develop, and sometimes the original goals or processes for reaching those goals prove unachievable. The best way for you to be informed about what's going on, to help shape the plan, and to prevent unfortunate surprises along the way, is to get your family member's permission to attend the care planning meeting.

Because rehabs are all about optimizing your family member's ability to go about his daily routine, they have a unique structure and way of operating. If you understand the way they work (box 17.1), get to know the people who make up the interdisciplinary team and, ideally, participate in care planning meetings, you can help improve your relative's stay.

Box 17.1

How Rehabs Run

- Goal: improve function
- Structure: interdisciplinary team
  - Nurse
  - Physical and occupational therapists
  - Physician and/or physician assistant or nurse practitioner
  - Social worker
- Operation: care plan
  - Spells out specific goals
  - Lays out implementation strategy

CHAPTER 18

Your Role
in the Rehab

Daily life in the rehab facility (skilled nursing facility or SNF) is simultaneously very much like the acute care hospital and not at all like the hospital. The SNF is a medical institution that dictates when your family member gets up, what she eats, and what appointments she has. It often features shared rooms that lie along corridors radiating out from a nursing station, which serves as the control center for the entire operation. It's run by medical personnel. But since the main focus is on rehabilitation and returning home rather than cure, it's of necessity very concerned with your family member's life, not just her diseases. Both the hospital and the rehab care about measurable outcomes, but a typical outcome in the hospital is improvement in your family member's electrolytes (the level of sodium and chloride and other chemicals in her blood), while a symbol of success in the rehab is a higher Katz ADL score (how well she does on activities such as washing and dressing; see chapter 2, "Ingredients of the Underlying Health State"). Because the rehab operates differently from the hospital, your strategy for involvement has to differ as well.

I already discussed getting to know the principal personnel and participating in care planning meetings, but there are other specific ways you can help.

Much of the care in the rehab is episodic—the physical therapist may only be there part of the day, ditto for the nurse practitioner, and the physician may only be on site once a week—so your best bet, if you have a complaint, a concern, or a question, is to go through the nurse. The nurse will typically have an eight-hour shift (though some work four ten-hour shifts per week). See if she can address your issue and if not, ask her how best to contact whoever it is you need to speak with, whether the physical therapist (PT), the nurse practitioner (NP), or the MD. Leave a number where you can be reached and a window during which you will be available.

A rehab stay provides a good opportunity for you to get some hands-on training. The physical therapist will often be delighted to teach you how to help get your family member into a car or how to transfer her from the bed to the chair (figure 18.1). The therapist may have a series of exercises that he wants your family member to do once

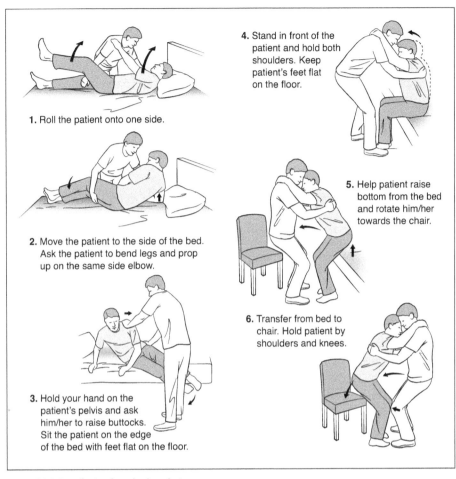

1. Roll the patient onto one side.

2. Move the patient to the side of the bed. Ask the patient to bend legs and prop up on the same side elbow.

3. Hold your hand on the patient's pelvis and ask him/her to raise buttocks. Sit the patient on the edge of the bed with feet flat on the floor.

4. Stand in front of the patient and hold both shoulders. Keep patient's feet flat on the floor.

5. Help patient raise bottom from the bed and rotate him/her towards the chair.

6. Transfer from bed to chair. Hold patient by shoulders and knees.

Figure 18.1. Transferring from bed to chair

she gets home and would love for you to be able to monitor that she's doing them correctly. If there's a nursing task to be performed at home, whether changing a dressing or giving an injection or administering artificial nutrition through a tube in your family member's stomach, this is your chance to watch someone else complete the task and to be supervised doing it yourself.

Rehab is potentially an excellent site for your family member to have a comprehensive geriatric assessment.

We talked about this interdisciplinary evaluation earlier (see chapter 9, "What a Geriatric Assessment Is and When to Ask for One"), but at rehab you won't need to make a special appointment or assemble the various component pieces: they are all present already. In principle, the rehab is routinely supposed to assess your relative, but often the staff focus narrowly on how to help her recovery from a recent acute event rather than taking the opportunity to evaluate all aspects of your relative's health and functioning. Tell the staff how great it is that they are looking at your family member from so many vantage points and say that you are looking forward to hearing their thoughts about her overall condition and what they hope can be achieved over time.

A helpful way to think about how best to remain informed and contribute during your family member's time in a rehab is to focus on various critical nodes or turning points during what may be a several-week period. The first critical period is admission.

Admission to Rehab

We've already talked a bit about admission, about meeting the evening nurse and, if possible, the day nurse, as well as the NP or physician assistant (PA), the primary certified nursing assistant, the physical therapist, and perhaps the physician (see chapter 17, "How Rehab Runs"). Admission is also a time to make sure the facility has your contact information. It's a chance to make sure the facility knows who is your family member's health-care proxy (hopefully, it's you and you have a piece of paper to prove it), her preferences about attempted cardiopulmonary resuscitation, and basic information about her home situation. You will also have another chance to meet the team and share information at the first comprehensive care planning meeting that typically takes place within a few days of admission.

When Your Relative Develops an Acute Problem

Another crucial moment in the course of a rehab stay occurs if your family member develops a new medical problem: if she becomes acutely ill or she falls or she is suddenly confused. At that moment, the rehab staff have to decide what approach to take to address this new problem; they can no longer be guided by the plan sent over from the hospital or by the recommendations of the physical therapist. In particular, they may have to choose whether to try to care for your relative within the rehab or send her back to the hospital. It seems to me there are two ways you want to be involved at such times. First, you want to be informed that there *is* a new medical problem.

You really don't want to learn that your family member fell and hit her head *after* she's been to the hospital emergency department, had a head computerized tomography (CT) scan, and been diagnosed with a subdural hematoma (blood around the brain). Far better to hear there's a problem from the nurse practitioner at the rehab than from the neurosurgeon at the hospital. You have a lot to contribute when something new develops—if, for example, the nurse's aide reported your family member wasn't her usual self this morning, she kept trying to put toothpaste on her hairbrush instead of on her toothbrush and she wanted to know when checkout was at "this hotel"—you might be able to report that the same thing happened several times before and the cause always turned out to be a bladder infection. Or you might ask about any new medications that had been started recently and let the staff know, for example, that your family member always gets confused after taking strong pain medications. Second, you should discuss, if you haven't already, whether your family member should have a "do not hospitalize" status.

Physicians devote an inordinate amount of time to discussing whether or not to attempt cardiopulmonary resuscitation if your family member's heart stops beating and she stops breathing. I say inordinate because the truth is that we can go through the steps involved in cardiopulmonary resuscitation (CPR)—delivering electric shocks, inserting a breathing tube, injecting potent cardiac stimulating medications—but the effort is almost never successful in individuals who are old and debilitated by multiple medical problems. The amount of time spent discussing a do-not-resuscitate (DNR) order tends to make people think that those three letters mean far more than engaging in an almost certainly futile exercise after death has effectively occurred; they assume, understandably, that the physician is talking about all kinds of other potentially life-preserving treatments, whether dialysis or blood transfusions or chemotherapy. But DNR just means do-not-resuscitate or, as I and many other physicians prefer, do-not-attempt-resuscitation (DNAR). A DNAR status is selected if this particular procedure—comprised of chest compressions, establishing an airway, and breathing for the patient—is deemed too aggressive, too potentially harmful, and of insufficient benefit to warrant its use. Do-not-hospitalize is another matter altogether.

We talked at some length earlier about the hazards of hospitalization (see chapter 10, "The Perils of Hospitalization"). If your family member is in rehab, she was probably recently in the hospital. She wasn't ready to go home after the hospital discharged her so she's in a facility for rehabilitation. Now there's a new problem or perhaps a recurrence of an old problem, or maybe an exacerbation of a problem that's been present all along. Is the best way to deal with the situation to send your family member back to the hospital and expose her to additional risks in exchange for added technological and medical sophistication? In many cases, the answer will be "it depends." It depends on just what the nature of the problem is and whether the rehab is equipped to handle it. It depends on whether it's something your family member would want "handled," or at least handled in the intensive, technological style of the acute care hospital. In other cases, the answer is a resounding "no." Your family member may be at a point in her life at which she doesn't want hospital-level care. That doesn't mean she wants the nurses and doctors to focus exclusively on her comfort. She might be quite willing to take pills for her heart condition or her infection. She might be willing to receive intravenous medication for a few days. She may be eager to have an oxygen mask and to undergo blood tests, an electrocardiogram, or a chest x-ray. Your family member might want exactly the level of sophistication available at the rehab, with its lower risk of side effects and complications. A change in your family member's condition that prompts consideration of hospital transfer is a good time to think about whether hospital care makes most sense for her or whether to invoke a previous discussion about "DNH" (do-not-hospitalize).

Discharge from Rehab

A third critical node during a rehab stay involves the decision to discharge your family member. Often, the same interdisciplinary team that held a comprehensive care planning meeting shortly after admission will meet again to review your family member's progress and discuss next steps. As with the phone call about hospital transfer, what you don't want is to first learn that discharge is in the works when you get a call informing you that your family member is going home tomorrow. The staff will collectively determine if they think the rehab is still important for your family member's recovery. If not, if she's no longer benefiting from ongoing physical therapy and nursing care, or if she has met whatever targets were set early on in her stay, then it's time for discharge. The Medicare allowance of one hundred days at a skilled nursing facility (what I'm calling "rehab") care "per beneficiary period" means a *maximum* of one hundred days (actually, only the first twenty days are fully covered; any remaining days are subject to a copay, which, in 2019, is $170.50 per day). You can appeal the decision if you feel that your family member is still deriving benefit. It's also important for you to know that the longstanding policy of insisting that your family member be improving to warrant staying on was challenged in court and was not held to be valid. In practice, however, someone who has reached a plateau, who is no longer getting better but may still benefit from "maintenance therapy" to consolidate what gains she has made, can often safely be discharged home. Physical therapy can be continued in the home setting and doesn't always require an institutional environment.

Where you can help, assuming it really is time to leave, is with designing the transition plan, in figuring out what your family member will need *after* discharge, both in terms of services and equipment. The nurse, therapists, and social worker at the rehab may have a pretty good idea of what they have to set up. They know that your family member didn't have a walker before, but now she needs one, and they also know that Medicare will pay for it. They know it would be really helpful to send a visiting nurse to make sure all the old medications are disposed of and that the new ones are being taken correctly. They know that your family member is eligible for Meals on Wheels and for subsidized transportation to go to medical appointments. But what you might know is that your family member is too polite to say no to Meals on Wheels but won't eat whatever they bring. You may know that the Ride in your neighborhood is unreliable and, in any event,

they don't provide door-to-door service, which is what your family member needs—they provide curbside service rather than escorting her from inside her home to inside her destination. Whether the rehab appreciates it or not, it is passing the baton to you, not to your family member's primary care doctor or the visiting nurse or anyone else. That handoff has to be well-executed if the transition is to work. As any track coach will tell you, the hand-off can make or break a relay race.

At last, your family member is back home. You worked with the facility staff, you navigated the tricky waters of the admissions process, acute medical problems, and discharge. If her experience at rehab wasn't what you hoped for, you will know what site to avoid next time. If it was generally good, you will want to make sure she goes back to the same facility if she needs rehab in the future.

Box 18.1

Your Role at Rehab

- Admission: meet staff, participate in care planning
- Routine care: get hands-on training, encourage comprehensive assessment
- Acute medical problem: clarify goals of care, discuss rehab versus transfer to hospital
- Discharge: help design transition

CHAPTER 19

Hospital-Lite— Another Role for Rehab

We've been talking about the rehab facility (skilled nursing facility or SNF) as a site for "post-acute care," for recovery and rehabilitation after a hospitalization. That's the main function of a SNF: caring for the approximately 20 percent of people enrolled in Medicare who go to rehab after hospitalization and the even greater percent of frail, very elderly people who go to rehab before returning home. But rehabs sometimes play other roles, chiefly serving as an alternative to hospitalization or as a site for end-of-life care. Rehabs also have the potential to provide other functions that they aren't normally thought of as offering, such as comprehensive geriatric assessment, advance care planning, or palliative care.

Let's begin with thinking about rehab *instead of* the acute care hospital, rather than *after* the acute care hospital. I've spent a lot of time talking with you about the hazards of hospitalization and have made the case that sometimes home is superior to hospital as a site of care, despite the many attractions of

the hospital, simply because it doesn't come with so many risks. I realize that home may not be a viable alternative for your family member, even if he doesn't need a lot of the sophisticated technology available in the hospital. He may need someone around to help him and check in on him around the clock and you might understandably feel that you cannot play that role. Your family member's home may not physically be set up to accommodate caring for him during an acute illness if he needs a hospital bed because he cannot sit up on his own. Maybe he's on the second floor of a walk-up, making it impossible for a portable x-ray machine to reach him. Or perhaps the problem is that there is no organized program in your family member's neighborhood that is equipped to provide what the Johns Hopkins Hospital at Home program offers—comprehensive home medical treatment for relatively straightforward problems such as pneumonia or urinary tract infection.

The default in these situations is hospitalization. This often seems like the only option that has a ghost of a chance of making your family member better. You figure you'll take all those steps we discussed earlier—advocate use of an acute care for elders (ACE) unit or request a geriatric consultation or say "no" to a transfer to the intensive care unit (see chapter 14, "Acute Care for the Elderly Units"). But sometimes there's another possibility and that is *direct admission* to rehab.

Rehab Instead of Hospitalization

You are already wrinkling your forehead—doesn't Medicare require a three-day hospital stay before it will pay for a skilled nursing facility admission? A rehab charges on the order of $500 or $600 a day, if you have to pay privately, while Medicare pays in full for the first twenty days of authorized skilled nursing facility care, so you aren't very likely to ignore Medicare rules. That regulation may change soon, but in the meantime, a number of Medicare Advantage plans have contracted with Medicare to allow them to bypass the "three-day rule." Originally designed to prevent inappropriate use of rehab, the rule doesn't make much sense in an era when rehabs can do much of what a hospital does for half the price. If your family member has been diagnosed with pneumonia or a urinary tract infection, or some other straightforward problem that requires correspondingly simple treatment, and if he needs a supervised setting in which to receive care, rehab may fit the bill perfectly. The physician in the office or the emergency department or in the "urgent care" clinic performs the necessary tests, makes the arrangements, and writes the medical orders. She specifies a seven-day course of intravenous antibiotics, for example, and use of an oxygen mask whenever your family member's blood oxygen level—which is to be checked three times a day—falls below a specified level. Your family member will have around-the-clock nursing care, a certified nursing assistant (CNA) to help with personal care, and visits from the rehab facility's nurse practitioner or physician every few days. Barring any complications, treatment can be carried out effortlessly and your relative will be back home in a week.

Care at rehab still involves your family member going to an unfamiliar place outside the home and being taken care of by people who don't know him. It's associated with some of the same risks as the acute care hospital, such as falls from tripping in a strange room and confusion from sleep medication given because he has trouble sleeping away from home. But your family member is not going to get a computerized tomography (CT) scan for the question of a spot on his lung, a spot that might turn out to be nothing or might prove to be something that he wouldn't want treated, because there's no CT scanner at rehab. He's not going to be evaluated by a cardiologist for the heart murmur he's had for years, a doctor almost certain to order a cardiac echo and perhaps recommend an angiogram, because there are no cardiologists who make rounds in the SNF. He's not going to languish in bed for the duration of his stay because he's in a facility devoted to rehabilitation—the physical therapist is in the habit of seeing every patient at the SNF and the nursing staff routinely tries to get everyone up and about.

Of course, there is a downside as well. Your family member might develop complications—his "straightforward" pneumonia or urinary tract infection may become far from routine if he goes into kidney failure from the antibiotic used to treat him or if bacteria travel through the bloodstream and take up residence on a heart valve.

He may develop a new problem altogether, one that is beyond the ability of the facility to handle, such as an acute gastrointestinal bleed (rehab facilities are generally not able to provide blood transfusions, an essential component of care for an active bleeding problem). A doctor is not as readily available as in the hospital and, if she does come to see your family member in a timely fashion, she may advocate transfer to the hospital to have access to precisely those tests and procedures that the rehab doesn't have which made it so appealing in the first place. The bottom line is that *some* rehab admissions will end up with transfer to the hospital, but even if a third of them do, that still means that two-thirds do not. As always, there are pluses and minuses to substituting rehab care for hospital care, but it's a possibility you should consider. At the very least, find out if your family member's health insurance plan includes the option.

Rehab as a Site for Geriatric Assessment

I've already alluded to the rehab as an ideal environment for comprehensive geriatric assessment. It's mandated by law to provide something like this in order to design a plan of action for every patient—what Medicare calls a "comprehensive care plan." But this interdisciplinary assessment is performed early on during the rehab stay and is geared to helping staff members figure out what to do with your family member to help him recover from his acute illness. By definition, he's not at his best at the beginning of his time at rehab. What you really want is a similar evaluation carried out towards the end of the rehab stay, when your family member *is* at his best, to determine just what he's going to need later on. As it turns out, the rehab is also required to engage in discharge planning—but to do that well, it ought to act as though it had to create a second comprehensive care plan. This is where geriatric assessment comes in. If you can persuade all the people who participated in the initial planning process, the nurse, the physical therapist, the occupational therapist, the physician, and perhaps others, to update their evaluations and to develop a coordinated set of recommendations for future care, you will effectively have recreated a comprehensive geriatric assessment.

What makes rehab uniquely well-suited to this sort of endeavor is that it has already gathered all the relevant professionals in one place. They are accustomed to working together as a team. In fact, they are already required to collect much of the data that should go into a comprehensive assessment: any SNF receiving Medicare funding, which is almost all of them, must complete the "Minimum Data Set," a lengthy compendium of information about your family member's diagnoses, physical function, mental status, medications, and emotional state. As an added plus, your family member doesn't have to go anywhere to have the evaluation performed; he's already on site. And if he's too tired to have all the component parts done on one day—a potential problem with outpatient geriatric assessment—which is often an exhausting, intensive, multi-hour ordeal for your family member—it can easily be spread over several days.

The purpose of this sort of assessment is to prepare for the future, which makes it the ideal foundation for advance care planning. Advance care planning, in turn, is a process for laying out an approximate road map for the future. It entails considering some of the "what ifs" that are most likely to arise in the next months or years. If you haven't undertaken this process with your family member, or if his status has changed sufficiently that it's time for reviewing your earlier plan, the tail end of a rehab admission is a good time to proceed.

Advance Care Planning at Rehab

The starting point for advance care planning involves considering what your family member's overall goals are. Is he principally concerned with prolonging his life, whatever the cost? Is he primarily worried about maintaining the abilities he has to function on a day-to-day basis? Or is he at a point where he wants to focus mainly on remaining as comfortable as possible? The answer to these questions, in turn, will shape planning for future health care. To make the leap into the future, you need to push the rehab staff to go one more step beyond the assessment that underlies discharge planning.

Instead of just asking, "What services will my family member need (and what is he eligible to receive) next week, after he goes home?," you want to raise the question of how to respond if he gets sick again. Obviously, nobody can predict the future and there's always the possibility that your family member will develop a new problem, something he's never before experienced. But if he has a number of chronic conditions, odds are that one of them will flare up. He might, for example, have been hospitalized for an exacerbation of his chronic obstructive lung disease or of his congestive heart failure. There's a good chance he will develop shortness of breath again in the future and that it will be due to a recurrence of what he had last time. Is there a series of steps he and you might go through that will help him improve without immediately going the hospital route?

Advance care planning can also consider the possibility of further functional decline in light of your family member's goals. Suppose that at the discharge planning meeting, you figure out that your family member needs additional home health aide assistance to get by at home and you make the necessary arrangements with help from the rehab staff. But suppose you also realize that his underlying neurological condition, say Parkinson's disease, is progressive and that just a little more deterioration, and he won't be able to live independently any more—he'll either need a live-in caregiver or he will have to move to a nursing home. Which option is right for him will depend on his goals as well as on the layout of his home, on his resources, and on the kind and amount of help you can commit to. If his main goal is to be as independent as possible, he may be willing to accept a plan that sacrifices some degree of safety in exchange for staying at home. If his chief concern is living as long as he can, he may prefer the more secure environment of a nursing home. The interdisciplinary team might have a sense of how quickly the current arrangements are likely to unravel and of what steps to take now to plan for that eventuality.

Palliative Care at Rehab

Depending on the nature of your family member's medical problems, he might also be an excellent candidate for a palliative care consultation and the rehab may be the ideal place for such an evaluation. Palliative care, with its focus on symptom management, advance care planning, and psycho- social support (for you as well as for your family member), is another route to laying the groundwork for future care (see chapter 15, "Hospital-Based Palliative Care"). If pain or constipation or nausea is getting in the way of your family member's quality of life and the hospital was much too busy attending to what the physicians regarded as the only important problems, those that were potentially life-threatening, a palliative care specialist may be the best person to find a solution. In fact, symptoms such as pain are one of the major impediments to your relative's regaining his baseline state: unless his pain comes under control, he's never going to be able to walk very far or do much for himself. Physical therapists know that a patient recovering from knee replacement surgery, for instance, often needs to take a dose of pain medication half an hour before starting his therapy session or he won't be able to tolerate the prescribed exercises. But a physician needs to order the pain medicine and sometimes it's tricky to find an effective drug that doesn't produce adverse effects. Palliative care consultants are familiar with pain regimens that may be foreign to orthopedists and general internists, including lidocaine patches and fentanyl patches. They know about the various types of pain, such as nerve pain, that don't respond to conventional analgesics but that may improve with antiseizure medication or antidepressants.

A palliative care team will also recognize that providing care to your family member means taking *your* needs, abilities, and preferences into consideration as well, a perspective different from the typical individualistic attitude of physicians. The team members will understand that a plan that sounds wonderful to your family member may impose an unacceptable burden on you—and that you shouldn't feel guilty if you aren't prepared to do "whatever it takes" to make your family member happy. They can help negotiate a solution that takes into consideration both your family member's desires and the realities of his situation.

Finally, palliative care specialists can tackle advance care planning. They are experts on eliciting goals of care and helping your family member prioritize what's most important to him. If nobody else has already done this, they can then work with you to translate those goals into a plan of care, whether by signing an out-of-hospital do-not-resuscitate (DNR) form, completing a Physician Orders for Life-Sustaining Treatment (POLST) document, or by delineating the overall approach in the medical record.

In principle, all of these strategies—comprehensive geriatric assessment, advance care planning, and palliative care consultation—can be pursued in other settings. But their availability in the outpatient world is often theoretical: many if not most communities do not offer palliative care or geriatric consultation, and most primary care physicians don't routinely engage in advance care planning with their patients. Likewise, they rarely happen in the hospital unless there is a crisis, either because patients are too sick to dwell on anything other than the immediate situation or, if they are well enough to think about the future, they are usually far too busy with tests and procedures. The pace in the hospital is just not conducive to what is often a fairly long process that is best conducted in stages. The rehab isn't usually used this way, but it has the potential to fill a tremendously important gap.

Box 19.1

Potential Uses for a Skilled Nursing Facility

- An alternative to hospitalization for acute illness
- A site for palliative care
- A locale for comprehensive geriatric assessment
- An opportunity for advance care planning

CHAPTER 20

Discharge Home

Your family member is finally back home after her hospitalization, perhaps after hospitalization plus a rehab stay. It's probably been a long haul for her. For you, all those days or weeks away from home may have provided a bit of a respite. Not that you weren't involved in what happened, but you had fewer responsibilities. You may have had the comforting feeling that someone else was in charge, allowing you to relax ever so slightly. Now your family member is back and whatever problem she went to the hospital with is supposedly all better, or at least under control. How very misleading!

Right away when you walk in, you may notice that your family member seems exhausted. The past few weeks have decidedly not been a vacation for her. She may look as though she has lost weight, which is not entirely surprising since she might have spent a few days in the hospital "NPO," which is Latin for "nothing by mouth," whether in anticipation of a procedure or surgery, as part of the treatment for gastrointestinal bleeding, or while she was being evaluated for "aspiration," or food going down the wrong way. Once she was able to eat, she might have had trouble extracting the food from the plastic in which it was wrapped or found it difficult to eat propped up in bed.

When she gets up and begins walking around, you may notice that she is weak and unsteady. The physical therapist in the rehab facility assured you she was "back on her feet," which you took to mean something approximating her baseline. Maybe the issue is that she feels anxious now that there is no physical therapist or nurse or certified nursing assistant around to help her, but she appears quite insecure. You rush over to give her your arm and wonder fleetingly whether she needs to be in a nursing home or should have a private aide a few hours a day or at the very least should have stayed longer at rehab.

Your family member shows you her new medication list and you realize with a sinking heart that you are going to have to cut short your visit and head over to the pharmacy with the new prescriptions. After you return with her pills, you will need to go through her medicine chest and get rid of all the old drugs that she isn't supposed to take any more and put the new pills—all nine of them—into her special daily pill dispenser. You flip through the prescriptions and realize there are at least three medications you've never heard of before. That means you'll need to read up on them so you can familiarize yourself with their side effects and other idiosyncrasies, such as whether they have to be taken on an empty stomach or a full stomach, in the morning or at night, once daily or multiple times a day. If they are brand name drugs, drugs relatively new to the market and not just to you, they are probably "Tier 3" or even "Tier 4," which means a sizable co-pay for your family member.

The Risk of Readmission to the Hospital

If you are worried that your family member doesn't look well, you are right to be concerned: as many as one in five Medicare fee-for-service patients is readmitted to the hospital within thirty days of discharge. Medicare believes that many of these readmissions are preventable—either by staying longer in the hospital, by planning better for discharge, or through a "transitional care program" that smooths the way to home care. Medicare is sufficiently concerned about avoidable readmissions that it has an elaborate program, the Medicare Readmissions Reduction Program, to try to remedy the problem and, incidentally, save as much as $17 billion each year. Much of the "program" is actually a system of penalties for hospitals that readmit more patients than Medicare feels they should, with the penalties running as high as a three percent cut in reimbursement for the offenders. Hospitals, for their part, don't want to incur that penalty so they have introduced special transitional care programs that your family member might benefit from— assuming she went directly home from the hospital. The simplest such program consists of telephone check-ins by a nurse to make sure your relative has her new medications, is scheduled for a follow-up medical appointment, and is generally doing all right. If your family member is especially fortunate, the hospital where she was admitted or the medical practice to which her primary care physician belongs will have a more robust transitional care program that involves a nurse (or nurse practitioner) who makes home visits. This clinician will come in-person and check whether your relative truly is doing all right, will make sure she is taking the correct medications, and will assess any symptoms she might be experiencing.

Hospital readmission rates are also high during or after a rehab stay. Although rehabs are themselves medical facilities and have a great deal more in the way of nursing care and diagnostic and treatment capacity than you do at home, they provide for some of the frailest and oldest patients. This sort of person, and your family member may be one of them, is often very precariously balanced between sickness and health. It's not surprising that a seemingly mild upper respiratory infection or too much (or too little) medication could tip the balance, and suddenly she is too sick to be cared for at rehab.

One strategy that might decrease the chance of a readmission is a follow-up visit to her primary physician. Most transitional care programs make a big deal of ensuring that follow-up has been arranged; some even levy penalties if a patient isn't seen by the primary care doctor within a few days of returning home. While there's no evidence that this practice actually makes a difference, it is one way of ensuring that your relative's primary care doctor knows that she was in the hospital (and perhaps rehab as well) and sees her new medication list. On the other hand, a faxed discharge summary from the hospital to the physician should also be effective and requires less effort for you and your relative. Your family member has just gotten back home and may find it burdensome to travel to the physician's office just so he can check off a box indicating she's had a follow-up visit within three days of discharge. If she's developing symptoms, either the same ones that sent her to the hospital initially or something new, however, she should definitely be evaluated. If not, she may

be just fine with a nurse coming to see her rather than traveling to the physician. If she is one of the rare individuals whose primary care physician makes house calls, then she has the best of all worlds.

Another step you can take is to spend more time with your family member than you did before she was hospitalized. Not indefinitely—just for a few days, perhaps a week, to allow you to observe her closely. If, after that time, she still seems fragile, perhaps more confused than usual, maybe more unsteady on her feet, perhaps short of breath after exertion, you may need to arrange for more help for her. She might need an aide several hours every day, either arranged through a home care agency such as the Visiting Nurse Association (VNA), if she is eligible for this service, or privately. She might need someone to go to the grocery store for her or to prepare meals. And keep your eyes peeled for signs of depression: apathy, poor appetite, insomnia, or trouble finding pleasure in life. Depression is always a risk among frail older people, but the period of hospitalization and its aftermath are especially treacherous times.

Advance Care Planning after Hospitalization

One more role to consider is advance care planning. If your family member didn't develop a new or more

detailed advance care plan while in the hospital or rehab, this is the time to do it. Whenever her clinical condition changes significantly, she should review her advance care plan. Having just been in the hospital, she's in an excellent position to think about whether she'd want to go back if the clinical situation warranted it. She's close enough to the experience to remember what it was like but has just enough distance to be able to appreciate the benefits it provided. In a few months, she may forget just how miserable she was in the hospital or, by contrast, how much of a relief it was to have twenty-four-hour nursing care.

She may also have a new diagnosis that she should take into consideration in thinking about the future. Before the hospitalization she might have had heart failure and arthritis, diabetes and early Parkinson's; now, she has all the same conditions plus atrial fibrillation or pulmonary fibrosis, breast cancer, or some other problem. Or one of her chronic conditions might have progressed: instead of mild heart failure, she now has moderately severe heart failure, putting her at high risk of relapse, of becoming short of breath and edematous; instead of early chronic lymphocytic leukemia, which is a smoldering condition rarely requiring treatment, she now has symptoms such as night sweats and low blood counts that indicate she would benefit from intervention. Whatever the situation, your family member needs to rethink her goals of care.

Depending on her primary goal at this juncture—living as long as possible, regardless of the consequences; maintaining her current level of functioning; or being physically comfortable—she will make different choices about treat-

ment. In particular, she should have a plan for what to do if she develops one of the acute medical conditions that is most likely in light of her diagnoses. If she feels short of breath, should she head straight for the emergency department? Or should she take an extra dose of furosemide—her diuretic pill—put on an oxygen mask, and see how she does? If oxygen and furosemide don't help, is the next step the hospital or should she take a small dose of morphine under the tongue?

As always, your family member might develop a new problem that she's never had before, but at least three-quarters of the time she's going to get something predictable. Planning a course of action for the foreseeable situations is sufficient to guide her—and your—response in most situations. When the crisis comes, it's also possible that the agreed-upon strategy will suddenly seems like a very bad idea. Your relative can always change her mind in the heat of the moment, but if she isn't prepared she won't have whatever medicines or equipment she needs to try the remedy she previously favored.

You and your family member shouldn't try to work out the details of an advance care plan alone: you need the input of the primary care physician or nurse practitioner. If the strategy you come up with is anything other than call 911 or head straight for the hospital, you will benefit from having a clinician to talk to, to walk you through the situation, and to provide additional guidance if the first maneuver is unsuccessful. You and your family member will find support from the medical professionals extremely helpful, whether in the form of telephonic reassurance, a home visit, or a guarantee that they will do their part by prescribing the necessary medication and arranging for other supplies such as oxygen or a bedside commode. But you can be the nudge, the person who pipes up at a follow-up medical appointment that you'd like to go over the advance care plan. If you want to be prepared for the next crisis, you might have to get the ball rolling now.

Eventually—it might take a week and it might take a month—you will find that you are providing chronic care rather than subacute or acute care.

Your relative's condition will have more or less stabilized: She may be much the way she was before the hospitalization, she may be a notch worse off, or she may find herself substantially different from her earlier condition (rarely better, though sometimes she will turn out to have been suffering from some undiagnosed or inadequately treated malady for a long time and now, after definitive intervention, she is greatly improved). But she's no longer changing day to day: the time has come for chronic home care. How to provide the best care in that situation is where we turn next.

Comprehensive Home Care

From a medical perspective, let me say at the outset that the ideal for frail older people is *comprehensive home care.* In such a system, both routine, maintenance care and acute care are provided at home to your family member by an interdisciplinary team. A typical team is made up of a nurse practitioner and a social worker, with a physician providing backup and occasional home visits. These teams are sophisticated in their knowledge of what kinds of services and devices your family member needs and how to arrange for them—a boon to your family member's health that will also make your life a great deal easier. The nurse practitioner can teach you how to draw up insulin in a syringe and how to administer it if that's something you need to know how to do. She will show you how to change

a dressing rather than leaving it to you to decipher the obscure instructions on the package insert or resort to a YouTube video. She will demonstrate how to transfer your family member from bed to chair or onto the toilet seat and supervise you as you try to do it yourself. Above all, the members of the team will serve as sources of support to you so that when you aren't sure what to make of a symptom or problem your family member has developed, they can help. A good home care team doesn't take caregivers for granted and its members understand that they need to partner with you to optimize care.

A small but growing number of programs provide this kind of comprehensive care. The oldest is the Program of All-Inclusive Care for the Elderly (PACE), which is mainly for people who are Medicare and Medicaid eligible and are impaired enough to qualify for chronic nursing home care. Much of the care is provided in an adult day health center, where physical therapy, occupational therapy, and social work services are offered. As of 2019, there are 129 PACE programs in thirty-one states, caring for over fifty thousand patients.

If you live in Indianapolis or a few other locations, your family member might qualify for Geriatric Resources for the Assessment and Care of Elders (GRACE), a program for low-income elders, many of whom receive both Medicaid and Medicare, and almost all of whom have multiple, chronic problems. Another program is Guided Care, which is available in scattered sites across the country and features a nurse who works with a group of four or five office-based physicians. Guided Care relies to a greater extent on telephone contact and office visits than some of the other programs such as GRACE, but it includes an initial, in-home assessment and some home-based follow-up along with a healthy dose of coordination and continuity. In both cases, as well as in the Independence at Home Demonstration project, initiated by the Centers for Medicare and Medicaid (CMS) Innovation Center to promote primary care at home for older people with multiple chronic conditions, caregivers are recognized as crucial members of the team. You can expect education, training, support, and access to the care team. Definitely something worth looking into.

If your family member cannot or does not want to avail herself of a comprehensive home care program, greater responsibility will fall on your shoulders. I will discuss management of chronic medical problems in part V and acute symptoms in part VI.

Box 20.1

After Discharge

- Anticipate possible decline in physical functioning after the hospitalization
- Watch for recurrence of previous medical problems or development of new ones
- Revisit goals of care in light of any new diagnoses
- Plan for future care

Chronic Care at Home

A s a caregiver, you will need to be comfortable with the day-to-day management of chronic conditions. Your family member, like most older people, probably has multiple chronic conditions. The older he gets, the more chronic conditions he is apt to have. If your relative is between age sixty-five and seventy-four, there's a slightly better than fifty-fifty chance that he has between two and five chronic conditions and just under a 10 percent chance that he has six or more chronic conditions. But if he's over eighty-five, he has a two out of three chance of having between two and five diseases, and a 25 percent chance of having six or more problems. His quality of life and his ability to function independently are strongly affected by his chronic conditions.

If your family member is reasonably mentally intact, he will be able to participate in the management of his chronic diseases and ideally, his physician will comanage the various problems with the two of you. In any case, you will want to know something about the most common conditions older people develop and basic strategies for care.

The ten leading chronic disease diagnoses among people over age sixty-five are

1. Hypertension (High Blood Pressure): 58 percent
2. High Cholesterol: 47 percent
3. Arthritis: 31 percent
4. Ischemic Heart Disease (Coronary Heart Disease): 29 percent
5. Diabetes: 27 percent
6. Chronic Kidney Disease: 18 percent
7. Heart Failure: 14 percent
8. Depression: 14 percent
9. Alzheimer's Disease and Dementia: 11 percent
10. Chronic Obstructive Lung Disease: 11 percent

CHAPTER 21

Your Medical Bag

To help manage your family member's medical problems, you are going to rely mainly on listening, asking questions, and observing. You will also benefit from a few simple instruments and medical supplies. Many of the techniques that you will need to deal with chronic conditions will also be useful in responding to acute medical problems (see part VI, "Acute Care at Home").

To begin with, you can ask your family member what he's experiencing. For decades, medical students have been taught that a good history—listening to the patient's story—will lead to a diagnosis 80 percent of the time. You won't need to make a diagnosis, but the message is the same: you can learn a great deal by listening. Just knowing that your relative has chest pain or diarrhea, for how long he has had it, and what exactly it feels like, is a useful beginning. You can learn even more by asking what brings the symptom on and what makes it better. You can also gather valuable information by watching whether your relative grimaces when he moves or by noticing if, for example, his lips are bluish. Together with a little knowledge about the most common medical conditions—both the ones he has and the ones he's likely to develop—these basic techniques will go

a long way to helping you manage his medical problems.

To supplement listening, you will find that a few pieces of equipment can help. Some will be familiar to you, such as a thermometer. Others may be familiar, such as a machine measuring blood pressure (sphygmomanometer) or the blood oxygen level (oximeter), but using them yourself will not be. Much of this equipment is readily available, inexpensive, and user-friendly: it is intended to be used by patients who are self-managing their chronic conditions. When self-management is not practical for your family member, you will have to take on this responsibility on his behalf.

Two types of gadgets may be especially useful: those for measuring bodily functions and those for treating them. In each case, you may want to review with your relative's primary care physician or nurse practitioner which type to purchase and how best to use the device. I will discuss separately equipment that aids mobility or compensates for limitations in function (see chapter 24, "Arthritis"). Let's talk first about measurement.

The most basic device you should have is a thermometer. Today's thermometers are digital: they differ from the mercury-containing thermometers you may remember from your own childhood or that of your kids (figure 21.1). You might also recall that thermometers used to come in two varieties, oral and rectal. Those are still options today, but in addition you can take the temperature reasonably accurately on the ear lobe or the forehead. Your family member's preferences and ability to tolerate the device should dictate what you choose.

You might also want to have the ability to measure blood pressure. This is particularly useful if your family member is being treated for high blood pressure. Recent guidelines issued by the American Heart Association advocate a new, lower cut-off for defining high blood pressure, a threshold that may not make sense for your family member if he is frail and has multiple other problems (see chapter 22, "High Blood Pressure"). Those same guidelines also call for home monitoring, both to diagnose and to treat high blood pressure—with the result that there are many reasonably priced, easy to use models available. As shown in figure 21.2, the actual monitor has several parts, a cuff to wrap around the arm (or in some models, the wrist) and the machine itself, plus a power source (either batteries or an electric cord).

To get an accurate blood pressure reading, you should follow the steps recommended by the American Heart Association (figure 21.3).

You may also find measuring blood pressure helpful if your family member does not have a diagnosis of hypertension but he's on medication for other problems that has the side effect of lowering blood pressure. In this setting,

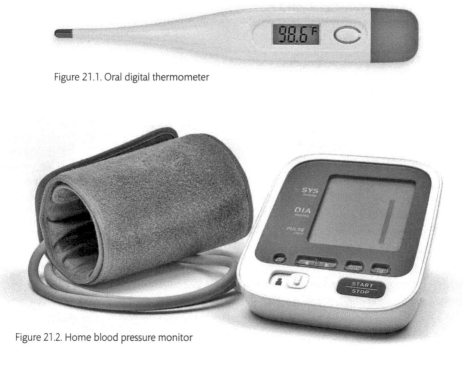

Figure 21.1. Oral digital thermometer

Figure 21.2. Home blood pressure monitor

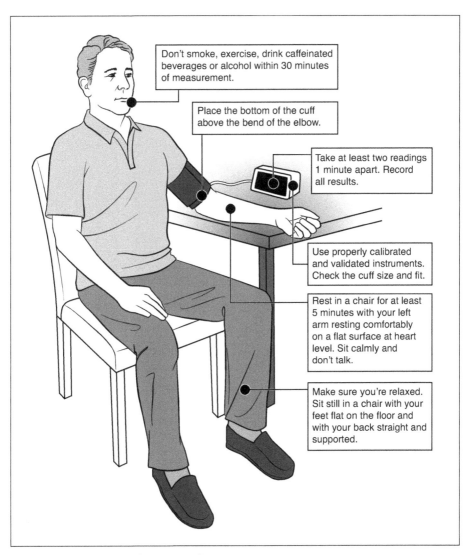

Don't smoke, exercise, drink caffeinated beverages or alcohol within 30 minutes of measurement.

Place the bottom of the cuff above the bend of the elbow.

Take at least two readings 1 minute apart. Record all results.

Use properly calibrated and validated instruments. Check the cuff size and fit.

Rest in a chair for at least 5 minutes with your left arm resting comfortably on a flat surface at heart level. Sit calmly and don't talk.

Make sure you're relaxed. Sit still in a chair with your feet flat on the floor and with your back straight and supported.

Figure 21.3. How to take blood pressure readings

you will want to be sure his pressure doesn't get dangerously low. If your family member has a history of fainting or falling, which can stem from low blood pressure, you will find the ability to the check blood pressure particularly useful.

Another device you might choose to purchase if your family member has a history of heart or lung problems is an oximeter, a gadget for measuring the amount of oxygen in his blood (figure 21.4). You may be familiar with these from the hospital: a small clip is typically placed over a fingertip and the clip is connected to a monitor that reads out the oxygen level. These devices usually also measure the pulse.

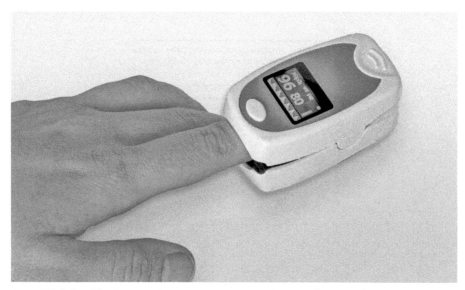

Figure 21.4. Pulse oximeter

Monitoring the oxygen saturation, as the reading is known, can help you figure out how serious a problem your relative has: a normal oxygen saturation level is greater than 98 percent. If your family member has developed a respiratory infection—cough, fever, and some trouble breathing—a low oxygen level might mean he has pneumonia. If you know he has a lung condition such as asthma or chronic obstructive lung disease, a marked decrease in the oximeter reading can signal that the exacerbation he's experiencing is serious. If your family member has home oxygen (provided via an oxygen concentrator), whether for a heart or a lung condition, a fall in the oxygen level often means you need to turn up the dial on the concentrator to increase the amount of oxygen he's getting.

The final measuring device you should consider is a scale (see figure 21.5). Measuring the weight is espe-cially useful in people with heart failure (see chapter 28, "Heart Failure"). When the heart doesn't pump properly, fluid builds up in all sorts of places where it doesn't belong, such as the ankles, the abdomen, and the lungs. The net effect is that your family member will gain weight. Keeping track of his weight is

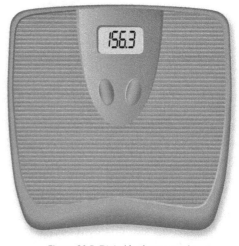

Figure 21.5. Digital bathroom scale

an excellent way to detect when heart failure is getting out of control—often before your family member experiences shortness of breath or noticeable leg edema. Monitoring your relative's weight is also important as a way to watch for an inadequate diet. If he has a poor appetite or is forgetful, he might neglect to eat and lose weight. The more weight he loses, the weaker he will get.

While everyone knows how to use a simple bathroom scale, getting your wobbly family member on and off the scale safely isn't so easy. You should hold on to him while he gets on the scale and help him off. My recommendation is that you don't keep the scale in the bathroom. The hard bathroom floor is the worst surface on which to fall and the risk of hitting his head on the porcelain sink or the bathtub on the way down makes it all the more dangerous. Putting the scale on a softer surface is safer, provided it's an even surface such as linoleum tiles. You will also want to be sure the scale has a large, bright, digital readout so the weight is readily apparent.

In addition to monitoring chronic conditions, you may also have occasion to treat some simple problems. I will mention many of the strategies you should use later, in the context of addressing acute care, but day-to-day chronic management and acute management often overlap. In any case, you should have adequate first aid equipment on hand. In addition to an assortment of bandaids, you will want to have some gauze and a roll of nonallergenic tape in case there's a larger cut or burn that needs attention. The reason for the special tape is that some people have very sensitive skin and develop a rash whenever regular tape is used.

Accidents are one of the leading reasons for trips to the emergency department: not only is your relative at risk of falling, but the older he is, the more likely he is to have paper-thin, very fragile skin that tears easily. If you can clean the wound, bandage it, and make sure your family member keeps it dry while it's healing, you can potentially spare him the anxiety and unpleasantness of hospital care. Contemporary emergency room physicians often apply what is essentially sterile super glue to many cuts that, just a few years ago, they would have sutured closed. The technique is safe and painless; it works by creating a seal that keeps bacteria and dirt out and allows the cut to heal. You can get the same product employed by physicians over the counter.

Alternatively, you can use a powder—also available over the counter—that works by producing a blood clot to seal the cut. Normally, bleeding stops when the body sends chemicals to the site of the cut that produce a clot, a process that may take some time. Wound powders react directly with a substance in the blood to form a clot. This approach is a little messier to use but is also dramatically effective. You should also have a tube of antibiotic ointment to apply to a wound before you cover it up with a bandage. Triple antibiotic preparations are the most common, but a single antibiotic such as bacitracin is adequate if your family member has an allergy to one of the ingredients of the three-drug ointment.

Along with antibiotic ointment, you may want to have a few other over-the-counter medications on hand. Acetaminophen is your basic drug against fever and pain: it comes in regular strength (325 mg) and extra strength (500 mg). You might also want an antacid such as Maalox or Mylanta (though be careful—these are to be avoided if your relative has chronic kidney disease).

That's it! Look, listen, and fill your medical bag with a few supplies (box 21.1). You already have the basic equipment necessary for outstanding caregiving.

Box 21.1

Medical Supplies

- Thermometer
- Blood pressure cuff
- Pulse oximeter
- Digital scale
- Bandages and tape
- Wound powder
- Over-the-counter medicines

CHAPTER 22

High Blood Pressure

More than three-fourths of older Americans have high blood pressure as defined by guidelines published in 2017 and endorsed by several professional groups. Blood pressure, or the amount of force generated as blood flows through the blood vessels, consists of two numbers: the systolic blood pressure—or upper number, which measures the amount of force exerted on the walls of the blood vessels when the heart contracts—and diastolic blood pressure—or the lower number, which measures the amount of force generated between contractions. According to the newest standards, either a systolic blood pressure of over 130 or a diastolic blood pressure of over 80 is too high. The reason for recommending that your family member's blood pressure remain below those cutoffs is that higher values are associated with a risk of cardiovascular events such as strokes and heart attacks, as well as death. In addition, high blood pressure is a factor in causing or worsening other conditions such as diabetes and dementia.

While people with lower blood pressure are, on average, better off, there's a cost to your family member of bringing her blood pressure down. When the strategy for lowering blood pressure is taking medication, that medication can cause serious side effects or interfere with other medications your relative may be taking. As a result, the new guidelines, while enthusiastic in principle about lowering blood pressure, advise caution. This is where you come in. The authorities recommend being certain that your family member *actually has* high blood pressure before embarking on a course of treatment. Since some people become anxious in the doctor's office and their blood pressure shoots up, you are advised to take your relative's blood pressure several times at home, in relaxed conditions, before considering starting medication. Mild elevations of blood pressure, for example, a systolic blood pressure between 130 and 140, which previously was considered normal, should be treated with diet before rushing to medicines. This means avoiding very salty foods and, if your relative is overweight, losing weight. Finally, the guidelines do not recommend a specific blood pressure goal—and by implication, suggest that treatment may not be warranted—for people who have an advanced illness with a limited life expectancy or those living in a nursing home. If your family member would benefit from treatment for high blood pressure, here are the main points you should know.

What Are the Symptoms of High Blood Pressure?

For the most part, none. That's what's so tricky about high blood pressure. Headaches rarely cause high blood pressure—the blood pressure has to be extraordinarily high, what's called "malignant hypertension," to cause acute symptoms. Looked at differently, the overwhelming majority of people who suffer from headaches develop them for some other reason, whether stress (probably the most common reason), the flu, a migraine, or some other reason.

What Problems Does Untreated High Blood Pressure Produce?

Longstanding, untreated high blood pressure is what will get your family member in trouble. The arteries that carry the blood from the heart to every part of the body are not designed to withstand the relentless pounding of continuous hypertension. As a result, the arterial lining, the smooth layer of tissue that comes in contact with the blood, is damaged. Once it's damaged, the lining becomes a setup for the formation of blood clots, it serves as a magnet for cholesterol, and over time the artery becomes narrowed. Whatever body part the artery feeds—a kidney or the brain or a leg—may not get enough blood. Starved for oxygen, which is carried by the blood, the affected body part develops "ischemia," which means lack of oxygen. Ischemia is painful and, if it persists, results in tissue death. Some of the major medical problems associated with high blood pressure are coronary heart disease (heart attack or angina), heart failure, stroke, and vascular dementia (one form of dementia). While lowering blood pressure to acceptable levels significantly reduces the chances of developing heart disease or a stroke, its benefits in preventing dementia are less well-established. Extremely high blood pressure that develops rapidly, what is called malignant hypertension, causes damage to organs such as the eyes and the kidneys. Treatment of this form of high blood pressure, involving readings of 180 over 120 or greater, is urgent.

How Do You Treat High Blood Pressure?

The initial response to consistently high blood pressure readings, if the decision is made to treat, should be exercise and diet along with smoking cessation. Exercise ideally involves thirty minutes of moderately intense aerobic exercise five days a week. Walking and swimming are two exercises that your relative may be able to engage in even if she is frail. Cycling (using a stationary bicycle) is also effective but may be problematic for your family member. Diet may mean weight loss; it also typically involves a decrease in salt intake. While the average person consumes 9 grams of salt a day or more, the World Health Organization recommends cutting this to below 5 grams. The U.S. National Heart Lung and Blood Institute recommends the "DASH" diet (Dietary Approaches to Stop Hypertension):

- Grains: 6–8 servings daily

- Vegetables: 4–5 servings daily

- Fruit: 4–5 servings daily

- Fat-free or low-fat dairy products: 2–3 servings daily

- Nuts, seeds, dry beans, and peas: 4–5 servings daily

- Fats and oils: 2–3 servings daily

- Meat, poultry, fish: 6 or less servings daily

- Sweets: 5 servings weekly or less

In addition to exercising and making changes in diet, your relative should be sure to stop smoking. (For more on these three lifestyle modifications, see chapter 32, "Prevention.")

If exercise and diet fail, the next step is medication. Several types or "classes" of medications are used to treat high blood pressure. The oldest, safest, and one of the most effective treatments is a diuretic or "fluid pill." If your family member takes a diuretic, she will probably be on a very low dose, for example 12.5 milligrams of the drug hydrochlorothiazide. If that proves insufficient, or if it has to be stopped because of side effects, then your relative's physician will probably move on to a different class of medication such as a beta blocker, an angiotensin-converting enzyme (ACE) inhibitor, or a calcium channel blocker. While all four types of medication are relatively safe, there's always the potential for side effects.

Diuretics cause trouble in two principle ways: one is by predisposing to dehydration, an issue that is especially of concern in very hot weather or if your relative has a fever; the other is by lowering the potassium, an essential chemical. One way to test for dehydration is by checking your family member's blood pressure when she is sitting down and then when she is standing up—if the systolic blood pressure is twenty or more points lower after she stands up, your relative has "orthostatic hypotension" and very likely needs to stop her diuretic. If she doesn't discontinue the medication, she's at risk of falling or fainting. A low potassium, which can cause an irregular heart rhythm, can only be diagnosed with a blood test. If your relative is on a diuretic, she will need to have her potassium level monitored periodically.

Beta blockers (medications such as metoprolol, atenolol, or labetalol) interact with (or "bind to") particular sites in the heart and blood vessels known, not surprisingly, as "beta receptors." The main side effect you will need to worry about is a slow heart rate due to the effect of beta blockers on the electrical system of the heart. You will probably be advised to check your relative's pulse periodically. This class of drugs is also potentially the cause of confusion or sluggishness.

Angiotensin-converting enzyme (ACE) inhibitors (medications such as captopril, enalapril, and lisinopril) cause blood vessels to relax, lowering blood pressure. They are called angiotensin-converting enzyme inhibitors because they prevent a certain enzyme from working, an enzyme that normally raises blood pressure by causing blood vessels to constrict. The major side effect of ACE inhibitors is impaired kidney function, which can only be diagnosed with a blood test that measures how well the kidneys are working. Usually, any impairment can be reversed by discontinuing the medication.

Calcium channel blockers (medications such as diltiazem, nifedipine, and amlodipine) also work by causing the muscles in the walls of blood vessels to relax. Two of the most common side effects of these drugs are ankle swelling and constipation. Your relative's physician may treat these complications with still other medications—or he may decide it would be prudent to discontinue the offending agent and try a different type of medication.

What Is Secondary Hypertension?

So far, we've been discussing the most common form of hypertension, what is called "primary hypertension." In this type of high blood pressure, the primary problem is the force generated by the blood as it flows through your relative's arteries. A rarer form of hypertension is "secondary hypertension." In these cases, the elevated blood pressure is due to some other problem entirely. A hormonal imbalance in which your relative produces too much of the chemical aldosterone can lead to high blood pressure, as can certain kidney problems (for example, the genetic condition, polycystic kidney disease) or a rare tumor of the adrenal gland, a pheochromocytoma, which results in excess production of the chemical epinephrine. Your relative's physician will only look for one of these conditions if medications are not working or if she has other symptoms suggestive of an unusual form of hypertension.

What Can Worsen High Blood Pressure?

As a caregiver managing your relative's hypertension, you should be aware that certain medications can cause her blood pressure to rise. One type of medication that has this effect is a steroid (medications such as prednisone); since it's a prescription drug, your family member's doctor should alert you to this possible complication and may ask you to take a few blood pressure readings. Several of the major offenders are over-the-counter medications. These include decongestants (for example, phenylephrine) and nonsteroidal anti-inflammatory medications (such as ibuprofen and naproxen). You may want to check with your relative's primary care physician before your relative uses either of these types of drugs.

Checking Blood Pressure at Home

The ability to check your family member's blood pressure is going to be particularly useful if she has hypertension—though as I mentioned earlier, it may be helpful in a variety of situations. A number of different, modestly priced home monitoring devices are available. Most of them resemble what you are familiar with from medical appointments and involve a cuff wrapped around the upper arm that is inflated and then gradually deflated (see chapter 21, "Your Medical Bag").

Other devices may be easier to use but not quite as accurate, such as one that goes around the wrist (figure 22.1).

You may wish to ask your relative's primary care physician or nurse practitioner for help selecting a device and guidance using it. Whatever device you choose, you will want to compare the reading you get with your equipment and the reading measured at the same time in the physician's office using a standard sphygmomanometer (blood pressure cuff).

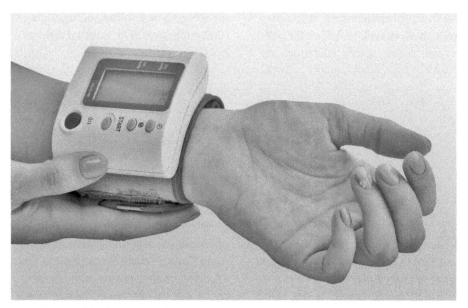

Figure 22.1. Wrist blood pressure device

How Often Should You Check Your Relative's Blood Pressure?

You probably have noticed that in the hospital, a nurse checks your family member's blood pressure at least once per shift, or every eight hours, sometimes more frequently. In the skilled nursing facility, too, nurses take frequent blood pressure readings, sometimes every time they give medication—and your relative may take certain medications three or four times a day. This approach makes sense if your family member is acutely ill and very unstable; in this situation, her blood pressure is apt to fluctuate. It also makes sense if her doctor has just started a new medicine and wants to be sure it is having the desired effect. In the home setting, however, there is rarely a need for such intensive monitoring. You will want to measure the blood pressure several times if the physician is trying to decide whether your family member has hypertension or not, and you will want to check the blood pressure if there's an acute problem (see part VI, "Acute Care at Home"). If your relative has been taking blood pressure medication for months or years and her pressure has been well-controlled, and if she isn't having any worrisome acute symptoms, then once a month is usually a satisfactory interval for blood pressure measurement.

High blood pressure is an example of a condition that you can manage almost entirely at home—with suitable input by the primary care physician, nurse practitioner, or physician assistant (box 22.1). That's good news for your family member, as you may be able to drastically limit the number of doctor visits and, at the same time, help stave off devastating conditions such as a stroke or heart attack.

Box 22.1

High Blood Pressure

- In general, produces no symptoms
- Over the long run, if untreated, leads to strokes, heart disease, and dementia
- Home measurement can aid in diagnosis and monitoring
- First line treatment involves diet and exercise
- When taking medications (diuretics, beta blockers, ACE inhibitors, calcium channel blockers), monitor for dehydration or slow pulse

CHAPTER 23

High Cholesterol

Elevated cholesterol is the second most common chronic medical condition among older people, so there is a good chance your family member carries this diagnosis. If he has high cholesterol, odds are that he's taking a medication to bring it down. You probably figure there's not much for you to do other than to make sure he's getting the medication from the pharmacy and taking it as prescribed. But in light of the risk of side effects, of interactions with other medications, and the cost you may want to question whether your family member benefits from treatment. The "Choosing Wisely" campaign, supported by a variety of professional medical associations, suggests that medications aren't always the answer for older people.

To think about the question of treatment, it's helpful to distinguish between people who have heart disease—who have had a heart attack or suffer from angina or heart failure—and those who don't. If your family member has a history of heart disease, it may be perfectly reasonable for him to take a variety of steps to keep it in check, including pills to lower his cholesterol.

If your relative doesn't have a history of heart disease, then the only reason for taking a statin is to try to prevent its development in the future.

It turns out that the older he is and the more other medical problems he has, the less likely a medication is to prevent him from getting first time heart trouble. To figure out whether taking medicine makes sense for your relative, you may have to know how much time he has left. That's a difficult question, both to ask and to answer, and you might feel as though it's disloyal to even contemplate the possibility your relative won't be around in five years. But you aren't doing him any favors letting him take a medication that is extremely unlikely to help, given that it will be years before the medication can be beneficial and that he doesn't have that much time. If your family member has high cholesterol but no history of heart disease, you may want to question the need for cholesterol-lowering medication simply because it would mean yet another pill. If he is already taking several medications—the average older person is on five or six medicines and many people take considerably more—adding another one can cause a drug-drug interaction, which is just what it sounds like. The statin itself may not cause a problem, but it might interfere with one of your family member's other pills, either preventing it from working or causing an excessively high level.

Medications for Lowering Cholesterol

Statins, whether atorvastatin, simvastatin, or pravastatin, or another similar drug ending in "statin," are far and away the most commonly used medications to lower cholesterol. In fact, according to the National Center for Health Statistics, just under half of all Americans age seventy-five and older take a statin. As of 2018, seven different statins are available in the United States. All except one are off-patent, which means you can find a generic version. They are all similar in how they work, in their effectiveness, and in their side effects. Some are far more potent than others, but that just means that 10 milligrams of one drug may be equivalent to 20 milligrams of another medication; it does not imply one is any better than the other.

Statins are reasonably safe, as medications go, but that doesn't mean they have no side effects. One of the most serious adverse reactions to statins is muscle damage. The milder form of this condition, myopathy, results in weakness and achy muscles; the more severe form, rhabdomyolysis, causes muscle breakdown, leading to dramatic weakness and potentially death. Another concerning side effect is liver failure: if your family member takes a statin, he will need periodic blood tests to detect evidence of liver malfunction. Other possible side effects include impaired memory and cataracts. Both of these

conditions are very common among older people, so it's difficult to tease out whether taking a statin makes them more likely.

Cholesterol-lowering medications also cost money. The single most widely used statin is Lipitor (atorvastatin), the brand name of a drug that, in its heyday, generated more than a billion dollars a year in revenue for its manufacturer. Now that it's off-patent, its price has come way down. Similarly, most of the other statins are relatively inexpensive, but drug costs add up. While drug plans are required by the Affordable Care Act to pay for "preventive medicines" without a co-pay or deductible, this provision will only help your family member if she is covered by a drug plan. The full price at area pharmacies for a three-month supply of an average dose of atorvastatin is $150 or $50 per month.

While statins are more common than other cholesterol-lowering medications, there are alternatives. The two drugs that have been around longest—niacin and cholestyramine—however, are associated with significant side effects and are seldom used.

Finally, there is an entirely new class of drugs, the PCSK9 inhibitors such as Repatha (generic name, evolocumab) and Praluent (generic name, alirocumab). These are extremely powerful—and very expensive—medications given by injection that are used primarily for people with a relatively rare genetic condition that makes it difficult to bring cholesterol levels down any other way. It would be extremely unusual for your relative to have survived to old age with this condition.

Other Ways to Reduce Risk

The point of taking a statin isn't really to lower cholesterol. The point is to lower the risk of developing heart disease (if your family member doesn't already have heart problems) or to lower the risk of developing a heart attack or stroke (if she does have known heart problems). The cholesterol level is a means to an end; it's not the end itself and there may be other ways to achieve that end. Giving up cigarette smoking is one strategy; exercise is still another; diet is a third. The problem is that it's easier to pop a pill than to get on an exercise bicycle every day or to quit smoking or to go from a high fat, meat-rich diet to a low-fat diet with fruits, vegetables, and lots of roughage. But what's important to realize is that physicians write prescriptions for medications, but you are the key to strategies that involve exercise, diet, or abandoning cigarettes.

What Is a Good Cholesterol Level?

If your family member does go on medication, what cholesterol level should he be shooting for? It turns out that this isn't exactly the right question to ask. The total cholesterol is the sum of two different molecules: cholesterol hooked to either of two transport proteins. When cholesterol is attached to one of these transport proteins, high density lipoprotein (HDL), it is on the way to the garbage heap. When cholesterol is attached to the other transport protein, low density lipoprotein (LDL), it is either on its way to the liver, where it will be used to manufacture other chemicals necessary for normal bodily function, or to a blood vessel, where it is apt to stir up trouble. The correct answer to the question about the "right" cholesterol level is that high levels of HDL are desirable, as are low levels of LDL. To complicate matters further, there's another type of fatty substance, triglycerides, that can also cause problems if your family member has a very high level. The National Heart, Lung, and Blood Institute has issued recommendations for target cholesterol levels in adults (table 23.1).

Treating high cholesterol is advisable for many older adults. Older people are at greater risk of heart problems than are younger people and may stand to benefit *more* from cholesterol-lowering medication than their younger counterparts. But for people such as your family member, who may have limited life expectancy, frailty, and multiple other chronic conditions, you will want to discuss with the primary care physician whether treatment makes sense, particularly if he does not carry a diagnosis of heart disease. Just as we discussed asking the right question about any diagnostic procedure in chapter 13, "The Technological Imperative"—What will it take to make a diagnosis and what difference will it make?—there's an analogous question for medical treatment: What are the benefits of treatment, what are the risks, and is there another alternative?

Table 23.1
Target Cholesterol Levels in Adults

	Total cholesterol	HDL cholesterol	LDL cholesterol	Triglycerides
Good	Less than 200	40 or higher	Less than 100	Less than 149
Borderline	200–239	n/a	130–159	150–199
High	240 or higher	n/a	160 or higher	200 or higher

Box 23.1

Cholesterol

- Lowering cholesterol may prevent the development of heart disease or its symptoms

- High density lipoprotein (HDL) rather than total cholesterol is the usual target

- Medications, primarily statins, are the mainstay of treatment

- Side effects of statins: liver problems, muscle weakness

- In frail elderly people, treatment may not be warranted

CHAPTER 24

Arthritis

Unlike high blood pressure and high cholesterol, the first two diagnoses in the list of the top ten chronic conditions found in older people, arthritis does produce symptoms. It causes pain and it interferes with mobility, two good reasons to want to do something about it. "It," by the way, can take a variety of forms, but the most common by far is osteoarthritis (OA), otherwise known as degenerative joint disease (DJD) because it results from wear and tear of the joints. In terms of its effect on quality of life, arthritis looms large.

What you need to know as a caregiver is both what *treatments* are available for arthritis and what *assistive devices*, things like canes and braces, can help your family member compensate for arthritis.

Treatments for Arthritis

Arthritis typically affects large joints such as knees and hips; the joints of the spine are also large joints. Not surprisingly, the main arthritic problems your family member is likely to experience are knee pain, hip pain, and back pain. Pain in all these areas can have a major effect on how well your relative can walk.

Simple interventions that can make a difference, especially in the setting of an acute worsening of pain, include mechanical measures such as a heating pad. While generally safe, with both electric and microwavable heating pads you need to be careful that your family member does not burn herself by making them too hot or leaving them on too long. A physical therapist may be able to prescribe exercises that can also help, sometimes indirectly by strengthening the muscles that are connected to the affected joints. One exercise that is particularly good for people with knee or hip arthritis is swimming: it's "non-weight-bearing," meaning your family member won't further traumatize the joints by walking on a hard surface.

Medications are what most people think of when they consider treatment of arthritis, and what physicians often resort to. They are of two basic types:

pain-relievers and anti-inflammatory medications. The most commonly used pain reliever is acetaminophen (Tylenol). If the pain is intermittent, it makes sense for your family member to take a pill whenever it acts up. If the pain is fairly constant, then it's a good idea to take medication around the clock. Pain relief is more effective if your family member has a consistent level of medication in her system rather than trying to play catch-up all the time. One caution with acetaminophen is that it's important not to take more than two extra-strength tablets three times a day. If your family member has a liver problem, she probably shouldn't take acetaminophen at all. It's always a good idea to check with the physician if a medication is going to be used over an extended period of time.

Pain relievers also include opioids such as morphine and its cousins (hydromorphone, oxycodone, and codeine are the ones most commonly used). These potent medicines should be reserved for severe pain that hasn't responded to other treatments because they have potential side effects including constipation and confusion; because they can cause addiction; and because they are at risk of being "diverted," which means getting into the hands of other people who either sell them or abuse them. On the other hand, if the pain is very bad and gets in the way of your family member doing her usual activities, if other medications haven't helped, if surgery is not an option, and if the physician recommends an opioid, you shouldn't reject it out of hand. You will need to make sure the medication is kept in a secure location and you'll

want to be sure your relative takes a laxative to counteract the constipating effects of chronic opioids.

Anti-inflammatory medication, while the mainstay of treatment for certain subtypes of arthritis such as rheumatoid arthritis, have a limited role in the more commonplace degenerative variant of arthritis. They are no more effective than acetaminophen, but have a more dangerous side effect profile: They can cause kidney malfunction, which can be quite insidious as it produces no symptoms and is only diagnosed with a blood test; and they can cause bleeding in the stomach or small intestine, which can be extremely dangerous. The risk of bleeding is especially high if your relative is also on a blood thinning medication such as warfarin. If your family member complains to her physician about joint pain and is told to take a nonsteroidal anti-inflammatory medication (ibuprofen, naproxen, or similar drugs)—or is given a prescription for an opioid (codeine, oxycodone, hydromorphone, or morphine), it's perfectly appropriate to ask whether he could recommend an alternative approach.

Finally, there's surgery. First introduced in the 1960s, hip replacement surgery has been called "the operation of the century" because it has had such an enormous impact on pain, mobility, and overall functioning. As the operation has become simpler and safer, it's been used in older and older people—just because your family member is over eighty doesn't mean she's not eligible for the surgery. Total knee replacement, which became widespread a decade or so later, is even more common today than is hip replacement. All told, over four hundred thousand Medicare patients undergo one or the other of these procedures every year—and that's only looking at first time surgery, not at the redo's (called revisions) that are sometimes needed.

If surgery is a possibility, your family member will need to have x-rays of the affected joint. Then she will need to see an orthopedist to determine if she is a good candidate for the procedure. If she has significant heart or lung disease, she may need to see a specialist to assess just how risky the procedure would be.

The hospital stay for either procedure is very short, usually only a couple of days. Medicare is even considering allowing joint replacement surgery in ambulatory surgery centers, which would mean patients wouldn't stay overnight after the procedure. While it was once routine for anyone who had had joint replacement surgery to be discharged to inpatient rehab, more and more commonly patients go straight home to have physical therapy at home. If your family member has multiple other medical problems, she may still benefit from spending time in rehab before coming home, particularly if she has had complications while she was in the hospital.

Compensating for Arthritis

An important strategy in dealing with arthritis is to compensate for your family member's difficulties. Often this involves using clever and fairly inexpensive gadgets to make routine tasks a little easier. Let's say your relative has arthritis of her *wrists*, which makes it hard for her to open cans or jars. You'll want to be sure she has an electric can opener and either an ergonomic or an electric jar opener if she uses cans or jars (figure 24.1).

If your family member has arthritis involving her *fingers* and has difficulty gripping things, she may benefit from special utensils—spoons, forks, and knives—for eating (figure 24.2). These often have thick rubber padding around the handles that make them easy to grasp and use. Similarly, pens with a special adaptive grip can facilitate writing. An occupational therapist can advise you on what devices would be most useful.

If your family member has arthritis involving her *knees* or *hips*, she may benefit from a mobility aid such as a cane, walker, or wheelchair. Some people have all three: a cane for use around the house, a walker for going for short trips outside the house, and a wheelchair for longer expeditions or outings involving uneven terrain. A physical therapist can help determine which type of device would make most sense and what model to obtain. The Mayo Clinic has useful information regarding how to select and

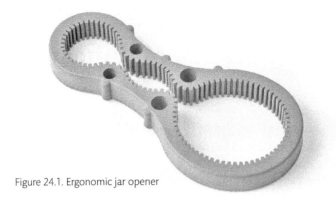

Figure 24.1. Ergonomic jar opener

use canes and walkers (visit https://www.mayoclinic.org/healthy-lifestyle/healthy-aging/multimedia/canes/sls-20077060 and https://www.mayoclinic.org/healthy-lifestyle/healthy-aging/multimedia/walker/sls-20076469).

Finally, it's worth noting that excess weight puts undesirable stress on the knee joints. Losing weight, while more challenging than popping a pill, can make a difference in the rate at which joints deteriorate. Extremely overweight people are also at high risk of complications if joint surgery is under consideration and may be advised to lose weight before having an operation. Unfortunately, your family member may find herself in a vicious circle: the heavier she is, the harder it is to exercise, and the less exercise she does, the more weight she gains.

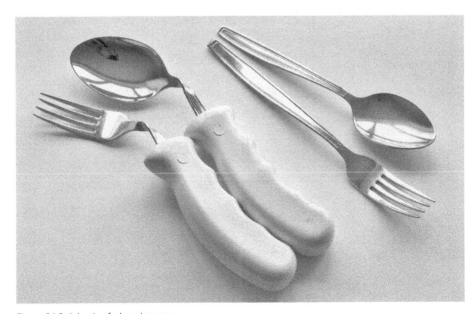

Figure 24.2. Adaptive fork and spoon

Environmental Modifications

So far, we have talked about interventions that focus on your family member: giving her medication to ease arthritic pain or a special device to help her get around or to open a jar. Sometimes, what makes most sense is to modify the *environment*. If your relative has trouble unlocking the front door, maybe the lock should be changed from the old-fashioned lock and key to a keypad lock, which requires pressing buttons rather than inserting and turning a key. If she has steps in her home that are difficult for her to navigate, perhaps she should have a stair lift installed (figure 24.3).

If your relative uses a wheelchair when she leaves the house, she may need a ramp to accommodate the wheelchair. A physical therapist can give you advice about what products are best suited to your family member's

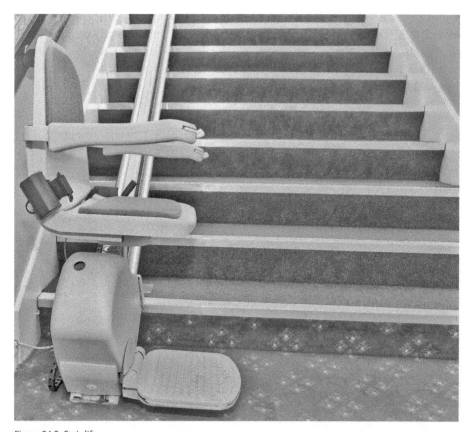

Figure 24.3. Stair lift

needs—and which ones Medicare considers "durable medical equipment" and will, therefore, pay for.

Your family member might live in a home that cannot be made accessible or comfortable for her. Perhaps she lives in an apartment that's a third story walk-up; maybe she has to climb over the side of an old porcelain bathtub to bathe. There may come a time when you simply are unable to manage her arthritis in her current location and your relative will have to move. A social worker can work with the two of you to identify a more appropriate living situation. The primary care physician may recommend a social worker or you could find someone through the local Area Agency on Aging (for more information about finding a social worker, see chapter 7, "What to Expect from Nurses, Social Workers, and Therapists").

Arthritis is another of those chronic conditions for which no cure is available (box 24.1). Nonetheless, with suitable medications, sometimes surgery, and a variety of adaptive devices, you are likely to be able to maximize your relative's functioning for a considerable period of time.

Box 24.1

Arthritis

- Treatment: pain medication, exercise, joint replacement
- Compensatory strategies: jar and can openers, adaptive pen, adaptive fork and spoon
- Environmental modifications: stair lift, keypad lock
- Prevention: weight control

CHAPTER 25

Coronary Heart Disease

Coronary heart disease ("coronary" refers to the heart), also called ischemic heart disease ("ischemia" means lack of blood flow), coronary artery disease (since it affects the blood vessels that nourish the heart), or simply coronary disease, is the leading cause of death in the United States in adults—regardless of age. Although we think of the heart as supplying blood to the rest of the body, the heart needs its own blood supply. Without oxygen and essential materials, the heart cannot function. The heart's own circulation is made up of a right coronary artery, a left coronary artery, and their branches (figure 25.1).

If any of the major coronary arteries or their branches do not permit blood to flow freely, for example, because they are narrowed and stiffened by cholesterol deposits, your family member may experience chest pain, or ischemia. Ischemia is especially common with exercise since the heart is working harder and, therefore, needs more blood to provide extra oxygen. If the blood vessels cannot accommodate the heart's needs, your relative may experience pain that he will typically describe as a heaviness or tightness in his chest.

When this kind of pain is short-lived, easing up with rest, the pain is known as angina. If the process continues for an extended period of time, the part of the heart muscle that isn't getting enough oxygen will die: that's a heart attack. Because angina tends to come on with exercise, whether mild exercise such as walking a few feet to the bathroom or more strenuous exercise such as going up a steep hill, physicians call

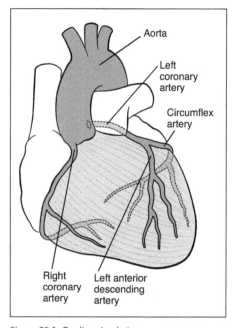

Figure 25.1. Cardiac circulation

it "exertional." Sometimes the narrowing of the coronary artery is so severe that chest pain occurs even at rest. "Rest angina" is a dangerous symptom, often a harbinger of a heart attack.

To help manage your family member's coronary heart disease, you should understand why blood vessels become stiff and narrow in the first place. The narrowing occurs when cholesterol and other undesirable material, collectively called a "plaque," builds up on the lining of the blood vessel in a process known as atherosclerosis. Plaques can cause damage not only by progressively blocking off an artery but also by bursting, or "rupturing." What's important for you to understand is that high cholesterol, cigarette smoking, high blood pressure, and diabetes *all* stimulate plaque formation. That's why they are considered "risk factors" for coronary heart disease.

Your role in the treatment of coronary heart disease, apart from addressing acute pain (which we will discuss in chapter 33, "Chest Pain") and lifestyle modification (which we will discuss in chapter 32, "Prevention") involves *chronic maintenance* and *repair*. With chronic maintenance, you are trying to prevent both angina (chest pain) and the further progression of the underlying disease process—plaque build-up resulting in narrowing of the coronary arteries. Repair involves improving blood flow to the heart by fixing or bypassing the narrowed section of the artery or arteries. It's accomplished by putting in a stent, a wire mesh that props the artery open, or by coronary artery bypass surgery, which substitutes a healthy segment of artery for the diseased one. Obviously, you aren't going to be putting in stents or performing a bypass—those are surgical procedures done by an "invasive cardiologist" and cardiac surgeon, respectively. Your role is helping your family member think through whether he is interested in one of these more invasive approaches to treatment, whether they are consistent with his goals of care, and to help support him if they are.

Chronic Maintenance

The mainstay of treatment for coronary heart disease is medications. These medications make it easier for the heart to function by lowering the demand for oxygen or by increasing the supply of oxygen. Either way, the imbalance between supply and demand is corrected and chest pain is less likely to develop. The principal types of medication that produce this effect are nitrates (drugs such as isosorbide or nitropaste), beta blockers (medicines such as atenolol or metoprolol), calcium channel blockers (for example nifedipine and amlodipine), and angiotensin-converting enzyme (ACE) inhibitors (drugs including enalapril and lisinopril) along with their cousins, angiotensin receptor blockers (such as losartan and valsartan). What you need to know about these forms of treatment is that they tend to lower blood pressure. This can be a problem if the blood pressure becomes so low that it leads to dizziness, falling, or fainting. You may be asked to check your family member's blood pressure from time to time to make sure the degree of blood pressure lowering is not excessive. Or, if he does fall or report that he's dizzy, you should check his blood pressure at that point so you can help determine, together with his physician, if the medication was part of the problem.

Beta blockers not only lower blood pressure but also heart rate. A very low heart rate means the heart is pumping slowly, decreasing the amount of blood that reaches your relative's organs each minute. If the heart rate is low enough that blood is not reaching the brain in sufficient quantities, your family member may become confused and disoriented. You may be asked to check his pulse periodically to make sure the beta blocker is not overly strong for him. Or, if he is confused or disoriented, you will want to measure his pulse so you can help the physician figure out if the beta blocker is likely responsible.

In addition to nitrates, beta blockers, calcium channel blockers, and ACE inhibitors, your family member may be taking a blood thinner to prevent blood clots from forming. Plaque build-up inside the coronary artery may trigger the body's natural clotting mechanism, just as a cut does. Often the best approach to preventing clotting is aspirin, and a baby aspirin once a day (81 milligrams) may be enough to do the job;

a related medication that is sometimes preferred is clopidogrel (brand name, Plavix). In select situations, for example when coronary heart disease is associated with a heart rhythm problem such as atrial fibrillation, the physician may prescribe a different type of blood thinner such as warfarin (brand name, Coumadin). To be effective, there has to be just enough warfarin in the system—but not too much, or there is a risk of bleeding. Warfarin is a trickier medication to take than aspirin, and your family member will need regular blood tests to check the level in his system. Missing a dose will affect the level and can trigger the physician's office to instruct your family member to increase the daily dose, which in turn can cause dangerously high levels, resulting in bruising or even bleeding in the stomach or the brain. You will want to be sure that there is a good system in place for being certain your family member is taking warfarin as prescribed—you don't have to be the one to hand him the pill and check off on a piece of paper that he took it, but you will want to check that someone is doing that. You should also be aware that your family member will tend to bleed easily and profusely if he cuts himself while on either aspirin or warfarin—a good reason for being prepared with appropriate supplies (for more about bandages, tape, and wound powder, see chapter 40, "Bleeding").

Prevention of the symptoms of coronary heart disease also involves a concerted effort to halt the process of atherosclerosis—of plaque formation. The principal way of doing this is by addressing the risk factors for developing plaque in the first place, medical disorders such as high blood pressure, high cholesterol, and diabetes (see chapter 22, "High Blood Pressure," chapter 23, "High Cholesterol," and chapter 26, "Diabetes"). Finally, cigarette smoking and a sedentary lifestyle are both bad for health in general and for the coronary arteries in particular. "Lifestyle modifications" can be beneficial for a variety of diseases, not just coronary disease (see chapter 32, "Prevention").

Repair

Repair involves mechanical interventions such as surgery or stents to improve blood flow through blocked or partially blocked blood vessels. Your role here is to help with the decision-making process. The best-established role for either surgery (the full name is coronary artery bypass graft or CABG, pronounced "cabbage," for short) or stenting (technically known as percutaneous coronary intervention, or PCI) is in the setting of a heart attack. Both these approaches can also be used in people who have coronary heart disease but are not in the middle of having a heart attack. Figuring out whether one or the other of these procedures would be useful for your family member depends on his exact situation and is far too complicated to discuss here. You may want to accompany your relative to the cardiologist's office to have the conversation. I will leave you with a few general thoughts.

Deciding on either CABG or PCI hinges on your family member's *underlying health state* and on his *goals of care* (see part I, "Underlying Health State"). Doing a CABG means performing open heart surgery. It's a major operation that typically takes three to four hours, longer if the surgeon is bypassing multiple blood vessels or if there are complications. To operate on the heart, the surgeon will need to induce a cardiac arrest and then put your family member on a cardiopulmonary bypass machine which temporarily takes over the functions of his heart and lungs. While the risk of the bypass machine causing long-term confusion has probably been overstated, frail older patients do stand a very good chance of developing delirium, or acute confusion (see chapter 38, "Confusion"). People with delirium are more likely to die than those who don't develop delirium, and delirium may persist for months. After a CABG, your relative will usually stay in the hospital about six days and then need up to three months to recover. Stroke, though relatively uncommon, remains a worrisome complication.

Bypass surgery can prolong life in selected situations—but the difference in effectiveness of surgery as opposed to medical therapy (medications, along with exercise and a good diet) is small. While far fewer bypass surgeries were performed in 2015 compared to ten years earlier, it's still one of the most common operations, with as many as four hundred thousand performed each year. You will want the cardiologist or cardiac surgeon to talk about just what the benefits are likely to be for your family member and what the risks are for someone in her condition. Then you'll need to assess whether the operation is warranted in light of whether your family member wishes to focus on comfort, quality of life, or living as long as possible.

A few words about PCI. This is a shorter procedure, typically lasting about an hour, that's done while your family member is awake. It involves threading a catheter from an artery in the groin through the circulation and into the coronary artery, injecting dye so the physician can see what she's doing, and then inflating a small balloon in the area of narrowing to open it up. The last stage of the procedure usually entails inserting a mesh stent into the blood vessel to prop it open. PCI can improve the quality of life for someone with angina who has not responded well despite medication. Just

because it is an invasive procedure doesn't mean that your family member shouldn't have it done, even if he is frail. In fact, the people who benefit the most from cardiac "revascularization," as both CABG and PCI are known because they effectively create a new, improved conduit for blood travelling to the heart, are those with the most serious disease. Over a million cases of PCI are performed yearly in the United States. You should know, however, that studies show it's a vastly overutilized procedure. People who receive stents often fare no better than people who are treated with medications alone in terms of the frequency with which they experience angina or their ability to go about their daily activities.

As a caregiver, you will want to avoid overtreatment *and* undertreatment. Both problems are common, especially in frail older people. The key to helping assure your family member gets the treatment that's right for him is to have a frank conversation with the relevant physician and to keep the underlying health state and the goals of care at the center of the discussion.

Complications of Coronary Disease

Managing coronary disease entails dealing with its complications as well as the underlying problem. The main complication I'd like to speak with you about is an abnormal heart rhythm. Sometimes the part of the heart that is affected by coronary disease is its elec-

trical circuitry, known as the conducting system. The heart is a muscle that pumps blood through the circulation; the signal that tells the heart when to pump is electrical. A smoothly functioning heart goes into action when the electrical system in one of the upper chambers (the right atrium) fires, telling both upper parts of the heart to contract and send blood into the lower chambers (the ventricles). The signal from the right atrium then alerts the corresponding electrical system that governs the ventricles to contract, sending blood to the rest of the body. If any part of the electrical circuit is disrupted, the result is an arrhythmia—an abnormal heart rhythm. You may be asked to take your relative's pulse to monitor his heartbeat.

Arrhythmias are of several varieties. They include a heartbeat that's too fast (tachycardia), a heartbeat that's too slow (bradycardia), or any of a variety of irregular heartbeats (for example, atrial fibrillation). All three types can lead to insufficient blood flow to critical parts of the body. If the area affected is the brain, dizziness, confusion, fainting, or even sudden death may result. The fix for these problems can involve medications, a pacemaker, or an implantable defibrillator. You might find yourself involved in a conversation about the wisdom of using one of these approaches, so I'm going to say a few words about each.

Adjusting medications is the simplest strategy. Sometimes the heartbeat is too slow *because* of a medication, and all that needs to be done to resolve the issue is to discontinue the offending medication. A beta blocker, for instance, might be the source of the problem. Sometimes a medication can be added to your relative's regimen to compensate for the electrical problem—that very same beta blocker that can

unduly slow the heart can also be used to curb a runaway electrical system. In other situations, such as chronic atrial fibrillation, the main potential danger might be the development of a blood clot that could travel to the brain, causing a stroke, and the recommended treatment might be a blood thinning medicine such as warfarin (Coumadin) or aspirin, as I discussed earlier.

Implanting a pacemaker is a way of compensating for an excessively slow heart rate that doesn't resolve after all potentially adverse medications are discontinued. A pacemaker is a small, battery-operated device that is placed under the skin of the chest, with wires (also called leads, or electrodes) that are threaded from the device into one of the large veins of the chest and from there into the heart (figure 25.2). Modern pacemakers weigh only a couple of ounces and are the size of two half dollars stacked on top of each other. The operation to insert a pacemaker is typically done under local anesthesia and your family member will be out of the hospital, barring complications, which are rare, in a day.

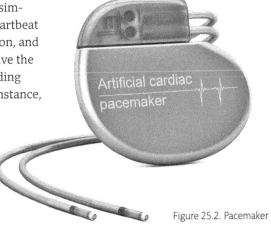

Artificial cardiac pacemaker

Figure 25.2. Pacemaker

The battery is usually made of lithium and typically lasts ten years. What I want to tell you about pacemakers is that while you may be skeptical about putting your relative through surgery, as procedures go, pacemaker implantation is relatively innocuous. Whether your family member's major goal is life prolongation, maintaining his independence, or maximizing comfort, a pacemaker may be very beneficial: it can sometimes prevent falling, fainting, and confusion.

An implantable cardioverter defibrillator (ICD), which is used to treat rapid, potentially life-threatening heart rhythms (ventricular tachycardia or ventricular fibrillation), is in a different category from a conventional pacemaker. This device is also inserted under the skin of the chest with wires threaded into the heart. Its job is to administer an electrical shock if it detects rapid firing by the ventricles. It functions much like the classic external defibrillator used in performing cardiopulmonary resuscitation, but the shock is delivered by the electrodes inside the heart rather than through paddles attached to a large machine outside the body. With increas-ing frequency, an ICD is recommended for people who have never had a life-threatening heart rhythm but *are at risk of developing one.* Your family member may be a candidate for an ICD, for example, if he had a major heart attack that left him with a heart that doesn't pump very well. What you need to know in thinking about whether to proceed with an ICD is that the much-vaunted improved survival with such a device hasn't panned out in people who are very old and have multiple chronic conditions. In such individuals, the device is more apt to go off by accident—giving your relative an extremely unpleasant jolt—than in response to a true problem. Moreover, every time the ICD fires, your family member is supposed to go to the hospital for evaluation. On balance, the technology may cause him more harm than good. One final note of caution: if your relative does have an ICD implanted, you should discuss with the cardiologist under what circumstances you would want it turned off. In a dying person, the device may fire repeatedly, simultaneously postponing the inevitable and creating intense suffering in the last days of life.

The Cardiologist's Role

Your family member will almost certainly have a cardiologist involved in his care if he has or is being considered for a pacemaker or an implantable defibrillator. He may well see a cardiologist if he has coronary heart disease, even without one of these devices. You might need to ask the cardiologist directly to comment on how advanced his condition is and what his options are. For more run-of-the-mill coronary disease, your relative's primary care physician should be able to provide satisfactory treatment. If you partner with her to supervise treatment and ensure that goals of care discussions enter into medical decision-making, the two of you should be able to provide excellent care.

Your role in managing coronary heart disease can range from making sure your relative takes her medications to engaging in decisions about technological interventions (box 25.1). The complexity of the disease and its treatment may seem daunting at times, but it's an example of where a little knowledge can go a long way.

Box 25.1

Caregiver Roles in Coronary Heart Disease

- Chronic maintenance: medication administration, principally nitrates and beta blockers
- Repair: decision-making about stents or bypass surgery
- Complications: decisions about a pacemaker or implantable defibrillator for treatment of irregular heart rhythms

CHAPTER 26

Diabetes

If your relative has diabetes that means she has difficulty processing sugar. Sugar, by the way, is a biochemical term that refers to a variety of different chemicals including glucose, lactose, and sucrose. In diabetes, the problem is handling the main type of sugar needed by cells, glucose, so when I say "sugar" I really mean "glucose." Now, the basis for your diabetic relative's problem is that she doesn't have enough insulin, the hormone that is responsible for transporting sugar (glucose) into cells. So, in effect, diabetes is really insulin-deficiency disease.

Why doesn't your family member have enough insulin? The main problem is typically that the pancreas, the organ responsible for making insulin, isn't working properly. A normally functioning pancreas is exquisitely sensitive to how much sugar is circulating in the bloodstream and adjusts the amount of insulin released into the bloodstream accordingly. As a result, the amount of sugar in the blood at any time is kept within a very narrow range in a normal person: on an empty stomach, the range is between 70 and 90 milligrams per deciliter (which both patients and doctors refer to as "seventy" or "ninety"), and two hours after eating, the normal value is below 140 milligrams per deciliter. In diabetics, the pancreas either is unable to make any insulin at all (Type 1 diabetes, which develops principally in children and young adults and is a lifelong problem) or not enough insulin to meet the demand (Type 2 diabetes, which typically occurs in people who are both overweight and middle-aged or older). If there's too little insulin, the result is rising blood sugar levels. The situation is further complicated because another feature of Type 2 diabetes is "insulin resistance" which just means that whatever insulin the body produces has difficulty transporting sugar into cells because the cells "resist" its effects.

The reason that glucose regulation matters is that your relative's cells need sugar to function properly. Moreover, both excessively high and abnormally low blood sugars produce serious symptoms. Very high blood sugar (levels of over 500 milligrams per deciliter) will cause her to be confused and weak: her body tries to get rid of the excess sugar in her urine, but that process sucks fluid out of her system, producing dehydration. It's the dehydration that causes weakness and confusion. If your family member has Type 1 diabetes, in which she cannot produce insulin at all and if her blood sugar reaches high levels, she will develop a life-threatening acidity of the blood that requires vigorous treatment in the hospital, often in an intensive care unit. Very low blood sugar, which isn't caused directly by diabetes but rather by treatment of diabetes that overshoots its target, will make your relative confused and dizzy: Her brain is effectively starved and cannot function; if the sugar gets low enough, she will pass out.

In addition to the symptoms that result from an abnormal sugar level, diabetes can cause problems by damaging blood vessels. This is a process that typically takes years to develop. If diabetes injures your family member's larger blood vessels, she may end up with heart disease or a stroke. If it injures smaller blood vessels, it may damage the kidneys, the nerves, and the eyes. These are all serious problems, making diabetes a nasty actor. Your role as caregiver is to be alert for symptoms indicating that the condition is out of whack, to help monitor the treatment, to promote a good diet, and to watch for complications.

Watching for Symptoms

If your family member has diabetes and she becomes confused—more disoriented, irrational, or incoherent than usual—you should wonder if her blood sugar is off, either too high or too low. Ideally, you will check her blood sugar on the spot with a glucometer. If that's not feasible, perhaps because you don't know how to use a monitor or maybe the two of you are outside and don't have a monitor along, give her a glass of orange juice to drink or a candy to suck on. If the issue was that her sugar was low, this simple step will likely rapidly reverse the problem; if the issue was that her sugar was too high, driving the sugar up a little further won't solve anything but neither will it make things substantially worse. The issue might not be her sugar at all— many problems other than an abnormal sugar can cause acute confusion—but it's worth thinking about in the setting of diabetes and it's easy and important to make a quick diagnosis.

Another symptom to watch for is frequent trips to the bathroom. If your relative has very high blood sugar, her kidneys are forced to make large amounts of urine, so she will have to go often. There are, of course, plenty of other reasons for her to run to the bathroom: She might have a bladder infection or she may be taking a fluid pill (diuretic) for a heart problem. But if she's a diabetic, think "high sugar." You have nothing to lose and everything to gain.

Lastly, think about adjusting her diabetes medications whenever your family member develops symptoms of some other acute medical problem, say a fever. A fever typically indicates there's an infection lurking somewhere and diabetes often acts up in the presence of an infection. Whether the problem is pneumonia or the flu or a bladder infection, odds are that your family member's usual dose of medication will need to be modified. Often, sugars go up in response to the infection, but if your relative is eating poorly because she doesn't feel well, the need for medication may decrease. To help guide treatment, her blood sugar should be checked, whether your family member does it with a home glucometer (figure 26.1), whether you do it, whether a visiting nurse measures it, or whether you bring your family member to the doctor's office.

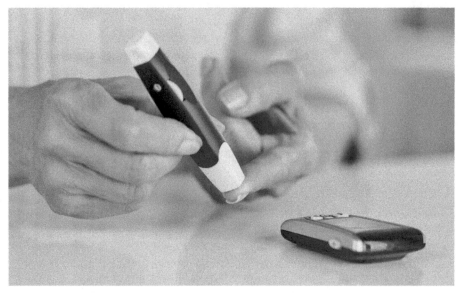

Figure 26.1. Glucometer

Monitoring Treatment

If your family member has diabetes, she is probably going to receive treatment in the form of medication (there are also people who are classified as "prediabetic," or who have "diet-controlled diabetes," but I am only going to talk about those with the full-fledged disorder). The medications are of two basic varieties: insulin to make up for the body's inability to produce enough on its own (given via injection) and pills that work either by stimulating the pancreas to make more insulin (sulfonylureas such as glyburide) or by lowering how much sugar gets into the system from the digestive tract (biguanides such as metformin). Your family member may be on several different medications simultaneously.

With both insulin injections and

oral hypoglycemics, as the pills are collectively called because they are taken by mouth and they lower the blood sugar, the first issue is taking the medication properly. Insulin presents a special challenge: the correct amount of liquid must be drawn up into a syringe and then injected under the skin. Most diabetics learn to self-administer insulin, but if your family member has impaired vision or poor cognition, self-administration can be problematic. It's possible to use an insulin pen, which makes use of a cartridge. These can be disposable (containing a prefilled cartridge) or reusable (the amount of insulin to be injected is set with a dial). In both cases, a new needle is attached for each use. Alternatively, syringes can be prefilled, either by a visiting nurse or by you.

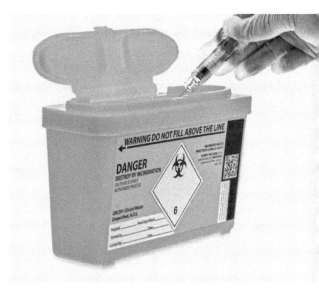

Figure 26.2. Sharps disposal container

Another challenge of using insulin is that your family member might take insulin once a day, twice a day, or many times over the course of the day, depending on her blood sugar. She might take both long- and short-acting types of insulin. Not only does the correct amount of insulin have to be measured out each time, and not only is a shot required, but the needles and syringes must be disposed of properly. To avoid injuring another person, it's essential to use a special "sharps disposal container" (figure 26.2).

Monitoring diabetes treatment generally requires keeping track of the sugar levels, on the one hand, and determining the right dose of medication, on the other. If your family member is taking pills, has been on a stable regimen for a while, and doesn't have any other acute problems going on that might rock the boat, then all that's necessary is a periodic check of the blood sugar. This job might fall to your relative, to you, to a visiting nurse, or may occur at the time of a periodic visit to the doctor's office. If your family member is on insulin, more frequent monitoring is desirable. Moreover, in many instances the dose of the insulin changes depending on the last blood sugar level. Some people check their sugars as often as three or four times a day. You may want to discuss with the physician what kind of system makes sense, given how "brittle" your family member's diabetes is, her capacity for self-management, and the home situation.

You will also want to talk over how tightly to control your relative's blood sugar. In many people, maintaining blood sugars as close to the normal range as possible is advisable: such a strategy prevents both short-term symptoms and long-term complications, such as the heart, kidney, and eye problems. The way physicians assess the adequacy of diabetes control is with a test called the hemoglobin A1c (HbA1c), which measures average blood sugars over the preceding three months. For frail older people, however, tight control of diabetes also brings with it the risk of low blood sugars, which, in turn, can cause falling and fainting. It may not make sense to significantly increase your family member's immediate chance of falling and breaking a hip just so she can lower her risk of kidney trouble in five or ten years. Experts recommend that the HbA1c be kept below 7.5 percent for otherwise healthy, diabetic older patients who have a life expectancy of greater than ten years. For older patients with many other medical conditions and a life expectancy of less than ten years, the target value is 8 percent. For frail older people, the target is 9 percent.

It's also worth considering that if your family member has trouble seeing and her memory isn't good, achieving tight control of her diabetes might require substantial nursing care, perhaps even a nursing home setting. Whether it makes sense to trade off her independence in exchange for better control of her diabetes depends on what is most important to her. Thinking about the big picture—your family member's underlying health state and her goals of care—is critical to figuring out how best to manage her diabetes.

Promoting a Good Diet

Everyone knows that diabetics are supposed to avoid sweets, particularly "concentrated sweets" such as cake or ice cream. These foods trigger a surge in blood glucose as they are broken down into their chemical components in the stomach and intestines and absorbed. But a good diet for a diabetic involves a great deal more than avoiding rich desserts. Your family member may know all this and have been cooking for herself appropriately for years. If she now relies on you, on Meals on Wheels, or on microwaveable prepared meals, eating properly presents a new challenge.

If you are doing the cooking, you may want to meet with a nutritionist to get advice on what to make for your family member. General guidelines include limiting the total amount of carbohydrates, avoiding food with a high glycemic index (foods such as ice cream that produce a rapid spike in blood sugar levels), and providing ample fiber from fruits, grains, and beans. If your family member is overweight, and many—though not all people—with Type 2 diabetes are overweight, you will want to try to help her lose weight or at least make sure she doesn't gain more weight.

Special diabetic meals are available through Meals on Wheels and at most adult day health centers and senior centers. If your relative lives in an assisted living facility or some other form of residence that provides meals, the kitchen staff should be notified that a special diet is required.

Observing for Complications

People with diabetes are prone to various other medical problems that you may want to be on the lookout for. I'm going to mention three of the most common: skin infections, impaired vision, and heart problems.

If your family member has diabetes, she is prone to skin infections on her legs and feet because of poor circulation (a common result of diabetes) combined with impaired ability to feel pain (due to neuropathy, another complication of diabetes). If unchecked, these infections can lead to hospitalization, intravenous antibiotics, and even amputation. You will want to inspect her feet periodically or make sure that a nurse or physician checks them, looking for signs of infection such as redness or unusually warm skin. You will also want to be sure she sees a podiatrist (foot doctor) regularly since good foot hygiene can prevent some of these complications. She may also need help cutting her toenails due to a combination of poor eyesight, neuropathy (nerve problems from diabetes) that impairs her ability to feel, and difficulty with mobility and coordination.

If your family member has visual problems, she might have cataracts (clouding of the lens of the eye), but she might also have a complication of her diabetes. The most serious of these is diabetic retinopathy, a complication of diabetes that results from damage to the blood vessels of the eyes resulting from chronically elevated sugar levels. When those blood vessels become blocked or leaky, the retina is damaged, the part of the eye where the nerve cells responsible for vision are located. If your family member experiences a change in her vision, she should see her eye doctor promptly. Laser treatments, which are done in the office and require only a local anesthetic, might improve her vision or prevent further deterioration from retinopathy. Alternatively, your relative may have hazy vision due to acutely elevated blood sugar levels—some of the excess sugar gets into the lens of the eye, causing blurred vision. In this case, vigorous treatment to lower your family member's sugar is warranted to improve her eyesight.

The final problem I'm going to mention is chest pain from coronary heart disease. Your relative is predisposed to developing coronary heart disease because diabetes affects the large blood vessels, including those to the heart (see chapter 25, "Coronary Heart Disease"). What makes diabetes especially tricky is that your family member may have atypical symptoms of heart disease. Instead of complaining of chest pain when she is in the middle of a heart attack, your family member might just report feeling sick to her stomach. Or she might get short of breath and her skin may be clammy. I don't mean to suggest that you should worry your relative is having a heart attack every time she says she's not feeling well, but you should realize that in the setting of diabetes, things may not be what they seem to be.

Diabetes is a complicated medical problem because it affects so many different parts of the body (box 26.1). Diabetes can interfere with your relative's mobility, her vision, her mental acuity and other functions. The good news is that knowing these simple tricks about managing the disease can make an enormous difference in her well-being.

Box 26.1

Caregiving in Diabetes

- Watch for symptoms of high or low blood sugar: confusion, frequent urination

- Monitor treatment: adjust medications (pills, insulin) based on sugar levels

- Promote good diet: fiber, limited concentrated sweets

- Look for complications: vision problems, foot infections

CHAPTER 27

Chronic Kidney Disease

C hronic kidney disease is one of those conditions that can sneak up on you unawares. You and your family member might not have known there was anything amiss until an abnormality showed up on a routine blood test. Perhaps you've been assured that it might be years before it becomes a significant problem. Alternatively, your family member may have been diagnosed with "end-stage renal disease" and is receiving dialysis three times a week, so you are all too well aware that he has chronic kidney disease and that it's far from benign. In between these two extremes lie various stages of kidney malfunction, which may have repercussions for your relative. What, exactly, do the kidneys do and what do you need to know about them to serve as an effective caregiver?

What the Kidneys Do

H ere is what the section of the National Institutes of Health has to say about these critical organs: "The kidneys are two bean-shaped organs, each about the size of a fist. They are located just below the rib cage, one on each side of the spine. Every day, the two kidneys filter about 120 to 150 quarts of blood to produce about 1 to 2 quarts of urine, composed of wastes and extra fluid" (figure 27.1).

The important words here are "wastes" and "extra fluid." The kidneys dispose of substances that would otherwise accumulate in the bloodstream; they also strive to maintain just the right amount of bodily fluid. The kidneys control, with extraordinary precision, the level of various important chemicals in the blood. By way of example, potassium is essential for many cellular activities, including the proper functioning of the heart cells. Its normal range is quite narrow, between 3.5 and 5 millimoles/liter. If the level falls between 3 and 3.5, your relative

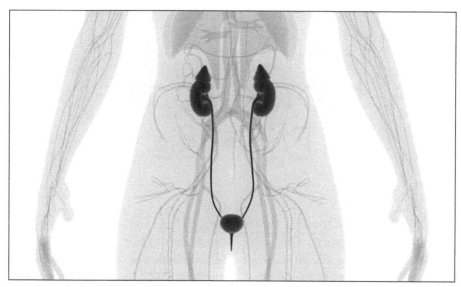

Figure 27.1. Location of kidneys

may feel weak or start to have muscle cramps. If the level rises between 5 and 6, he may have an irregular heartbeat. Below 3 or above 6 is the danger zone: the heart might stop beating entirely. The kidneys work tirelessly to keep the level in the normal range, no matter what your relative eats (bananas and spinach are notorious for containing potassium). Similarly, the kidneys keep the sodium level in the desired range. They also get rid of medications and the breakdown products of the body's normal metabolism. In addition, they seek to prevent both fluid overload (edema, in which excess fluid ends up in the lungs, the legs, or other places it doesn't belong) and dehydration (insufficient fluid leads to low blood pressure, fainting, and ultimately, collapse of the circulatory system).

The kidneys are so important and so efficient that even if they are functioning at only half strength, your family member won't notice anything is wrong. It helps that people normally have two kidneys, so there's ample reserve if something goes wrong with one of them. Nonetheless, a variety of different disorders can cause one or both kidneys to stop working. Usually it's a gradual process though some conditions, such as a severe narrowing of the main artery to the kidney, a tumor, or a blockage in the urinary system, can abruptly cause one or both kidneys to cease functioning entirely. In older people, the most common causes of kidney malfunction are atherosclerosis—the same process that causes coronary heart disease can also cause kidney problems—and diabetes. Aging itself can affect kidney function, with most people showing some evidence of decline over time. Regardless of the cause of the problem, you, as the caregiver, have an important role to play in the ongoing management of chronic kidney disease.

Your family member's physician might report that his creatinine, a chemical routinely measured in a simple blood test, is elevated. Creatinine is a byproduct of muscle breakdown and turns out to be a fairly reliable indicator of how well the kidneys are doing their job. What happens is that the body's repair system destroys old muscle fibers, ships the waste products to the kidneys for them to dispose of, and then makes new muscle. If the kidneys aren't functioning properly, the creatinine level will rise because the kidneys cannot dispose of it fast enough. A normal level, to give you some idea, is 0.6–1.2 milligrams per deciliter, and the level in a person whose kidneys have stopped working entirely may be around 10 milligrams per deciliter.

The creatinine level, while very easy to determine, is actually only a very approximate way of assessing kidney function. In some cases, it is only minimally elevated even though the kidneys are working poorly. What really matters is the glomerular filtration rate (GFR), a precise and reliable measure of how well the kidneys get rid of waste. Simple formulas allow physicians to estimate the GFR based on your family member's age, gender, race, and the serum creatinine. Doing this calculation shows that a slightly elevated creatinine of 2.0 translates into a GFR of 24 milliliters/minute, which is considered severe chronic kidney disease. It is stage four, the level just before dialysis is recommended (table 27.1).

You will have different responsibilities depending on whether your relative has mild-to-moderate or severe kidney disease.

Table 27.1
Stages of Kidney Disease

Stages	Description	GFR* mL/min/1.73m2
1	Slight kidney damage with normal or increased filtration	More than 90
2	Mild decrease in kidney function	60–89
3	Moderate decrease in kidney function	30–59
4	Severe decrease in kidney function	15–29
5	Kidney failure	Less than 15 (or dialysis)

* GFR is glomerular filtration rate, a measure of the kidney's function.

Your Role Managing Mild-to-Moderate Kidney Disease

With mild-to-moderate kidney disease, the main roles that you as a caregiver can play relate to *diet* and *medications*. Even though your family member is likely to be asymptomatic, he can get into trouble if he takes food or medications that his kidneys are unable to handle. What the kidneys do is metabolize chemicals (alter them in preparation for disposal), which you might think of as processing, and filter them from the bloodstream (remove them and dump them into the urine). As long as the kidneys are still working, they will continue to process and remove various components of food such as salt and potassium, as well as the drugs they usually metabolize and excrete. But they won't be able to process and remove with their usual speed, so certain chemicals will tend to build up. If your family member is taking a diuretic, for example, and is taking potassium supplements to counteract the potassium-lowering effects of the drug, or if he's taking an angiotensin-converting enzyme (ACE) inhibitor for his blood pressure, which tends to raise potassium levels, and suddenly his kidney function worsens, his potassium will shoot up. Even modest elevations of potassium can cause an abnormal heart rhythm. If your relative is taking the anti-seizure medication phenytoin (brand name, Dilantin), which is normally broken down by the kidneys, and his kidney function declines, his usual medication dose will produce higher than recommended drug levels. For this medication in particular, even modestly exceeding the target can cause confusion and other problems.

The way to avoid these difficulties is to restrict the amounts of certain foods in the diet, on the one hand, and to eliminate or decrease the dose of various drugs on the other. For dietary restrictions, you and your family member might want to consult a nutritionist. As a general rule of thumb, you will want to avoid or limit bananas and spinach and go easy on the protein. With medications, you'll want to check with your relative's physician about any over-the-counter medications your relative is taking or considering taking. The physician should be aware of the kidney condition and adjust prescription medications appropriately; it's principally the non-prescription medicines that you need to worry about. Because ibuprofen (brand name, Motrin), can further impair the kidneys' already limited processing capacity, for instance, many physicians recommend avoiding it entirely.

Your Role Managing Advanced Kidney Disease

In this stage, you will need to demonstrate even greater vigilance about food and medicines. Your family member is likely to be sent to a kidney specialist (nephrologist) for a consultation; you can be helpful by going to the appointment and participating in the discussion about next steps.

The next step you will need to talk about is dialysis. When stage five kidney disease is reached, the ability of the kidneys to do their job is so limited that physicians typically recommend using a machine to take over their function. This process is either done by cleaning the blood, or hemodialysis ("heme" refers to blood), or by relying on the movement of toxins from an area of high concentration to an area of low concentration with peritoneal dialysis. In hemodialysis, a surgeon inserts a special catheter called a fistula to connect an artery and a vein and that fistula is used to remove blood; the blood is passed through a filtering machine and then returned to the body, also through the fistula. Hemodialysis is normally carried out in a freestanding dialysis center or the hospital; the process typically takes about four hours and is usually done three times a week (figure 27.2). In peritoneal dialysis, a catheter is in-

serted into the abdominal cavity, where it remains. During dialysis, a special sterile solution travels into the abdomen through the catheter, bathes the intestines for a period of hours, and then the fluid is removed, taking with it the wastes that have built up in the body. Peritoneal dialysis is customarily carried out at home, by a family member. It's often done overnight.

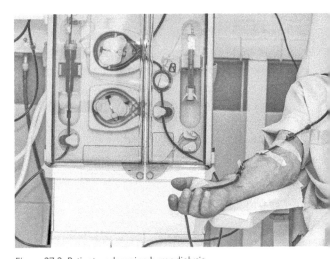

Figure 27.2. Patient undergoing hemodialysis

Dialysis is a major undertaking that requires careful, thoughtful consideration. You and your family member need to understand the pros and cons given his underlying health status and his preferences. You also need to understand the alternatives. The good news is that this complex decision typically doesn't need to be made abruptly;

ideally, you will meet with the kidney specialist when your family member reaches stage four disease or even earlier, giving you both time to mull things over.

You should note that for people who have many different chronic medical problems on top of their chronic kidney disease, as well as advanced age, dialysis has *not been shown to prolong life.* You should also recognize that it may be impossible to determine in advance what undergoing dialysis will be like for your family member. He has the option to start dialysis and then to decide to stop: in fact, about one-fifth of people who go on dialysis ultimately decide to discontinue it.

If your family member does go on dialysis—or is already on it when you start your caregiving role—you will have a different set of responsibilities. Unless your relative is getting peritoneal dialysis, he will need to go to a dialysis center at least three times a week. That means arranging for transportation. In many cases, the dialysis center will help set this up. But even if you do not regularly take your family member to and from dialysis, you may want to visit at least once to get a better handle on what goes on there and to meet the personnel.

The same concerns that mattered during the period of moderately severe (stage four) kidney disease continue to matter once your family member has started dialysis, but there are some additional wrinkles. Certain medications are routinely given at the time of dialysis, including erythropoietin, a medicine that stimulates red blood cell production to avoid the anemia that occurs with chronic kidney disease. The exact schedule for taking medications may need adjustment: since some drugs are removed from the system during dialysis, medications that used to be taken once a day, for example in the morning, might need to be taken after dialysis instead. The dose of other medications may be modified once dialysis has been initiated. The kidney doctor will go over all these changes: I just want to make sure you realize there will be schedule and dose changes once dialysis begins.

Your Role in Forgoing or Stopping Dialysis

Because dialysis is of limited benefit in people who are very elderly and have multiple chronic diseases, your family member may choose not to start it in the first place. Or, he may decide to give it a try but, at some point, might decide that going to a dialysis center three times a week for four hours is too burdensome and he will stop. How long your relative will live without dialysis depends on whether his kidneys are still functioning a little bit and on how well his other organs are working. If your family member is totally dependent on dialysis for getting rid of wastes, then chances are he will only survive a few weeks off dialysis. If he still makes a little urine, he might go for months or even longer.

You should be aware that your relative may qualify for hospice care if he has end-stage kidney disease and chooses to forgo dialysis. This service may enable him to stay at home with additional help—a hospice nurse, a home health aide, medications delivered to the home, and other forms of assistance (see chapter 51, "Home Hospice"). You should also recognize that several symptoms arise commonly with severe chronic kidney disease including itching, confusion, weakness, and shortness of breath. Medication or nonpharmacologic approaches such as oxygen and one-on-one attention can ameliorate these symptoms.

Whatever stage of kidney disease affects your family member, try to keep his primary care physician involved in his care. Often, especially with patients receiving dialysis, the kidney specialist effectively takes over all medical management. If dialysis is administered at a freestanding clinic, the supervising nephrologist may not be the same physician your family member saw in consultation in the earlier stages of the disease. This doctor had no relationship with your relative until he arrived at the dialysis center. If he travels by chair car to dialysis, you may never meet this doctor. Maintaining the involvement of the primary care physician can be helpful in managing symptoms of kidney failure, in guiding both of you through the difficult decision of whether to continue dialysis, and in ensuring that all your family member's other medical problems are not neglected.

Box 27.1

Chronic Kidney Disease

- Medication doses may need to be adjusted in each stage of kidney failure

- Dialysis does not prolong life in frail, very old people

- If dialysis is stopped or not started in advanced kidney failure, consider hospice

CHAPTER 28

Heart Failure

Y ou may be surprised to learn that your relative has heart failure. The name seems to imply that her heart isn't working at all, that it's stopped. Heart failure (or congestive heart failure, or CHF) means something else: it means that your family member's heart is not pumping blood efficiently. If it is only slightly impaired, CHF is mild; if the heart is functioning poorly, CHF is considered severe. In either case, she has a chronically weakened heart and is at risk both of gradual worsening of her condition and of an acute worsening, or flare of the disease. This is obviously very different from true stoppage of the heart, which is known as a cardiac arrest.

A variety of underlying problems can cause heart failure, of which the most common is inadequately treated, long-standing high blood pressure, which damages the heart muscle. Also common is coronary heart disease that has caused one or more heart attacks (see chapter 25, "Coronary Heart Disease"). When parts of the heart muscle die, as happens with a heart attack, the overall pump function is often weakened. Degeneration of the heart valves, which regulate blood flow between the chambers of the heart, can also result in heart failure. The mainstay of treatment, regardless of the cause of

the problem, is making the heart's job easier by lightening its load or easing some of the barriers it faces when it tries to pump blood through the circulation. Think of carrying rocks up a mountain: one way to make the task easier is to carry smaller rocks; another is to find a path that may be a bit longer but is less steep.

Heart failure is the sixth most common chronic disease in older people but it accounts for more hospitalizations than any other illness. As so often happens when frail older people are hospitalized, a hospital stay for your relative because of heart failure may lead to a generalized decline in function, with weakness, confusion, and heightened dependence on other people. Moreover, your family member may also have other medical problems such as kidney disease, heart rhythm abnormalities, or chronic lung disease. She is probably taking multiple medications for these assorted problems, further increasing the risk of adverse outcomes from hospitalization. Optimal home management of heart failure is key to keeping your relative out of the hospital.

Ideal cardiac care involves a team comprising your family member, you, and at least one clinician. Sometimes the clinician is the primary care physician; in other cases, it is a cardiologist. The best approach, when available, includes a nurse who works closely with the cardiologist to monitor and treat your family member in a special CHF disease management program. But whether you are partnering with a physician or a team of clinicians, your family member will be best served if you help with the ongoing management of her disease. That includes monitoring her condition, supervising administration of medications, and a few miscellaneous strategies ranging from using oxygen to planning for future care.

Monitoring

Any time your relative gains four or five pounds in a couple of days, the cause is probably excess fluid. It's hard to gain that much weight so fast any other way: even splurging on chocolate cake and ice cream won't do it. As a result, one excellent way to monitor heart failure is to watch for fluid gain, and the best way to track fluid gain is by following your family member's weight. I talked about choosing a good scale earlier (see chapter 21, "Your Medical Bag"), emphasizing that the scale should be digital, the numbers should be illuminated and easy to read, and measurements should be taken on a firm surface but not the bathroom floor with its hard tiles. You also want to be sure there is something to grab on to for balance near the scale and that your family member is weighed at roughly the same time each day.

Blood pressure is also useful to monitor, especially if your family member is taking extra doses of a fluid pill (diuretic) in an effort to get rid of fluid. If you overshoot—and it's easy to do that, particularly but not exclusively in someone whose kidneys aren't working perfectly—the blood will become overly concentrated as too much liquid is squeezed out. If there's too little blood volume, your relative's blood pressure will drop and she can become dizzy and faint. Checking the blood pressure—perhaps before giving that extra dose of diuretic—allows you, in conjunction with the physician or nurse, to decide whether or not to go ahead with the medication. (For using a blood pressure cuff at home, see chapter 21, "Your Medical Bag.")

Since one of the major—and most alarming—symptoms of a flare of heart failure is shortness of breath, you may find it useful to be able to measure your family member's *respiratory rate*. That's just how many times a minute she takes a breath. You don't need any special equipment other than a watch. Begin timing when your relative breathes in. Then count each time she takes another breath until you've been timing for 30 seconds. Multiply by two and you have the number of breaths per minute. A normal respiratory rate is between

12 and 20 breaths per minute. If your family member is breathing faster than that, especially if she's not anxious and if her usual rate is around 12, that's cause for concern and worth reporting to her physician. A respiratory rate over 30 is particularly worrisome.

Another simple and useful way to monitor heart failure is by taking your family member's pulse. If her heart is having difficulty pumping enough blood, it typically tries to compensate by beating more quickly. It's like pouring water into a pot when you're cooking. For example, suppose you want to measure out a quart of water and you have a one-cup measure. The most efficient strategy is to fill the cup four times. But if you only have a half-cup measure, the best you can do is to fill the half cup eight times. If you're in a hurry, you'll want to move twice as fast if you are using the smaller measure. Not quite the same as the heart pumping blood, but you get the idea. To measure the pulse, you again just need a watch. To find your family member's pulse, have her turn her hand palm side up and place your second and third fingers on the thumb side of her wrist. Once you feel the pulse, start timing. As with the respiratory rate, it's usually adequate to count how many beats you feel in 30 seconds and multiply by two. As an alternative, some home blood pressure cuffs record the heart rate along with the pressure. Most authorities say that a normal heart rate in an adult is between 60 and 100 beats per minute, but I think 60 to 90 is more realistic. Heart rates of over 120 or below 50 generally indicate trouble. In addition to monitoring your family member for a rate that's either very fast or very slow, you will want to take note if there is a change from her baseline. If her pulse usually runs between 70 and 80, then 100 is high for her and 60 is on the low side.

The final type of monitoring you may want to do relates to medications. Since medicines are such a critical part of the treatment of heart failure, I'm going to consider them separately.

Medications

Concern number one has to be with medication adherence—with whether your family member is taking the medicines she's supposed to be taking and in the correct doses. People with heart failure are often on quite a few medicines for this one diagnosis alone: your relative may be taking a diuretic to get rid of the extra fluid that tends to accumulate; she may be on a beta blocker such as metoprolol or atenolol to cut back on how hard the heart has to work; and she may be on an angiotensin-converting enzyme (ACE) inhibitor to relax the blood vessels so they are less stiff. Other medications that are sometimes used to treat heart failure include digoxin, nitrates, and blood thinners such as aspirin or warfarin. If your family member is taking multiple medications and administers her own pills, you may want to set the pills up in a special dispenser (figure 28.1).

Fortunately, most of the medications needed to treat heart failure are available as generic drugs so they are inexpensive, but occasionally your family member's physician might prescribe something new—and pricey. It's perfectly reasonable to ask him the cost of whatever medication he's prescribing and to question how much of a benefit the brand name drug confers over an older medicine. At the very least, when the open enrollment period for health insurance rolls around, you might want to check whether your relative's current medications are all covered and what "tier" they are in, which determines what the co-pay is, if any (see chapter 47, "Choosing a Health Plan").

Depending on which medications your family member is taking, you will have different side effects to watch for. For medicines in general and heart medicines in particular, you may want to find out from the physician what you should pay attention to. For example, if your family member is on a beta blocker, you may want to check her pulse now and then to make sure it's not too slow. Beta blockers are supposed to slow the heart rate, but if they slow it too much, your relative may become dizzy or confused. If she does get dizzy or confused, you will want to check her pulse to see if a slow heart rate is the problem, potentially implicating the beta blocker. If your family

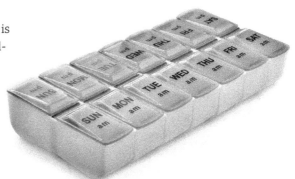

Figure 28.1. Pill dispenser

member is on a diuretic, and almost everyone with heart failure is on this class of medicine to get rid of excess fluid, the risk is that she will lose too much fluid and become dehydrated. You can sometimes detect this condition by noticing that her blood pressure has fallen. And you will certainly want to check the blood pressure if she becomes unsteady on her feet or if she feels faint to see if low pressure is the culprit. If your relative is on an ACE inhibitor she might be one of the many people who develop a dry, hacking cough. It's something to think about if she starts coughing but doesn't seem to be sick.

Most patients are given a chart showing their medications, what they are for, and when to take them. You might ask your family member's physician to add a column for the major possible side effects. The package insert that comes with a new bottle of pills will provide a list of side effects, but it's so comprehensive that you may not be able to focus on what's really important. In addition, the print on those inserts is so small that it's a challenge for anyone to read.

More Management Strategies

To optimally manage your family member's heart failure, you will also want to know something about the use of supplementary oxygen. In cases of severe heart failure, the oxygen level in the blood is chronically low and the physician may order home oxygen. The oxygen is provided by a supplier who will typically deliver a prefilled tank every week. Your family member can get around even if she needs to use oxygen all the time by carrying a portable oxygen concentrator with her. The oxygen supplier will educate your family member—and you, if you wish— on how to handle oxygen equipment (for more on supplementary oxygen, see chapter 30, "Chronic Obstructive Lung Disease").

Heart failure is a progressive, ultimately lethal disease, though optimal medical treatment can help control the symptoms and keep your family member going for a number of years. Input from a cardiologist may help as the disease advances, though keeping the primary care physician at the center of care is usually advisable (see chapter 8, "What to Expect from Medical Specialists"). There are also several, high-tech ways of treating very advanced heart failure, including a heart transplant and a left ventricular assist device, which is essentially a partial artificial heart. The vast majority of frail older people are not eligible for these approaches because they have too many other medical problems. What is

important as heart failure progresses is that you and your family member revisit the question of defining her goals of care. Once she's on the home stretch, she may want to have an approach to treatment that focuses more on comfort than on keeping her going. If she decides she wants to make every effort to prolong her life, she will have to recognize that there may be a price to pay in terms of her level of independence and her degree of comfort.

Whatever goal she settles on—and communicates to her physicians—she may wish to opt for a do-not-resuscitate status. Attempted cardiopulmonary resuscitation (CPR) in someone with advanced heart failure is just that—an attempt. It almost never succeeds. If your relative has a cardiac arrest and CPR is tried, and if she does not die while the doctors are trying to shock her heart back into functioning, all the while performing "chest compressions" (repeatedly pressing on her chest) to manually force the blood through the circulation and mechanically breathing for her, she is liable to linger for a few days or weeks in the intensive care unit—and then die. Even people who want every effort made to prolong their lives don't usually want interventions that are virtually guaranteed to fail.

It's not easy to have a conversation about dying and many physicians, including cardiologists, have a hard time initiating such a discussion. But you will be doing your family member a favor if you nudge the doctor to talk about prognosis. He can emphasize all the interventions that can make a difference while at the same time acknowledging that at the point when the heart stops altogether, it may be time to forgo measures that are uncomfortable and extremely unlikely to help. In the most advanced stage of heart failure, hospice care is an option that can help keep your family member comfortable and at home.

Whatever stage of heart failure your family member has reached, you should realize the condition is progressive and, other than a heart transplant, there is no cure. The net effect is that the disease may be more lethal than cancer. On the other hand, the enormous advances in understanding the underlying disease process and in developing treatments translate into a good quality of life for most patients for years after the diagnosis is made.

Box 28.1

Caregiver Roles in Heart Failure

- Monitor heart failure by weighing regularly

- Manage medications to assure correct dosage and schedule

- Plan for the future, consider a do-not-resuscitate (DNR) order

CHAPTER 29

Alzheimer's Disease and Other Dementias

Dementia is number nine in the list of the most common chronic conditions among older people, but for caregivers it may feel like number one. That's because it is the leading reason that family members become caregivers. For the many individuals with multiple chronic conditions, dementia is often the most challenging problem for families to deal with.

Managing dementia means supervising the *treatment* of the disorder and dealing with the *behavioral* symptoms that are part and parcel of the disease, symptoms such as restlessness, wandering, and paranoia, and planning for *future care*. But before we talk about management, let me clarify what dementia is.

What Is Dementia?

Dementia is a catch-all term for a progressive, irreversible, ultimately fatal neurological disease that causes problems with memory and other aspects of thinking, problems that are sufficiently severe to interfere with everyday life. Mild forgetfulness which does not get in the way of your family member's daily activities does not indicate dementia. The most common form is Alzheimer's disease, a condition first identified by the German pathologist and psychiatrist Alois Alzheimer in 1906.

Alzheimer's disease is a clinical diagnosis—there is no specific test other than a brain biopsy, which is typically not something done while your family member is alive. It's a disorder that progresses over a period of years, lasting on average five to seven years. Memory loss is a very prominent feature of Alzheimer's disease, but the disorder also affects language—not just the names of individual words, but also your relative's ability to express himself or understand complex speech. It commonly causes problems with what is known as visuospatial orientation, or the ability to perceive relationships in three dimensions—resulting in your family member getting lost, sometimes even inside your house. Some of its most devastating but often subtle effects include impaired judgment and difficulty problem-solving.

Vascular dementia is the second most common form of dementia. You can think of vascular dementia as resulting from multiple small strokes that effectively kill small amounts of tissue in various parts of the brain. Those small strokes, in turn, are caused by the same factors that cause other strokes: diabetes, cigarette smoking, high blood pressure, and high cholesterol. Vascular dementia differs from Alzheimer's disease in having a "step-wise progression"; each small stroke or cluster of small strokes results in a worsening of the symptoms of dementia. Alzheimer's, by contrast, classically has a slow but steady downhill course. With vascular dementia, people typically don't have quite so much trouble with their memory early on—it comes later— but may instead show evidence of "executive dysfunction," or difficulty problem-solving. If your relative has vascular dementia, he will commonly develop an abnormal gait, taking small shuffling steps.

Distinguishing between Alzheimer's and vascular dementia may be difficult, especially in the more ad-

vanced stages, when they look quite similar. Moreover, many people have "mixed dementia," which is to say they have *both* Alzheimer's disease and vascular dementia, which we know because of autopsy studies.

Finally, there are a variety of other less common forms of dementia (figure 29.1). Lewy body dementia resembles Alzheimer's but often comes with marked sleep disturbances, visual hallucinations, and a gait abnormality that looks like Parkinson's disease. What's important to recognize about this type of dementia is that the medications that are commonly used to treat hallucinations tend to make matters worse with Lewy body dementia, both in terms of their effects on cognition and on walking. Frontotemporal dementia, a still less common form of dementia,

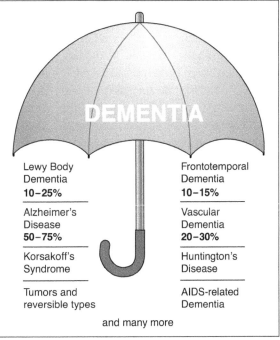

Figure 29.1. Types of dementia

DEMENTIA

Lewy Body Dementia 10–25%	Frontotemporal Dementia 10–15%
Alzheimer's Disease 50–75%	Vascular Dementia 20–30%
Korsakoff's Syndrome	Huntington's Disease
Tumors and reversible types	AIDS-related Dementia

and many more

includes a variety of subtypes sporting names such as progressive supranuclear palsy and Pick's disease. What's characteristic of frontotemporal dementia is a marked change in personality and behavior early in the course of the illness, with a sparing of memory until later on. Parkinson's disease, which is best known for affecting motor function (causing a tremor, difficulty initiating movement, and a slow, shuffling gait), also results in dementia in about one-third of cases. Diagnosing Parkinson's is important because there are medications for the motor symptoms of this disorder and because antipsychotic medications, which are sometimes used to treat the behavioral complications of dementia, tend to exacerbate the motor disorder.

Medications to Treat Dementia

The medical treatment of dementia depends on the underlying type. If your family member has Alzheimer's disease—diagnosed by taking a history, doing a physical examination, and excluding various other problems through simple blood tests and perhaps a computed tomography (CT) scan or a magnetic resonance imaging (MRI) scan of the brain—then his physician might prescribe a medication such as donepezil (Aricept). The technical name for this type of drug is an acetylcholinesterase inhibitor, which works by blocking one chemical that normally destroys a different chemical, with the net effect that there's more of the second chemical around. That second chemical (acetylcholine) is a neurotransmitter that people with Alzheimer's disease don't have in sufficient quantities. In any event, this type of medication is approved by the Food and Drug Administration (FDA) for use in mild to moderate Alzheimer's disease. While medication may improve your relative's memory and thinking a little, his faculties will continue declining at roughly the same rate as before. At best, treatment turns the clock back a bit but does nothing to keep it from ticking.

If your family member is taking a medication against Alzheimer's disease, whether donepezil or its cousins such as rivastigmine (Exelon) and galantamine (Reminyl), the most common side effects are gastrointestinal: either nausea or diarrhea. You should look out for these problems; your relative might not be able to explain that he's nauseated, but he might give you a clue by simply eating less than usual. If your relative has difficulty swallowing pills, a form of donepezil is available that doesn't have to be swallowed, it simply dissolves in the mouth.

Once your relative has been on a medication for Alzheimer's for a while, you might want to question whether it's time to stop. I'm all for a time-limited trial—your family member can take a medication for a defined period, say six weeks, and then be evaluated to see if there has been a measurable improvement in his cognitive function. If not, there's no point continuing. If he does show some benefit and continues to take the drug, reassess once a year to determine whether remaining on the medication makes sense. It's another pill to take and he may already be on many other medications. Even though the cholinesterase inhibitors are all available as generics now, the typical monthly cost ranges from $10 for donepezil to $60 for rivastigmine and $70 for galantamine.

If your family member has vascular dementia, there is no specific treatment. His diabetes and high blood pressure, which contributed to causing the disease in the first place, should continue being treated. There is some evidence that if these problems are poorly controlled, the dementia will get worse.

Drug treatment is available for Parkinson's disease but has no effect on the development of dementia. No specific medication exists for the other, rarer forms of dementia. But medications are often used, along with other techniques, to manage the behavioral symptoms of dementia, regardless of the cause of the disease.

Treating the Behavioral Symptoms of Dementia

Recognizing and responding to the behavioral manifestations of dementia is an enormous topic about which entire books have been written. I will touch on a few of the most common symptoms in the early, middle, and late stages of the disease and some ways to approach each of them.

In the *early* stage of dementia, you may find your relative is irritable. The repetitiveness that is taking its toll on you is also affecting him: he may be painfully aware that he is forgetful, that he cannot figure out how to solve various problems he encounters in daily life, and that he's just not as sharp as he once was. If he's irritable, it's likely that he is actually annoyed at himself. You can help by not rubbing in his deficits; instead of insisting that you already told him he has a doctor's appointment or your son is coming to visit when he denies knowing, just state the facts. You might be able to minimize the impact of the memory loss and resulting irritability by pinning notes about upcoming events to the refrigerator door or by providing information only on a need-to-know basis—telling him on the day of a visit that it's taking place.

Another symptom of early dementia is anxiety. Your relative may respond to his weakening sense of control over his life by feeling anxious. Physicians are often tempted to prescribe antianxiety medications in this setting, but these drugs can worsen confusion, cause falls, and make your family member sleepy. A preferable approach is to provide reassurance: if the anxiety occurs when your relative is alone, you might schedule a phone call at a set time or provide companionship, whether through adult day care or regular visits by aides, neighbors, friends, or volunteers. Distraction can also be effective, either by changing the subject, offering a cup of tea, or doing something such as going for a walk or looking at family photographs.

Another problem in early dementia that may become even more common as the disorder progresses to the *middle stage* is depression. If your family member is depressed, he may become withdrawn or apathetic. He does not seem to enjoy life, even those activities that previously gave him satisfaction. Distinguishing between dementia and depression may be difficult. Often the only way to tell is to treat for presumed depression and see if your relative responds, so you should alert his physician to your concern.

Sleep disturbances are also common in middle-stage depression. The most extreme is day-night reversal, in which your family member naps extensively during daylight and is wide awake and walking around at night. Caregiving is particularly difficult in this situation and providing meaningful activities almost impossible. The best way to combat this problem is to avoid coffee during the late afternoon or evening (as well as caffeine-containing medications such as the pain relievers Excedrin and Anacin) and to insist on an exercise regime during the day. Many caregivers are tempted to start sleeping medications at night to try to reverse the cycle, but these often cause worsening confusion as well as daytime sedation. Both over-the-counter preparations such as Sominex and Zzzquil (brand names for the antihistamine diphenhydramine) and prescription medications such as temazepam (brand name Restoril) and zolpidem (brand name Ambien) tend to cause side effects, especially if your relative has dementia.

As dementia progresses from middle to *late stage*, your family member may also have delusions (beliefs that are verifiably false) and hallucinations (hearing or seeing things that are not present). These can be very disturbing to both of you, especially if what your relative "sees" is threatening or hostile. You will want to discuss these symptoms with his physician as this is one of the few situations in which anti-psychotic medication may be useful in dementia.

Another behavioral problem as dementia advances is what is often called wandering. Your relative may leave the house and get lost; he may go out in the middle of the night, sometimes inappropriately dressed. The approach to this problem begins with working to identify what he is trying to do: Is he looking for someone or does he just enjoy walking? Sometimes satisfying his desire to go for walks can be met by going for regular walks—with supervision, during daylight, and wearing suitable clothes. Occasionally, strategies such as visiting his wife's grave may diminish his tendency to go out looking for her. In addition, however, you will need to ensure your family member is safe by locking the house door, by making sure he wears a medic-alert bracelet and, if necessary, by arranging for twenty-four-hour care.

One of the most disturbing behavioral symptoms of late stage dementia is agitation—pacing, yelling, or striking caregivers. Pacing, much like wandering, suggests the need to channel energy in a more constructive direction. Yelling usually indicates fear or an unmet need—is your relative in pain? Is he constipated? You can try to figure out what's bothering him and address the underlying problem. Hitting, biting, or otherwise "resisting care" typically occurs because your family member does not understand what the caregiver is trying to do or finds the action unpleasant. He might balk at taking a shower because the water is not warm enough or refuse to put on a shirt because he finds the sensation of a shirt over his face frightening. The solution, in these examples, may be as simple as adjusting the water temperature or using button-down shirts instead of pullovers.

Dealing with the behavioral symptoms of dementia is incredibly challenging. In addition to consulting with your relative's physician, you may want to read more on the subject or attend a support group. Other people who have experienced what you are going through can be a tremendous support and may have valuable tips for you.

Preventing Progression of Dementia

As a caregiver, you may be encouraged to work with your family member to keep assorted problems such as high blood pressure, diabetes, and high cholesterol under good control. Just as these disorders cause atherosclerosis of the blood vessels of the heart, similarly, they can lead to atherosclerosis of blood vessels in other parts of the body—including the brain. This process both causes vascular dementia and probably makes it worse once it has set in. Moreover, vascular changes also seem to exacerbate Alzheimer's disease. While tight control of these problems may not be warranted (see chapter 22, "High Blood Pressure," chapter 23, "High Cholesterol," and chapter 26, "Diabetes"), judicious treatment is advisable.

Another strategy that is sometimes recommended for preventing the development or progression of dementia is intellectual stimulation. We would all like to believe that memory games or crossword puzzles are helpful, but, unfortunately, the evidence of benefit is minimal. If such games or reading or playing a musical instrument are enjoyable for your family member, then you should certainly encourage these activities. As long as they might help, there's no harm trying (unless, of course, your relative finds these activities frustrating).

Finally, exercise is sometimes promoted as beneficial both as a treatment for dementia and as a preventive technique. As with memory games, the scientific evidence supporting this strategy is scant. However, exercise has many other positive effects, for example on mobility and weight, and as long as it's not burdensome or painful, it may be worth a try.

Advance Care Planning

Your family member's dementia will affect treatment decisions for whatever other medical problems he has. His degree of confusion and his behavioral symptoms should be considered in choosing medications, procedures, or surgery for disorders ranging from cataracts to coronary heart disease. You may also want to consider the likely future trajectory of his dementia in deciding how vigorous to be in treating concomitant problems. If the purpose of aggressive treatment of a heart condition, for example, is to extend life into the distant future, you will need to struggle with the hard question of whether that is in your relative's best interest, given that you would be increasing the likelihood that he will live to experience advanced dementia.

Finally, because dementia is progressive and caregiving needs multiply over time, you may want to lay the groundwork for future caregiving arrangements early in the course of the disease.

For instance, you might conclude that a continuing care retirement community that offers the full spectrum of living arrangements, from independent living to assisted living to nursing home care, is the best long-range solution for your family member—and for you.

If your relative is in the very earliest stages of dementia or, better yet, if he is cognitively intact, you might want to work with him on drawing up a living will to guide treatment if he does become demented. He may want to identify a different goal for each stage of the disease (box 29.1).

Modern medicine plays only a modest role in the management of dementia. As a caregiver, you have a correspondingly large role. Your involvement can make the difference between your relative remaining at home or entering a nursing home and between an aggressive or a more palliative approach to his other medical problems. In general, your care may well shape his overall quality of life (box 29.2).

Box 29.1

Advance Directive for Dementia
(choose one goal for each stage)

- To live as long as possible: full efforts to prolong life, including efforts to restart my heart if it stops

- To receive treatments to prolong life, but if my heart stops or I cannot breathe on my own, do not try CPR and do not place me on a breathing machine. Instead, allow me to die peacefully.

- To receive care only in the place where I am living. Do not send me to the hospital or attempt CPR. If treatments such as antibiotics might keep me alive and can be given where I live, I would want such care.

- To receive comfort-oriented care only, focusing on relieving pain, anxiety, breathlessness, or other symptoms of suffering. I would not want care that is focused only on keeping me alive.

Source: B. Gaster, E. Larson, and J. R. Curtis, "Advance Directives for Dementia," *JAMA* 318 (2017): 2175–2176, available at https://static1.squarespace.com/static/5a0128cf8fd4d22ca11a405d/t/5ab55969562fa77d1761c62a/1521834345937/dementia-directive.pdf.

Box 29.2

Caregiver Roles in Dementia

- Supervise medications: watch for side effects, discuss if and when to stop

- Deal with behavioral symptoms:
  - *Early stage dementia*—distraction, use memos and phone calls as reminders
  - *Middle stage dementia*—use daytime exercise, night time hot chocolate for sleep disturbance, inform MD of depression
  - *Late stage dementia*—respond to agitation, wandering by identifying and treating triggers

- Plan for the future: goal-specific plan for each dementia stage

CHAPTER 30

Chronic Obstructive Lung Disease

A variety of lung conditions are found in older people, but the most common is chronic obstructive lung disease (COLD), also called chronic obstructive pulmonary disease (COPD). "Chronic," "lung," and "disease" are self-explanatory; the "obstructive" part refers to impaired air flow through the passages that make up the respiratory system. To understand your relative's symptoms and how to manage them, it's helpful to know just a little bit about the structure of the respiratory system and a smidgeon about what goes wrong in COLD.

The respiratory system is made up of the trachea, or windpipe, the lungs, and the bronchial tree (figure 30.1). The bronchial tree, in turn, is composed of branches from the trachea to each lung (bronchi) that are subdivided into smaller and smaller tubes (bronchioles) that ultimately reach the air sacs (alveoli). The alveoli are where "gas exchange" takes place: they transmit oxygen directly to the blood vessels and receive carbon dioxide in return, which is then expelled from the lungs.

Chronic obstructive lung disease is usually brought on by a long period of exposure to inhaled toxins—most commonly cigarette smoke. The toxins cause trouble in two ways: they produce chronic bronchitis and they cause emphysema. If your family member has chronic bronchitis, the toxins have affected her lungs by causing chronic inflammation of the airways. This irritation stimulates her to cough, in a vain attempt to expel the irritants. If your relative has emphysema, the toxins have affected her lungs by gradually destroying the alveoli, making it hard to take in oxygen and get rid of carbon dioxide. Most COLD sufferers have components of both emphysema and

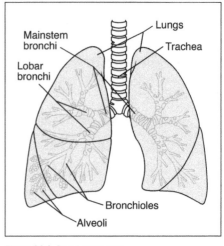

Figure 30.1. Respiratory tree

chronic bronchitis, although in varying proportions. The net effect is that your family member has a chronic cough and is short of breath. She is also at high risk of respiratory infections such as acute bronchitis and pneumonia—which, in turn, worsen her cough and sputum production.

As a caregiver, you will need to be concerned with the ongoing management of your family member's COLD as well as with episodes of acute worsening of her symptoms. Acute management will be addressed in chapter 34, "Shortness of Breath." Chronic management is intended to control symptoms and to stave off an exacerbation of the disease. Typically, it involves medications and, depending on the severity of the condition, oxygen. Other preventive measures such as vaccinations and smoking cessation will be discussed in chapter 32, "Prevention." Let's start with medications, the territory that's probably most familiar to you.

Medications for the Chronic Treatment of COLD

As with medication management for other chronic conditions, your first responsibility may involve obtaining the drugs from the pharmacy. Your relative may be especially dependent on you for this task if she gets short of breath with any kind of exertion. Buying medications will directly involve you in paying for them, so you may find you need to question the physician about the specific drugs he is recommending and request a generic version, if available.

Once the drugs are safely in your family's medicine cabinet, you may play a role in making sure she takes them as directed. The special wrinkle here is that the medications for COLD are often neither pills nor liquid; rather, they are inhaled directly into the lungs by using a device called an inhaler. You may need to learn how this is done if you are to make sure your relative is using her medications correctly. Often when patients use an inhaler, the medicine never reaches the lungs—it ends up in the back of the throat where it doesn't do any good and may result in a sore throat. It can even adversely affect your relative's vocal chords, causing hoarseness. The way to ensure that the medication gets to her lungs is for her to use a device called a spacer (figure 30.2). Not all physicians prescribe this routinely, so it's good to ask about it. A nurse, either in the physician's office or a visiting nurse, is the best person to teach your family member how to use the spacer.

The medications used to help the airways stay open in COLD are of several types, most with regrettably long

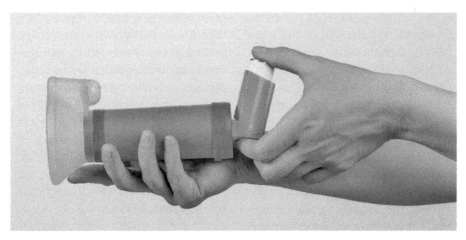

Figure 30.2. Spacer

and technical names: anti-muscarinic drugs, beta agonists, steroids, and methylxanthines. In addition, each type of medication comes as a short-acting and a long-acting preparation (see figure 30.3). I'm just going to say a few words about each of the major classes.

The *anti-muscarinic drugs* are currently among the most popular of the many agents used to treat COLD. They are also referred to as anticholinergic medicines because they block a naturally occurring chemical called acetylcholine, which tends to cause airway constriction. By counteracting the effect of this airway narrowing chemical, they open up the airways. A widely used long-acting drug (long-acting anti-muscarinic or LAMA) is tiotropium (brand name Spiriva) and a commonly used short-acting drug (SAMA) is ipratropium (brand name Atrovent). Because these are inhaled rather than taken as pills, their effects are concentrated in the lungs, limiting the side effects that result from oral medication. Relatively little of the medication gets

into your relative's system; to the extent that it does, it may cause a dry mouth.

Another popular category is *beta agonist drugs*, which work by relaxing the muscles lining the airways, helping them stay open. An example of the long-acting variety (long-acting beta agonists or LABA) is salmeterol (brand name Serevent) and an example of the short-acting variety (short-acting beta agonists or SABA) is salbutamol (Albuterol). These drugs have the potential for significant side effects, including a rapid heart rate. LABAs are generally used in combination with another type of medication, either a LAMA or a steroid, and frequent use of SABAs is to be avoided.

The *methylxanthines* such as theophylline were the mainstay of treatment for COLD many years ago but have largely been replaced by LABAs and SABAs. Theophylline is an oral medication that must be given in just the right dose to avoid side effects: too much causes a rapid heart rate and can trigger heart failure, angina, or even a heart

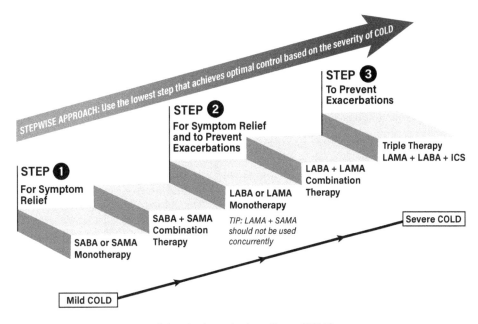

Figure 30.3. Stepwise treatment of chronic obstructive lung disease (COLD)

attack. However, it may be useful if your family member has trouble with the other types of drugs.

Inhaled corticosteroids or ICS (medications such as budesonide, brand name Pulmicort, and fluticasone, brand name Flovent) are more commonly used to treat asthma, a disease characterized by reversible airway obstruction, than they are to treat COLD, in which there's permanent obstruction.

If your family member experiences frequent flares of her COLD, her doctor may opt for a steroid inhaler. The side effects include oral fungus (a yeast infection known as candidiasis) and occasionally, a hoarse voice.

Finally, your family member might be on a *chronic antibiotic* such as erythromycin or azithromycin. These medications significantly decrease the likelihood of acute flares of COLD.

Oxygen in the Treatment of COLD

Depending on the severity of her condition, your relative may need oxygen in addition to medications. Some people only use oxygen at night, a time when the amount of oxygen

in the bloodstream tends to be at its lowest—a level that may be too low for the heart and the brain to function well. Other people only use oxygen if they are having a flare of their COLD, and still others need to use oxygen all the time. Using oxygen means having a source of oxygen, typically a tank, that is connected to either a mask or a nasal cannula (prongs) via a plastic tube. You or your family member will need to arrange for a supplier to bring in a new oxygen tank and take away the used one on a regular basis. She will also need a small, portable oxygen tank so she can leave the house (figure 30.4). You will also need to worry about her tripping over the cord, the plastic tubing, when walking around at home. Having oxygen means absolutely *no* smoking or candles—oxygen is highly combustible. The good news is that Medicare pays for oxygen therapy, the tank, the cannula, and so forth, provided your relative meets certain criteria that typically have to do with her average oxygen level.

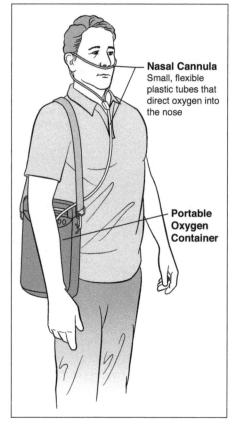

Nasal Cannula
Small, flexible plastic tubes that direct oxygen into the nose

Portable Oxygen Container

Figure 30.4. Patient with portable oxygen (tubing and small container)

Progression of COLD

Over time, your relative will probably experience a gradual worsening of her symptoms. If she deteriorates suddenly, the cause is probably a treatable condition such as bronchitis or pneumonia. In these cases, she will most likely have shortness of breath, worsening cough, or a fever. I will discuss management of *acute* symptoms later (see chapter 34, "Shortness of Breath," chapter 35, "Cough," and chapter 42, "Fever"). If, on the contrary, she is slowly getting worse, you may need to fine tune her medications and her oxygen. You might simply need to dial up the amount of oxygen she is getting—every oxygen tank comes with a *regulator* that controls the oxygen flow. A typical flow rate might be 2 liters per minute. If your family member is short of breath, you might turn this up to 2.5 or 3 liters per minute. It's important to check with your relative's physician about what oxygen flow rates are acceptable for her—some people with COLD cannot tolerate even a small increase because their brain is so accustomed to low oxygen levels that it will misinterpret any increase as a reason to breathe infrequently, which can be dangerous. If the acute worsening of her symptoms is associated with audible wheezing, she is likely to benefit from extra doses of short acting bronchodilator medication through her hand-held nebulizer (and a spacer). You may want to work out with the physician, ideally in advance of any actual problem, what drugs to use and in what doses.

If your family member's COLD is clearly progressing, this is a good time to revisit the issue of her goals of care—or to address it for the first time, if you, your relative, and her physician have not previously talked about this. What is most important to her, given the limitations caused by her chronic lung disease? What approach to medical treatment makes most sense, in light of her goals? You will want to talk about whether she would want artificial ventilation using a breathing machine if she deteriorates further.

Use of a Ventilator in COLD

A respirator, or ventilator as it is also called, is a machine that can be used to take over the function of breathing for your family member if she cannot breathe adequately on her own—despite an oxygen mask and medication. It is normally used in a hospital, typically in an intensive care unit and is attached to your relative via a tube (an endotracheal tube) that is passed through her nose or mouth into the lungs. The machine is also connected to an oxygen source and it rhythmically pumps oxygen into the lungs, at whatever rate and concentration the physician orders. The net effect is that your relative will get oxygen but is unable to speak or eat and will need to depend on other means of communication and nutrition.

The respirator is a descendant of the iron lung that was used to compensate for the weak muscles of respiration found in polio victims. Like the iron lung, it was designed as a stop-gap measure, a way to provide your relative with sufficient quantities of oxygen to keep all her organs working as she recovers from a short-term problem such as severe pneumonia or a drug overdose or, in principal, a sudden worsening of COLD. But modern medicine has discovered that it's possible to maintain a person on a ventilator for very long periods of time, essentially indefinitely. To remain on a ventilator long-term, a surgeon will need to perform a tracheostomy, a small incision in the trachea (the part of the body connecting the back of the throat to the lungs), through which he will insert a tube that joins up with the ventilator (figure 30.5). This tube then replaces the endotracheal tube.

What you and your relative need to understand, if she has advanced COLD, is that there will come a time when her breathing will have deteriorated to the point where she cannot get enough oxygen to sustain life—unless she's attached to such a machine. The question you should face together, preferably before confronted with a crisis, is whether she favors use of a ventilator at all. She might, for example, decide that she wouldn't under any circumstances want to be attached to such a machine. She would prefer, if she was breathing very poorly, to control the sense of shortness of breath with morphine or similar medications. Or, she might

decide she would want to be put on a ventilator in the hope that it would tide her over until her infection, if she had one, came under control. In this case, you should discuss what she would want if it turned out that she could not successfully be withdrawn from the respirator, or in medical jargon, "weaned" from it. Would she be willing to remain on a respirator indefinitely—perhaps for weeks or months or longer? She might, instead, opt for a "limited trial": giving the respirator a specified amount of time, say a week or two, to determine if it was proving useful, and then disconnecting it if it was not helping. This is always a difficult decision to make, which is why it's useful to talk about it in advance. There is no obligation to continue a treatment that's not working, but you have to be sure you have clearly defined what "working" means.

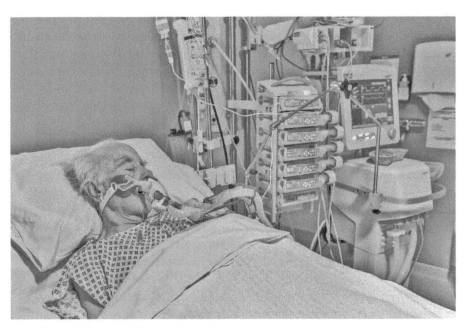

Figure 30.5. Patient intubated and using a ventilator

Remember that you are not a bad person if you call a halt to ineffective treatment; you are just doing what your family member wanted at a time when she may not be able to speak for herself.

Your role in helping manage your family member's chronic lung disease may evolve as her disease progresses. In mild disease, you may find she can take care of herself—assuming she does not have a condition such as dementia on top of her lung problems—or perhaps you just help by picking up medication from the pharmacy. In moderately severe disease, you might have greater involvement as your relative experiences more flares of her condition and more episodes of bronchitis or pneumonia. By the time the disease becomes very advanced, you may find yourself involved in discussions about the use of ventilators and ICU care as well as with low-tech approaches to decreasing symptoms such as a fan or relaxation exercises (see chapter 34, "Shortness of Breath").

Box 30.1

Chronic Obstructive Lung Disease

- COLD includes both emphysema and chronic bronchitis

- The backbone of chronic treatment is a long-acting, inhaled medication, best used with a spacer

- As COLD progresses, it can lead to respiratory failure

- Discuss in advance whether your family member would want treatment with a ventilator (breathing machine) or symptomatic relief (with opioid medication) in the setting of respiratory failure

---

CHAPTER 31

Depression

We all experience the symptoms of depression from time to time: We feel sad, we don't feel like doing much of anything, and we can't imagine things are going to get better any time soon. What differentiates those feelings from true depression, a medical disorder that can be effectively treated, is the depth and duration of those feelings. To be diagnosed with depression, your family member must have had at least five symptoms for at least two weeks. The symptoms may include

- Sadness
- Loss of interest in life
- Loss of interest in enjoyable activities
- Loss of appetite
- Feelings of anxiety
- Avoidance of people
- Problems sleeping
- Low confidence level
- Feelings of unworthiness or guilt
- Thoughts of suicide

Diagnosing depression in your family member may be tricky because he probably has several chronic diseases that individually or collectively cause some of the same symptoms as are found with depression, such as fatigue or poor appetite. But your job as a caregiver is not to make the diagnosis; rather, it's to be alert to the possibility of depression and to raise the issue with your family member's physician if you are concerned. Many people put on a good show for the doctor; they dress neatly, they seem alert and engaged, and they deny that anything's bothering them. It's as though they can make their problems disappear by pulling the wool over their physician's eyes. You are far more likely to see your relative as he really is—and if what you see is someone who sleeps all the time, who feels helpless and hopeless, and who isn't able to take pleasure in anything anymore, that's an extremely important observation that should be communicated to his physician.

Effects of Depression

If your relative has depression, he may experience further impairment of his already limited ability to perform the basic tasks necessary to get by day to day; he may pay even less attention than usual to his appearance and to personal hygiene and become withdrawn from social activities. He's miserable and his caregiving needs have multiplied. The good news is that more than three-quarters of older people who are diagnosed as depressed can be successfully treated with resulting improvement in their self-care, their personal relationships, and their mood. Although depression is very common, affecting at least 10 percent of older people, and despite its profound, debilitating effects, it often goes unrecognized and under-treated.

Medications to Treat Depression

If your relative *is* diagnosed with depression and is started on treatment, what do you need to know to be an effective caregiver? Chances are, he will be started on an antidepressant medication, typically a selective serotonin reuptake inhibitor (SSRI) such as fluoxetine (brand name Prozac), citalopram (brand name Celexa), or paroxetine (brand name Paxil), though other antidepressants may also be used. These are very effective and relatively nontoxic drugs but, like all medications, they sometimes do have side effects. The most common are agitation with associated difficulty sleeping, and nausea. One side effect that is found almost exclusively in older people is a low sodium level in the bloodstream, which can make your relative confused. Your relative's physician will need to obtain a blood test to determine if the sodium is abnormal.

The physician may well choose which drug to use based on its side effects. Trying to take advantage of a medication's side effects is an old geriatric trick. For example, if your relative is having trouble sleeping, a reasonable choice for an antidepressant is mirtazapine (brand name Remeron) because it tends to make people sleepy. If he needs to gain weight, his physician might select paroxetine because it's been associated with weight gain.

As with other types of medications, you may be concerned about cost. There are plenty of antidepressants available as generics, so if your relative's physician prescribes an expensive new medication, it's perfectly reasonable to ask why. A thirty-day supply of citalopram, for example, costs on the order of $7. A thirty-day supply of vilazodone (brand name Vibryd) costs around $220, or over thirty times as much. Is there a convincing reason for choosing the pricier drug? Has your family member tried another, cheaper alternative first?

Treatment does not take effect right away. Medicines usually kick in after two or more weeks. That means weeks of dealing with someone who may be apathetic and poorly motivated to attend to his hygiene or take his pills, even if he normally takes care of these tasks himself. It means having to continue worrying about whether he's suicidal. Suicide is alarmingly common in older people in general and in older white men in particular, and elderly, depressed people have the highest suicide rate of any subgroup of the population. You cannot be expected to guarantee your relative's safety, but you can make sure there are no guns in his home. If you haven't thought about this issue, start thinking about it. This has nothing to do with what you think about guns in general, or the Second Amendment, or gun control legislation. It has everything to do with preventing your family member from killing himself. A sobering statistic, if you need a sobering statistic to be convinced, is that more than 60 percent of the gun-related deaths in the United States are suicides. Here's another one: just about twice as many firearm deaths are due to suicide as are due to homicide (other firearm deaths are due to accidents, to law enforcement, or their cause is unclear). So, here's one case where I'm going to tell you what I think you ought to do: remove any and all guns from your family member's residence.

Nonpharmaceutical Treatment of Depression

Medications are the most commonly used treatment because, in general, we prefer taking a pill over other more complicated strategies. That's why, as a society, Americans would rather decrease the risk of heart disease by taking a pill to lower cholesterol than exercise half an hour a day, several times a week. But there are other ways to treat depression, including psychotherapy (talk therapy) and cognitive behavioral therapy (devising an action plan intended to damp out various negative emotions). Sometimes these therapies are utilized in conjunction with medications. If your family member develops severe side effects to several medications, these alternatives may be tried on their own.

You should also know that electroconvulsive therapy, or shock therapy (ECT), is an option for very depressed individuals. Sometimes you can't afford to wait weeks for medication to work—your relative may be so weak and eating so poorly that his life is in danger. Shock therapy got a bad reputation from films such as *One Flew Over the Cuckoo's Nest*; in fact, shock therapy today looks very different from the portrayal in the movies. It is done under anesthesia so your relative will not be awake and it is commonly done on one side of the brain, not both sides, vastly decreasing the risk he will have memory problems afterwards. It is a low-risk, very effective procedure that should not be rejected out of hand.

A new, noninvasive treatment that can be considered if your family member does not tolerate medications or they are ineffective is transcranial magnetic stimulation. This procedure uses magnetic fields to stimulate nerve cells in the brain. It involves placing an electromagnetic coil against the scalp near your relative's forehead. How this works is unclear but preliminary studies are promising. The procedure is very low risk—assuming your relative is not frightened by the equipment.

Your family member will need a specially trained clinician if he is going to receive psychotherapy, cognitive behavioral therapy, transcranial magnetic stimulation, or electric shock treatment. This raises the more general question: should you be urging him to see a psychiatrist?

When to See a Psychiatrist

Bear in mind that there's a stigma associated with psychiatry in the minds of many older individuals. Your family member may think you only see a psychiatrist if you're crazy. You should also realize that board certified geriatric psychiatrists, physicians who specialize in the psychiatric problems of older people, are rare. Many communities don't have a single geriatric psychiatrist, nor do they have a geriatric psychiatric unit in the local hospital. The good news is that, in most cases, depression can be diagnosed and treated by your relative's primary care physician. My rule of thumb is that if two different antidepressants prove ineffective, or if there is any suggestion that your family member is thinking of committing suicide, he should be referred to a psychiatrist.

If your relative does need a psychiatrist, try to find someone who is interested in and experienced with treating depressed, older patients. If what you are looking for is psychotherapy, you should certainly consider a non-physician as a therapist. Many social workers and clinical psychologists are skilled and experienced therapists. They may also charge less than psychiatrists—which may be relevant because the mental health benefits under many health insurance plans, including Medicaid, are limited. Medicare is more generous in its coverage of outpatient mental health services, but many psychiatrists opt out of Medicare (they don't accept Medicare reimbursement). If your relative sees a mental health provider who does not take Medicare, he will be responsible for the entire bill himself.

Interaction of Depression and Other Disorders

If your relative has depression, your role in managing the care of all his other medical problems will be greater than usual. He may need more help with dressing and bathing and more reminders to take his medications. He may forget or neglect medical appointments. And because depression often impairs judgment, expecting your family member to make decisions about his health may be inappropriate. If, for instance, he happens to need surgery for his gallbladder while his depression is not under control, he may not be in a position to give consent for the operation. This role will fall to you as his health-care proxy.

Not only does depression make your family member feel sad; it affects everyone around him. *You* may feel sad or discouraged. You may start to become depressed yourself. But remember, depression is a treatable disease. Your relative may need to stay on medication a good long time—because the condition tends to recur, some physicians advise remaining on medication indefinitely—but he has an excellent chance of complete recovery.

Box 31.1

Depression

- Symptoms: loss of interest in life, poor appetite, trouble sleeping
- Treatment: medication (principally selective serotonin reuptake inhibitors or SSRIs), electroconvulsive therapy (ECT), psychotherapy, cognitive behavioral therapy
- Effects: mood, physical functioning, demands on caregivers

CHAPTER 32

Prevention

Lest you think that prevention is a panacea for all ills, let me be clear up front: your family member will almost definitely develop diseases that you could not possibly have prevented. Some of those conditions have been years in the making, perhaps due to a lifetime of bad habits (such as lung cancer caused by cigarette smoking); some are due to genetic factors that mysteriously only cause problems in older age; and some are due to bad luck. The boundary between true prevention—taking steps to prevent a condition from developing in the first place—and chronic disease management—monitoring an existing condition and adjusting the treatment in response—is often hazy. Many true preventive strategies will be initiated and implemented by your relative's physician, such as vaccinations or mammograms, but you can play a critical role as well.

Nutrition

Underweight and overweight are important issues among older people. Both contribute to poor health and to mobility problems: if your family member is very thin and ill-nourished, she will lose muscle mass, adversely affecting both strength and balance. If she is very overweight, she is particularly prone to developing arthritis in her knees and may have trouble walking. You can figure out whether she is overweight or underweight by measuring her body mass index (BMI). This is just the weight in kilograms divided by the height in meters squared (see table 32.1). Or, if you measure the weight in pounds and the height in inches, you take the weight divided by the square of the height and multiply by 703.

The standard definition of normal is between 18.5 and 24.9, although some authorities revise the upper end to 23 for people over age sixty-five.

The total number of calories needed per day generally falls with age due to a decline in muscle mass and to lower activity levels. The recommended number of calories varies depending on gender, age, and how active your family member is (see box 32.1).

Table 32.1

BMI (Body Mass Index)

$$BMI = \frac{Weight\ (kg)}{(Height\ (m))^2} \quad or \quad BMI = \frac{Weight\ (lb)}{(Height\ (in))^2} \times 703$$

Weight Categories	BMI
Underweight	Less than 18.5
Perfect Weight	18.5–24.9
Overweight	25–29.9
Obese	More than 30

Note: BMI is a measure of body fat based on your weight and height

Box 32.1

Recommended Caloric Intake

Moderately active woman over 70:	1800 calories/day
Moderately active man over 70:	2200 calories/day
Sedentary woman over 70:	1600 calories/day
Sedentary man over 70:	2000 calories/day

Source: U.S. Department of Health and Human Services and U.S. Department of Agriculture, "2015–2020 Dietary Guidelines for Americans: 8th Edition," last modified December 2015, http://health.gov/dietaryguidelines/2015/guidelines/.

What Is a Good Diet?

A good diet for an older person is essentially the same as a good diet for any adult. It should include adequate protein, essential for maintaining muscles and for making the body's chemicals, typically about 1.5 grams for every 2.2 pounds, or 70 grams for a 110-pound woman. High protein foods that are easy to eat include hard boiled eggs and peanut butter sandwiches. Particularly important for your relative is adequate intake of vitamin D and calcium, both of which are essential to maintain strong bones. The recommendation for both older men and women is at least 1,200 milligrams of calcium each day. This can be supplied through milk (a full 8-ounce glass contains 300 mg), yogurt, cheese and, for a non-dairy source, fortified orange juice or fortified cereals. These same foods also are a rich source of vitamin D.

Also important is fiber, which helps avoid constipation. To get enough fiber, your family member should eat four or five servings of fruits and vegetables each day. Breakfast cereals that contain bran are also a good way to get fiber.

Special Challenges

Your family member may have trouble getting food in the first place. If she lives on her own, you may have to do the shopping for her or arrange for food delivery. The market for home grocery delivery is becoming quite competitive; depending on where your relative lives, there may be a number of options (table 32.2).

Your family member may need help preparing as well as obtaining food. In that case, she may benefit from a service such as Meals on Wheels, a program authorized by the Older Americans Act, that delivers ready-to-eat hot meals to over 2 million American seniors. A sliding scale is available if your relative cannot afford the standard $7.10 per meal price. More expensive options are home delivery by area restaurants and ready-to-cook kits that include fresh ingredients in all the right quantities. It's a burgeoning market, with new offerings appearing regularly. Some of these new options, such as Martha's Senior Gourmet (with delivery

Table 32.2
Sample Home Delivery Services (2018)

Name	Cost	Features	Minimum purchase	Restrictions
Google Express	Free	Many stores	$25/store	No perishables
Instacart	$3.99/delivery; free with membership	Many stores, 1-hr service	$35	
Amazon Fresh	$14.99/month	Prime members only	$40	
Peapod	$6.95–$7.95/ delivery	Online shopping list	$60	Next day delivery

in major cities in California, Texas, and Arizona), advertise themselves as specially geared to older people.

A variety of medical difficulties can make eating challenging, even if the meal has been prepared and is in principle ready to eat. Your relative may not have any teeth, which makes chewing a problem. If she has dentures, she may still need to eat soft foods. She may also have difficulty swallowing because of a neurological condition such as stroke, Parkinson's disease, or dementia. Or, she may have trouble swallowing because she suffers from a dry mouth, in many instances caused by medication. If you recognize that a dry mouth is making it hard for your family member to eat, you should notify her physician. He may modify her medications or prescribe artificial saliva.

Your relative might not eat well because she has a poor appetite. Appetite is affected by a variety of medical conditions, ranging from depression to cancer. Her sense of taste may be impaired, often because of a loss of her sense of smell (the two are related), adversely affecting her appetite. Sometimes there's a reversible medical cause for the loss of smell; more often, the best solution is to eat spicier foods. If your family member has dementia, she might no longer be able to use a fork and knife, in which case you should focus on finger foods. Even if she can handle utensils properly, she may find a plate with multiple different foods on it overwhelming and will do better if she is served one food at a time.

Finally, eating together with others is a good way for your relative to remain socially engaged. Whether that means eating with you and your family, having lunch at the local senior center, or eating in a communal dining room at an assisted living facility or nursing home, you may find your relative eats more if she's not eating alone.

Dental Hygiene

I mentioned teeth and dentures in connection with eating; it turns out that good oral health is important for other reasons as well. Your family member needs her teeth—or well-fitting dentures—to speak clearly. Speaking is obviously a critical component of communication; if she's difficult to understand, she will not be able to articulate her needs and may have trouble interacting socially. Ideally, your relative will make regular visits to the dentist for cleanings, filling cavities, and the detection and treatment of gum disease. Geriatric dentists, who specialize in the problems of older patients and are experienced in treating people despite cognitive and/or hearing difficulties, are a rarity but are the ideal solution. Not surprisingly, given the equipment they usually use, dentists who make home visits are even more scarce than physicians who make home visits.

Poor oral health turns out to increase the risk of pneumonia, especially in nursing home residents, but potentially in other frail older people as well. Bacteria accumulate in plaques and may end up traveling from the mouth to the lungs, where they set up shop. The best way to prevent this phenomenon is with good tooth-brushing. Your family member may not have the dexterity or the cognitive capacity to do a good job brushing her teeth. An electric toothbrush can help or she may require the assistance of another person—either you or a home health aide.

Recent studies have found poor oral health to be associated with diabetes, heart disease and, more generally, with frailty. What's not entirely clear is whether poor dentition *causes* these various medical problems (or at least is one of multiple risk factors) or whether it's simply a *marker* of things to come. Perhaps the same people who have problems with their teeth or gums are also people who are destined to get dementia. You could imagine that an early sign of cognitive difficulties might be failure to brush one's teeth properly. Over time, the cognitive difficulties may well progress to full-fledged dementia—and the inadequate dental hygiene will lead to cavities. Or you could imagine that someone who eats large quantities of sweets and becomes overweight will develop diabetes—and tooth decay. But the evidence that the mouth matters is growing. Paying attention to your family member's teeth seems prudent.

Exercise

Exercise is not a panacea; it can't prevent all the various medical problems your relative might develop, but it has a role to play in keeping her as healthy and functional as possible, even if she is frail. Exercise comes in several varieties: aerobic, resistance exercise, and flexibility and balance exercise. Each is helpful in a different way.

Aerobic exercise refers to any activity that uses large muscle groups and can be carried out for extended periods of time. If your family member is frail, tennis and running are unlikely to be realistic options, but brisk walking, pedaling on an exercise bicycle, or using a treadmill may be feasible. Whatever the modality, your relative will need to work hard enough to increase her heart rate and to sustain it for at least twenty minutes. Regularly engaging in this kind of activity may help stave off heart disease and can sometimes lessen the symptoms of depression.

Resistance exercise involves repetitive weight lifting or analogous activity until the point of fatigue. Strengthening the upper extremities may make it possible for your family member to carry a bag of groceries, for example, while strengthening the lower extremities may make it easier for her to go up a flight of stairs or a hill.

Balance exercises are not precisely defined, but include Tai Chi, a form of Chinese martial arts. These exercises are mainly recommended to prevent falls, and Tai Chi is modestly effective in this regard. Formal instruction is generally necessary at first, although your family member can then continue on her own.

There is some evidence that your relative may benefit from an exercise program that includes balance, strength, and endurance (aerobic) exercises. In the Frailty Intervention Trial (FIT), the combination of all three forms of exercise led to improvement in mobility and diminished frailty. If exercise can truly improve function, enabling your relative to do more for herself, to be more independent in general and more mobile in particular, it's a good idea (box 32.2).

A major challenge for many older people is finding a place to exercise. Unless she lives in a building with its own gym, your family member will have to travel to a suitable facility. Using a swimming pool is even more complicated and time-consuming, as she will have to change and shower to make use of it. Motivation, or rather lack of it, is another obstacle. Unless your relative has exercised on a regular basis for

Box 32.2

Exercise Recommendations for Frail Older Adults

Aerobic Exercise
Moderate to vigorous activity enough to raise the pulse rate to 70–80 percent of the maximum heart rate. Activity performed for a minimum of 20–30 minutes at least three days per week.

Resistance Exercise
The progressive resistance program should involve all major muscle groups of the upper and lower extremities and trunk. One set of 8–10 different exercises, with 10–15 repetitions per set, performed 2–3 nonconsecutive days per week. Moderate-high intensity training is recommended, in which moderate intensity is 5 or 6 on a 0–10 scale.

Flexibility and Balance Exercise
Stretching to the point of tightness and holding the position for a few seconds. Flexibility activities are performed on all days that aerobic or muscle strengthening activity is performed. Balance training exercise 2–3 times per week.

Source: L. Aguirre and D. Villareal, "Physical Exercise as Therapy for Frailty," *Nestle Nutrition Institute Workshop Series* 83 (2015): 83–92, https://www.ncbi.nlm.nih.gov/pmc/articles/PMC4712448/.

much of her adult life, starting when she's eighty-five and has multiple medical problems can be intimidating. One approach that works for some people is to join a class. Exercising then has a social dimension as well as a medical benefit. In select circumstances, physicians will prescribe an exercise regimen: Cardiac rehabilitation is common after a heart attack and pulmonary rehab has been shown to be helpful for people with chronic obstructive lung disease (COLD).

No Smoking!

In general, I think it's reasonable to ease many stringent guidelines when prescribing for frail older people. If quality of life is what matters most to your family member and she derives pleasure from chocolate, let her eat chocolate. Not so much chocolate that she spoils her appetite for dinner or begins gaining a great deal of weight, but perhaps more than you would eat. In a similar vein, if she has diabetes, then tight control of her blood sugars is seldom warranted (see chapter 26, "Diabetes"). In this case, the issue isn't so much quality of life, but rather that she's unlikely to live long enough to benefit from tight control—and might well get dizzy and fall if her blood sugar is too low. But my laissez-faire attitude, if you want to call it that, doesn't apply to smoking. It seems to me that if you want to take effective preventive measures, the place to start is by getting your relative to stop smoking. Smoking is a safety risk, it causes health problems, *and* it's expensive.

The safety issue has to do with fires. If your family member is forgetful or tends to doze off, she shouldn't be smoking. Cigarettes are the single largest cause of fires in the home and 40 percent of the victims of home fires are over 65, though this age group only accounts for 13 percent of the population. If your relative is over 85 her risk of dying in a fire is 3.4 times higher than the risk in the general population. And as I mentioned in the discussion of supplemental oxygen for people with chronic lung or heart disease, oxygen tanks can burst into flames, so smoking is absolutely out of the question if your relative uses oxygen.

As far as health is concerned, cigarette smoking continues to wreak havoc with health as long as your family member continues to smoke. Moreover, if she has smoked for years and quits, and if she doesn't already have heart disease, her risk of developing heart problems will actually *fall*. In the case of chronic obstructive lung disease, by contrast, much of the damage from cigarettes is irreversible. Nonetheless, your family member will experience fewer symptoms such as cough or shortness of breath if she stops smoking. More generally, cigarettes are a major contributor to the development of atherosclerosis, whether the affected arteries deliver oxygen and other nutrients to the brain or the heart or the kidneys. If your family member stops smoking, she will prevent further damage to those critical blood vessels, potentially avoiding or at least delaying the onset of a stroke, a heart attack, or kidney failure.

Quitting is no easier in an old person than in someone younger because cigarettes contain nicotine which is addictive. But there are more aids to quitting today than formerly and they are often effective. Encouragement and advice from your relative's primary care physician matters. If her doctor doesn't ask about smoking, you might want to mention that it's an issue. Behavioral therapy can help and has the great advantage that it does not involve medications. If medication is used, you should be aware that bupropion (brand name Wellbutrin) is an antidepressant that is fairly well-tolerated in older people—and that is also helpful in decreasing the craving for cigarettes. Nicotine patches, while available over the counter, may cause problems in older people so you should be sure your family member discusses the advisability of using them with her physician.

Vaccinations

Vaccination is one of the most effective public health interventions of all time. In general, your family member's primary care physician will recommend and administer vaccines. But I want to say a few words about the three major ones—influenza vaccine, pneumonia vaccine, and the shingles vaccine—because you may be critically important in assuring your relative gets them.

Influenza, which is a viral illness, is a potentially serious disease in older people: it may cause viral pneumonia or be complicated by the development of bacterial pneumonia, and it can trigger a worsening of other medical problems such as heart disease. The vaccine must be given every year because the virus that causes the flu mutates frequently, necessitating annual tweaks to the vaccine. It's often available at your local pharmacy or senior center, which may be more convenient than taking your relative to the doctor in the early fall. You should make sure she gets the special high dose vaccine for older individuals. Some older people resist getting the shot, insisting that it "gave them the flu" in the past. Influenza vaccine can cause a little pain at the injection site for a day and may result in very minor aches and pains and a low grade fever, but it *does not cause influenza*. What is true is that it's not perfect at preventing the disease and it has no effect on preventing colds and other viral respiratory illnesses. Unfortunately, the people who need it the most are at risk of receiving only partial protection from the shot, but vaccination lowers the risk of getting the flu, and if your family member does get the flu, it's apt to be a mild case.

Pneumonia and influenza together are the eighth most common cause of death in older people. The good news is that the most common form of pneumonia in the community, pneumococcal pneumonia, is in at least large measure preventable with the Pneumovax vaccine. This is something your relative's primary care physician should recommend and administer. But what you need to know is that until a few years ago, the available vaccine protected people from thirteen different strains of bacteria; today, there's a new vaccine that protects against twenty-three strains. So even though in principle, the pneumonia vaccine needs to be given only once, if your relative got the original vaccine when she turned 65, she should get a second vaccination with the newer version.

Finally, you should be aware that there's a very effective vaccine against shingles (herpes zoster), an extremely painful and sometimes dangerous condition that results from "reawakening" of the chicken pox virus that may have lain dormant in your family member for years. As with the pneumonia vaccine, there's a new version of the shingles vaccine. The new one, Shingrix, is far more effective than the old one, Zostavax, so the Centers for Disease Control and Prevention advise getting the new vaccine even if your family member already received the first one. You may not want to wait until she has her regularly scheduled checkup but arrange for a visit to get the new vaccine, which is given as two shots, as soon as possible.

From taking your family member for a flu shot to helping her brush her teeth, there are many preventive strategies with the potential for significant impact (box 32.3). You will find mention of still other approaches to prevention scattered through this book in the relevant sections. Chapter 22, "High Blood Pressure," and chapter 23, "High Cholesterol," include suggestions about prevention as well as ongoing treatment of those conditions. Chapter 3, "Thinking like a Geriatrician: Geriatric Syndromes," includes material on falls and delirium—and how to prevent them.

Box 32.3

Preventive Strategies

- Nutrition is affected by appetite, dental care, availability of food, and social context

- Exercise can help stave off frailty

- Balance exercises help prevent falls

- Vaccinations against influenza, pneumonia, and shingles are safe and effective

PART VI

Acute Care at Home

As a family caregiver, you will often discover that your family member has something wrong and you will be expected to do something about it. If it looks like a medical problem of some kind, you are going to have to figure out whether you should call the physician or go to the emergency department or start treatment yourself. To decide, you'll need to know a bit about evaluating your family member. Because he will manifest disease with a symptom—he will say he's feeling short of breath, not that he's having a flare of his congestive heart failure, or he will have a cough but won't announce that he's developed pneumonia—I'm going to organize this section by symptom. You are not expected to develop the expertise of a nurse or a physician, and you shouldn't feel alone in taking care of someone who is sick. But you can become familiar with the basics and learn how best to respond to your family member's symptoms depending, in part, on his goals of care as well as on the severity of his symptoms.

CHAPTER 33

Chest Pain

One symptom that you may find especially alarming in your family member is chest pain. You will no doubt immediately worry about heart trouble. It's true that if the heart doesn't get enough oxygen, usually because there is a narrowing or blockage of one of the blood vessels feeding the heart, the result is chest pain: either angina (short-lived cardiac pain) or a heart attack (myocardial infarction, the actual death of part of the heart muscle). But if you visualize the chest for a moment, you will quickly realize that your relative might be having chest pain for an entirely different reason.

Starting with the outside of the chest, you will discover bones connected by muscles (figure 33.1). Go inside the chest and you will find the heart (inside a sac called the pericardium), blood vessels, the trachea, and the lungs (figure 33.2).

Inside the lungs is the bronchial tree: the trachea (the tube connecting the nose to the lungs) and its branches, the bronchi, and their branches, the bronchioles, which end in air sacs. The chest cavity also includes the esophagus, or tube linking the mouth to the stomach, which is part of the gastrointestinal system. Not surprisingly, the main causes of chest pain reflect problems in

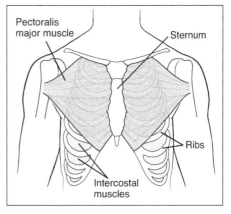

Figure 33.1. Chest wall

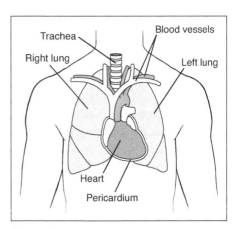

Figure 33.2. Chest cavity organs

the heart (or its blood vessels), the lungs (or associated parts of the respiratory tree), the esophagus, or the musculoskeletal scaffolding. If this sounds daunting, it's not as bad as it seems. Chest pain emanating from each of these sources has its own characteristics and associated symptoms. But your job is not to diagnose the problem—that's what physicians do. Your job is to assess the severity of the problem, collect some basic relevant information, and then act, taking into consideration your family member's history and preferences for care.

How Severe Is the Pain?

The first step in this process is to figure out how severe the problem is. If your relative's chest pain is very severe—the classic description is "it feels like there's an elephant on my chest"—or if he is very pale and is breaking out in a cold sweat, you will want to get medical attention right away. Even without any of these telltale signs of a severe problem, chest pain can be serious.

Physicians commonly ask patients to rate their pain on a scale from one to ten, where one is very mild and ten is the worst pain ever. Showing your relative a series of faces and asking him to pick which one best represents his situation is a good approach for people who have trouble quantifying their pain (figure 33.3).

To help figure out how serious the problem is, you may want to check your family member's vital signs (for more information about assessing vital signs, see chapter 21, "Your Medical Bag"). Begin with the pulse: if his heart is going at over 120 beats a minute, his condition is likely to be severe. If you know how to take his blood pressure, this is a good time to do so. You should be concerned if the top number, the systolic blood pressure, is less than 90 or more than 180. If you have an oximeter, the device for measuring the amount of oxygen in your family member's system, you will want to take a

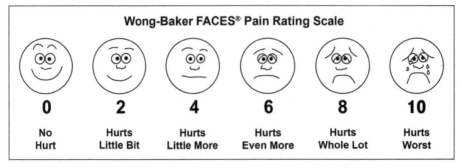

Figure 33.3. Wong-Baker FACES® Pain Rating Scale. © Wong-Baker FACES Foundation (2019). Retrieved February 21, 2019, with permission from http://www.WongBaker FACES.org.

reading. The cutoff for worrying varies from person to person; if you plan to use an oximeter, your family member's physician should specify a threshold for normal. Below that level, the problem is apt to be severe. In any of these situations—the sensation of a weight on the chest, very pale complexion, very elevated pulse, either very low or very high blood pressure, or an inadequate oxygen level—you probably want to call your family member's physician office without delay.

What Is the Pain Like?

If the pain isn't quite so severe, you have time to collect additional information that will help guide the next steps. If your family member is able to communicate what he's feeling, you can ask a few basic questions. What is the pain like? What brings it on? What, if anything, makes it better? If the pain first came on when your relative was walking or lifting something and it got better when he sat down, that may well be heart pain. If the pain starts whenever he takes a deep breath, it is called pleuritic. Pleuritic pain, in turn, can be caused by a variety of different problems, ranging from blood clots to the lungs (a serious condition) to irritation of the nerves in the chest wall (an unpleasant but not dangerous musculoskeletal problem). If the pain starts after eating, it may be due to acid (produced by the stomach in response to eating) flowing up into the esophagus, a common problem known as reflux. Your family member may already have taken a spoonful of antacid and can tell you if that helped.

Other Associated Symptoms

Just a few more questions, this time about other symptoms that accompany the chest pain. Medical problems often produce a constellation of symptoms, so information about what else is going on is very helpful. Is your family member experiencing nausea—is he sick to his stomach? While that doesn't definitively pinpoint the problem to the gastrointestinal system—some heart attacks are associated with nausea—it's helpful to know about. What about shortness of breath? Is that a problem? Again, several sources of chest pain also cause difficulty breathing, including pulmonary emboli, pneumonia, and a heart attack, but not, for example, acid reflux. One other specific symptom to ask about is cough. Chest pain due to a heart attack or to inflammation of the ribs isn't usually associated with a cough.

You already have a great deal of information: you know how severe the pain is and, if it's not terribly severe, you know what it's like, what brings it on, what makes it better, and what other symptoms your family member reports. If you are in the room with him, you may have measured his heart rate, his blood pressure, and perhaps his oxygen saturation. At this point, you are almost ready to speak with the physician or nurse practitioner about the situation. Before you do, you'll want to have a list of your family member's medications handy. You will also want to have a list of his medical problems in front of you when you call: knowing that he's had a heart attack in the past and has a history of angina is very useful; similarly, if he has a diagnosis of heart failure or has had multiple bouts of pneumonia in the past, that's also relevant.

Deciding What to Do Next

It's time for action. Whether that action is calling your family member's physician, taking him to the emergency room, or initiating treatment yourself will depend not only on how severe the pain is and on its most likely cause, but also on his *goals of care*. Let's say you and your family member have previously agreed that the primary goal of care is *living as long as possible*. In this situation, your relative will probably need to be examined by his physician, though how severe the pain is affects whether you can take him to the doctor's office, whether you need to head to the emergency department of the nearest hospital, or whether you can start with a telephone consultation.

If you've established that the most important goal of care is *remaining comfortable*, you might decide to try some simple treatments at home, preferably based on a plan you previously devised together with the physician. Your family member might, for example, have chest pain when he walks more than a few feet, but with no shortness of breath or nausea. The pain feels a lot like his usual angina and this kind of pain has responded well to nitroglycerin tablets in the past. You feel comfortable advising him to take nitroglycerin and to seek medical input only if the pain doesn't go away. Or, suppose he has a history of reflux and says his chest pain is unrelated to exercise, though he's not sure if it's associated with eating. He already takes a proton pump inhibitor (a medicine such as omeprazole, brand name Prilosec) for this problem. You might suggest that he try a tablespoon of antacid and see if the pain eases up.

The other possibility is that your family member has said his principal goal of care is to *remain as independent as possible*, to keep on doing the things he enjoys. He is interested in life-prolonging medical treatment, but only if the price isn't a lot of painful tests, and he'd rather avoid being hospitalized if there is a reasonable alternative because he knows that being in the hospital takes a lot out of him. In this case, you will probably want to speak with the physician about your family member's symptoms, mentioning any other symptoms he's having and reporting his vital signs. Together with the physician, you can decide whether the next step is to try a medication at home or to bring your family member to the office.

You shouldn't be playing doctor—even if you are a physician or nurse, you shouldn't be serving as your family member's physician. Nor should you embark on home treatment if you feel uncomfortable with this approach. But just as parents learn when they need to take their children to the pediatrician and when they can treat them at home, just as they learn to recognize certain recurring conditions, so, too, can you learn enough about your family member's medical problems to initiate treatment at home.

Box 33.1

> ## Evaluating Chest Pain
>
> - Determine the severity of the pain
> - Find out what makes it better or worse
> - Measure heart rate, blood pressure, respiratory rate
> - Assemble medications and list of diagnoses, then call MD
> - Consider empiric treatment, home therapy, office appointment, or trip to emergency room, depending on severity of symptoms and goals of care

CHAPTER 34

Shortness of Breath

I f chest pain instills fear in you, the caregiver, shortness of breath generates fear in your family member. Pain, nausea, and itching are all unpleasant, but shortness of breath is especially distressing. In its most severe form, your family member feels as though she's suffocating. We are hardwired to respond to threats from the outside world: Pain is a neurologic trigger telling us something is very wrong and we should take immediate action (for example, we should take our hand away from the hot stove); and nausea is the body's way of alerting us to a toxin that we should avoid (for instance, those mushrooms are poisonous, don't eat any more of them!); but breathlessness is the most basic of all because it's a response to a lack of oxygen. And if we don't have enough air, we will die.

What Causes Shortness of Breath?

S hortness of breath (the medical term is dyspnea) often stems from a problem in the lungs, whether emphysema or an infection such as pneumonia. Other disease processes that can affect the lungs are cancer (either a primary lung tumor or metastases to the lungs) and pulmonary emboli, or blood clots that travel from elsewhere in the circulation to the lungs. Shortness of breath can also develop from a condition that arises in another organ, such as the heart, but secondarily produces effects in the lungs. In heart failure, for instance, the heart doesn't pump blood normally, resulting in fluid backing up into the lungs.

Common causes of shortness of breath can include

- Chronic obstructive lung disease (COLD)

- Bronchitis

- Asthma

- Pneumonia

- Blood clot in the lung and other heart and lung problems

How Severe is the Shortness of Breath?

If your family member reports she is short of breath, your first step is to figure out how severe the problem is, much as we discussed for chest pain. If the shortness of breath is very severe, you don't have time to proceed leisurely and systematically to evaluate the problem—your family member needs help immediately. One way to assess severity is to notice if your relative's lips are blue: if they are, she doesn't have enough oxygen in her bloodstream. Another way is to watch her breathe: if she's working so hard to catch her breath that you can see her neck muscles contract, her breathing problem is severe. If you have a pulse oximeter, a device you place on the fingertip to measure the amount of oxygen in your family member's blood (see chapter 21, "Your Medical Bag"), and the reading is low, lower than whatever level the physician indicated is normal for your relative, then you have to take steps right away.

Other Symptoms

The next step is to find out if there are other symptoms that have developed along with the breathing problem. If the breathing problem is related to an infection (bronchitis, the flu, or pneumonia), your family member will probably be coughing. If she's coughing, find out if she's bringing up sputum (phlegm). If so, is it clear or is it yellow or green? Is it blood-tinged? Infection is often, though not always, associated with fever. Has your relative felt feverish? Has she had a shaking chill? When the body temperature is on its way up, the brain will mistakenly tell your relative that she's cold; she will then start shivering.

If the breathing problem is due to heart failure, your relative will probably have excess fluid somewhere else besides her lungs, such as the lower legs. You will, therefore, want to inquire about—or look yourself—for ankle swelling. The heart failure, in turn, might have been triggered by other heart problems: you should ask your family member if she has had any chest pain or palpitations.

You may want to ask a couple of the questions that will help your relative's physician make a diagnosis. He will want to know how long she's had the difficulty, what makes it better, and what makes it worse. If the problem started very suddenly, it could be caused by a blood clot to the lungs (a pulmonary embolism), which is a serious condition that needs to be addressed right away. On the other hand, if it's been developing gradually, and if your family member has also been losing weight and coughing, the problem could be due to a pleural effusion, an accumulation of fluid in the sac surrounding the lungs, possibly stemming from cancer. If the breathing gets worse when your relative lies down, her problem could be related to heart failure—fluid build-up in the lungs is increased when gravity isn't available to help out.

Useful Tests You Can Perform

At this point, you may want to take a few more measurements, using some of the tools in your medical bag (see chapter 21, "Your Medical Bag"). Take your family member's temperature with your digital thermometer. A temperature of 101°F, or warmer usually means inflammation, most commonly (though not always) infection. If you have a blood pressure cuff, use it. Blood pressure that is either very high or very low raises a red flag. You will also want to measure her pulse, which can either be done manually or with the automatic blood pressure cuff. Typically, her heart rate will go up with fever, but an extremely elevated heart rate, even if it's an expected consequence of the high temperature, is itself risky in a frail older person.

Chronic Medical Problems

The final step is to think about which of your relative's chronic medical problems might be acting up. Perhaps she has chronic lung disease or asthma. Has she been wheezing? Has she been taking her lung medications, such as bronchodilators? Maybe she has chronic heart failure, in which case you will want to weigh her. An exacerbation of heart failure is associated with fluid gain, whether in the lungs (causing shortness of breath), in the legs (producing ankle edema), or in the abdomen (causing ascites), and you can estimate the magnitude of the fluid build-up by seeing how much weight your family member has gained. Knowing what infections are going around is also helpful: if you are in the midst of a flu epidemic and half the other people who attend the same adult day health program as your relative are home with the flu, and if your family member now has a fever and runny nose along with shortness of breath, odds are that she also has the flu.

Initiating Treatment

Once you've finished your investigation, you are ready to act. What exactly you will do depends on the severity of your relative's symptoms, on what you've learned from the information you gathered, and on your family member's *goals of care.* As usual, the extreme situations are easiest to handle. Suppose your relative is *severely* short of breath and has clearly indicated that her number one priority is living as long as possible, no matter what it takes. In this situation, what's needed is prompt medical evaluation; the only question is whether to call the physician's office or take your relative directly to the nearest hospital emergency department. If, by contrast, your family member has chronic obstructive lung disease and her symptoms are just a bit worse than usual, and if she has stated unequivocally that she wants simple medical treatments focused on keeping her as comfortable and independent as possible, then it would be entirely reasonable to encourage her to take an extra couple of puffs of her bronchodilator medication using her inhaler.

The in-between situations are more challenging. Ideally, you will discuss what you have learned with your relative's primary care physician or affiliated nurse practitioner and come up with a plan. You will want to remind the physician of your family member's goals as well as reporting her temperature and respiratory rate. In some cases, the two of you—or the three of you, if your relative was able to participate in the discussion—will already have devised a plan for what to do in just this sort of a situation. If your relative has a history of heart failure and takes a daily dose of a fluid pill, and if all the evidence points to her now having a slight worsening of her heart failure, the plan might be to double the dose of her diuretic and monitor her weight. If she has chronic lung disease and uses oxygen on a regular basis, the plan might be to give her an extra dose of inhaler and increase her oxygen rate from 2 liters/minute to 3 liters/minute. Or perhaps she has chronic lung disease and gets bronchitis several times a year. Each time, the course is entirely predictable: she starts coughing more than usual and she begins to bring up yellow sputum, and after a couple of days she feels increasingly short of breath. Her primary care physician prescribes a week of antibiotics and a short course of oral steroids whenever this happens. You may already have the necessary prescriptions or even a supply of antibiotics and of prednisone so that you can initiate the usual regimen promptly.

Other Strategies to Control Symptoms

Your relative might have an advanced condition that causes shortness of breath, whether cancer, heart failure, or chronic lung disease. If the decision is to focus exclusively on comfort, you should know about a few other strategies that can help alleviate symptoms. Even though the problem may be in the lungs, the discomfort your family member feels—air hunger or chest tightness or anxiety—often results from signals the brain sends out in response to a low oxygen level. Treatment may be directed against the underlying problem, for example excess fluid in the lungs or an infection, but it may also target the symptom rather than the cause. Your relative might feel more comfortable and breathe more easily if she has a fan blowing air at her. She may respond well to antianxiety medication such as low dose lorazepam. In select situations, morphine can be very helpful by relaxing both the mind and blood vessels, though not all physicians are comfortable with prescribing opioids in this situation. You may also want to try alternative approaches to produce relaxation such as acupuncture or Reiki, a Japanese stress reduction technique.

Shortness of breath must always be taken seriously (box 34.1). Because it usually connotes a serious problem, you may want to discuss the situation with your relative's primary care physician sooner rather than later. But you have a role to play in helping the physician make a diagnosis as well as in administering treatment and keeping your family member comfortable.

Box 34.1

Evaluating Acute Shortness of Breath

- How severe is it?

- What other symptoms are present?

- What are the vital signs (heart rate, respiratory rate, and temperature)?

- Which chronic diseases have been diagnosed?

CHAPTER 35

Cough

Many of the symptoms your relative might develop are beyond your personal experience. You may never have had chest pain or acute confusion or thrown up blood. But everyone has had a cough.

Most of the time, a cough is a symptom of the common cold. Sometimes, it means something else and as a caregiver, you will want to know when to worry and what to do about your family member's cough.

Infectious Causes of Cough

Since you are most familiar with a cough that is a symptom of a respiratory infection, a good place to begin is by trying to figure out if the cough is infectious. If the cough comes with a runny nose, a low-grade temperature (less than 101°F), and a sore throat, your family member most likely has a cold. If his temperature is somewhat higher (101°F or above) and he aches all over and feels really miserable, the cough may be a symptom of influenza or some other viral upper respiratory infection. If the cough is associated with sputum production (phlegm), the problem may be bronchitis or pneu-

monia. You will want to be in touch with your relative's physician if fever of over 101°F is present or if the cough is accompanied by shortness of breath. Otherwise, you can probably manage the symptoms just the way you would if you were similarly afflicted.

If you are fairly certain that your family member's cough is not from an infection, then you are faced with a wide variety of other possibilities. You can make considerable headway in determining the actual cause by a process of elimination. Let's start with some of the simplest possible explanations.

Noninfectious Causes of Cough

One of the more surprising causes of cough is a drug reaction. The angiotensin-converting enzyme (ACE) inhibitors, drugs such as enalapril and lisinopril that are widely used to treat high blood pressure, cause a chronic cough in at least 10 percent of users—some studies report the rate as high as 35 percent. If this annoying side effect occurs, it will happen early on, not a year or two after the medication is started. That means that you should check whether your relative has recently started a drug in this class. If he has, let the primary care physician know; she will discontinue the medication and find a different type of treatment.

Another somewhat surprising cause of cough is gastroesophageal reflux disease (GERD). It's not entirely clear how this works, but one theory is that when acid backs up into the esophagus—that's what the "reflux" refers to in gastroesophageal reflux—it triggers a cough response. At least 25 percent of cases of chronic cough are attributable to GERD. What makes this a tricky diagnosis is that you may not know that your relative has GERD. In fact, the first symptom might be a chronic cough! But if you do know that your family member has a history of GERD and if he has not been taking a proton pump inhibitor (PPI) such as omeprazole (Prilosec), lansoprazole (Prevacid), or pantoprazole (Protonix), it may be worth going back on one of these medications. Both omeprazole and lansoprazole are available over the counter.

If your family member suffers from allergic rhinitis, he might develop a cough from postnasal drip. He will normally be aware that his nose is running. In many cases, successful treatment of the allergy, typically with an over-the-counter antihistamine, will greatly decrease the postnasal drip—and indirectly, the cough.

Another commonplace problem that can lead to cough is dry air. Many homes are very dry in winter when the heat is turned on. Excessively dry air can cause all sorts of problems, ranging from nosebleeds to itchy skin to cough. The fix is to use a humidifier (figure 35.1). Ear, nose, and throat physicians usually recommend a cool mist humidifier. The size will vary depending on

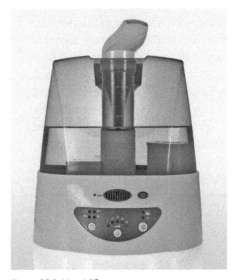

Figure 35.1. Humidifier

the size of the room. They are generally simple to operate, but it's important to change the filter on some of these devices and you may have to take charge of refilling the humidifier when the water level gets low.

Still another noninfectious cause is cancer. Often, lung cancer will be associated with additional symptoms such as shortness of breath or weight loss, and in many cases, your relative will be coughing up bloody sputum. But a chronic cough that isn't from an ACE inhibitor or GERD and that can't be blamed on dry air or postnasal drip warrants further investigation. Your family member's physician will probably want to get a chest x-ray to look for evidence of a tumor or perhaps a pleu-ral effusion, fluid in the sac encasing the lungs—assuming this kind of evaluation is consistent with your relative's goals of care. Remember that making a definitive diagnosis of lung cancer usually requires a biopsy, done either at the time of bronchoscopy (passing a special instrument through the mouth or nose and into the airways of the lungs) or via a surgical procedure, though sometimes removing fluid surrounding the lungs with a needle can lead to a diagnosis. These are all at least moderately invasive procedures. Treatment for lung cancer, if that turns out to be the diagnosis, is often very burdensome and not terribly effective, although oral targeted chemotherapy drugs are an option in a minority of cases.

Symptomatic Treatment

While treating the underlying cause of the cough is advisable whenever feasible, you may want to try various simple remedies to try to improve this annoying symptom. Everyone knows about cough drops. The most popular ingredients in cough drops are honey and menthol. But do they work? Nobody has definitively shown that either of them works—but neither has anyone shown that they don't work. If your family member has an infection producing his cough, he may find it soothing to take cough drops for a few days. If he has a noninfectious cause of the cough and the cough has lasted for days or even weeks, it will become evident that cough drops are not doing the job.

Two medications that are supposed to suppress coughing by their effect on the brain are codeine (available as a stand-alone medicine or in combination with acetaminophen as Tylenol #2 and Tylenol #3) and dextromethorphan (the active ingredient of brand name over-the-counter medications such as Robitussin). Codeine is an opioid medication that, like all opioids, is addictive and has many potential side effects, especially in older people: it is notorious for causing constipation and confusion. Moreover, it is a controlled substance, available only by prescription. This is a concern, not so much because I worry that your relative will become an addict and will start holding people up for cash to buy drugs, an unlikely outcome if the drug is prescribed for a short period of time, but rather because of the risk of *diversion*. Not long after the opioid epidemic was first identified in the United States, physicians, regulators, and public health officials realized that many legitimately prescribed medications end up in the hands of people for whom they have not been described, individuals who are themselves addicted and use the drug or who sell it to others. Whenever a medication such as codeine (a relatively weak opioid, but an opioid nonetheless) is prescribed for your relative, you will want to be very careful to restrict its use to your family member. For many years, codeine was thought to be an effective cough suppressant and was considered the "gold standard" by pharmacists and physicians. More recently, its effectiveness has been challenged. Since codeine is a potentially hazardous drug and it is not even clear that it works well to suppress coughing, I cannot recommend its routine use.

Dextromethorphan is available over the counter and has few side effects when taken in the recommended doses, but is a stimulant when taken in excessive quantities—and probably ineffective as a cough suppressant. If your family member wants to give it a try, you shouldn't expect much and you need to make sure he does not take more than the recommended amount of one teaspoon four times a day.

Another alleged cough suppressant is benzonatate (brand name Tessalon Perles), which works, to the extent that it does work, by numbing the respiratory passages, thus getting rid of the "tickle" that seems to stimulate coughing. The advantage of benzonatate is that it *isn't* an opioid and is not addictive. However, in high doses, it can cause seizures and an irregular heartbeat. In addition, the only group of patients in whom it's been shown to be at all effective is those with cancer. Tessalon Perles are available only by prescription, should be administered as directed, and should be kept out of the hands of children.

Many people are convinced that various herbal teas are helpful, especially when sweetened with honey. The evidence that this remedy actually works is scant, but it is the most harmless of all the symptomatic treatments. As long as your family member can boil water for tea safely and is able to pour the water without risking a burn—or if there is someone else to make the tea, and as long as he is able to drink a hot beverage from a cup, it's worth a try.

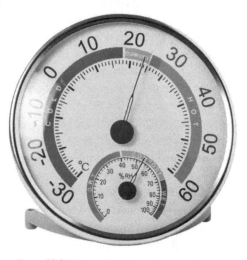

Figure 35.2. Hygrometer

Finally, as I mentioned earlier, you may want to use a humidifier in the winter when the heat is on. If you wish to know whether your family member's home is excessively dry, you can measure the humidity with a hygrometer (figure 35.2). This is a simple device that is often combined with a thermometer. The ideal degree of humidity is 40–50 percent.

Cough, in summary, can be a minor, self-limited nuisance, a sign of a serious medical problem, or something in between. Your job as a caregiver is to help sort out which it is and to find a way to soothe your family member's distress.

Box 35.1

Causes of Cough

- Infection (common cold, bronchitis, flu, pneumonia)
- Heart failure
- Lung cancer
- Medication side effect

Treatments for Cough

- Herbal remedies (honey, tea)
- Over-the-counter medications
- Opioids

CHAPTER 36

Nausea and Vomiting

As a caregiver, one of your main goals is to make your family member comfortable, and nausea and vomiting are decidedly unpleasant symptoms. Your first task when you learn that your relative has nausea or vomiting is to figure out whether she is having a serious problem that requires prompt medical attention or whether the condition is less dire, in which case you can start with home management.

How Serious Is the Nausea and Vomiting?

We have all experienced nausea and vomiting at some point in our lives. Aside from pregnancy, the most common cause is viral gastroenteritis, a self-limiting infection that spreads either through contaminated food or person to person. Even this source of nausea and vomiting can be serious in a frail older person if she cannot keep food or drink down, resulting in dehydration. If she throws up her medications, this can also have major consequences. Even if she is able to take her medicines, the doses may need to be adjusted if she is eating very little, as is the case with diabetes medication.

Another red flag is what is called "projectile vomiting," in which stomach contents are expelled violently and suddenly, often shooting out from your relative like a volcanic eruption. This symptom may be an indicator of an obstruction blocking the digested food from moving out of the stomach and into the small intestine. You should call the primary care doctor if you observe this phenomenon or if your family member describes her symptoms this way.

Nausea and vomiting are serious if your relative is throwing up bright red blood. She might also be throwing up material that looks like coffee grounds, which in fact is coagulated blood, blood that's been in the stomach for a while. In both instances, the problem requires prompt medical attention. Depending on your family member's goals of care, you may or may not want to go directly to the hospital, and if you do go to the hospital, you may or may not want treatment in an intensive care unit. But in any case, you will need to discuss the appropriate management with your relative's physician.

A prolonged period of vomiting—more than a couple of days—is another indicator that something serious may be going on. If your family member seems to have a viral gastroenteritis because the symptoms came on suddenly and she is able to eat toast and bananas and drink tea and clear juices, you might wait a couple of days to see how things go. But if after two days, she's no better, it's time to ask for professional input.

Finally, if your family member is having abdominal pain in addition to the nausea and vomiting, not just discomfort while she's in the process of throwing up, you should seek medical attention. In general, the additional symptoms she's having apart from the nausea and vomiting may provide the clue to what's going on.

What Other Symptoms Are Present?

I've already mentioned *abdominal pain*. If your family member has abdominal pain, even when she's not vomiting, you should bring this to the attention of her physician. If she has *fever*, this suggests an infectious process. Many run-of-the-mill cases of gastroenteritis are not associated with fever, and many older people who have an infection do not run a fever, but if your relative does have a fever, it points in the direction of an infection such as norovirus or rotavirus.

Another common accompaniment to nausea is *diarrhea*. When the two go together, the cause is often viral gastroenteritis. But if your relative is having both diarrhea and vomiting, she is losing fluids in two different ways, increasing her chance of dehydration. You will probably want to discuss what's happening with your family member's physician. He might want her to stop taking her fluid pill (diuretic) during this episode or to cut back on her diabetes medication.

When nausea is present without vomiting, a variety of other possible causes should be considered. Check whether your relative is having *chest pain* (heart attacks are sometimes associated with nausea). Ask about *dizziness*, which goes along with a variety of inner ear causes of nausea.

Once you've figured out how worried you should be and have asked about other symptoms, you are ready to begin to think about what might be causing the problem.

Triggers for Nausea

Nausea can be triggered by signals sent from the gastrointestinal tract, typically the stomach, by signals from the brain (the prosaically named "vomit center" or something called the "chemoreceptor trigger zone"), or from the inner ear (the vestibular or balance center) (figure 36.1).

In other words, nausea is perceived by your family member as a distinct

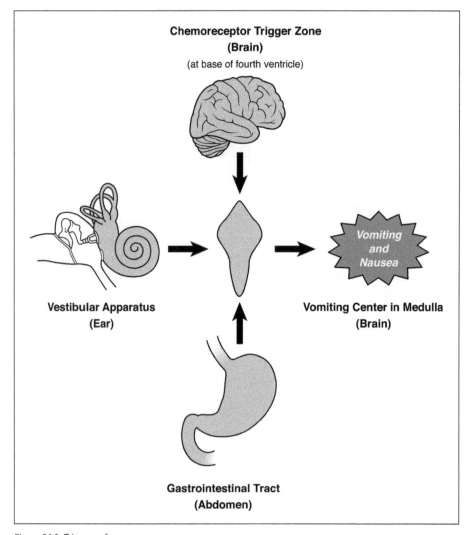

Chemoreceptor Trigger Zone (Brain)
(at base of fourth ventricle)

Vestibular Apparatus (Ear)

Vomiting and Nausea

Vomiting Center in Medulla (Brain)

Gastrointestinal Tract (Abdomen)

Figure 36.1. Triggers of nausea

sensation, but it may arise from an irritation in the stomach, from chemicals that trigger specific parts of the brain, or from a problem in the inner ear. Not surprisingly, a whole host of very different sorts of medical disorders result in nausea, and when the nausea is extreme, the effect is vomiting. The main *stomach problems* that can cause nausea are gastroenteritis (an infection) or gastritis (an inflammation of the lining of the stomach). Gastroenteritis, in turn, is either viral (outbreaks of norovirus and rotavirus are often in the news) or bacterial (Salmonella and E. coli are two common ones). Gastritis is typically due to a chemical irritant such as a nonsteroidal anti-inflammatory medication (either aspirin or a drug such as ibuprofen or naproxen) or alcohol. Also common is gastroparesis, which is delayed gastric emptying. In this condition, especially common in people with diabetes, food moves with difficulty from the stomach into the small intestine.

The most common *inner ear* causes of nausea arise from a problem with the balance organ, or vestibular system, that forms part of the inner ear along with the part devoted to hearing (the cochlea). Problems with the vestibular system include motion sickness, Ménière's disease, and acute labyrinthitis.

If your relative's nausea is due to a problem in the *brain*, what is referred to as central nausea (where the brain is the center and everything else is the periphery), the cause is likely to be medication or, far less commonly, a brain tumor.

There are also a number of other causes of nausea. I'll just mention one, and that's a heart attack. You may be starting to think that just about any symptom can indicate a heart attack—not just chest pain, but also shortness of breath, confusion, and now, apparently, nausea. That doesn't mean that every time your family member is a bit sick to her stomach, you should worry that she's having a heart attack. But it is a reason to pay attention to all the other symptoms your relative is experiencing as well as their severity.

According to fastmed.com, common causes of nausea and vomiting can be either internal or external.

Internal Causes

- Headaches

- Viral infections

- Heart attack

- Severe pain (from any source)

- Abdominal sources (appendicitis, hepatitis, kidney, or gallbladder issues)

- Pregnancy

External Causes

- Motion sickness

- Alcohol poisoning

- Food poisoning

- Medicines

Treatment of Nausea

Ideally, treatment of nausea involves eliminating the cause of the nausea. Viral gastroenteritis typically resolves on its own within a couple of days; motion sickness lasts only as long as your relative is in a car or on a boat, and nausea caused by medications is best addressed by stopping the offending drug. But you may want to provide short-term symptomatic relief while you are waiting for the underlying cause to resolve. What you need to realize is that there are different classes of medications that will prove useful, depending on whether the nausea arises from the stomach, the inner ear, or the brain. If the stomach problem is an ulcer or gastritis, in which pain results from acid irritating the lining of the stomach, the most effective treatment involves minimizing the amount of acid. That can be done by neutralizing existing acids with antacids or by decreasing the body's production of acid with a proton pump inhibitor, two of which are now available over the counter (lansoprazole, brand name Prevacid and omeprazole, brand name Prilosec).

If the stomach problem is due to gastroparesis, then a medication such as metoclopramide (brand name, Reglan) can stimulate the stomach muscles, pushing food along. This is a prescription medication and needs to be used with caution in older people as it can cause confusion and lethargy. Inner ear problems involving balance are often treated with meclizine, which is an antihistamine that has proved useful in this setting. An over-the-counter form is available as Bonine. Brain causes of nausea are sometimes treated with drugs such as haloperidol and droperidol, antipsychotic medications that are often used to treat nausea resulting from anesthetics or chemotherapy. These are potent medications with the potential for significant side effects and must be prescribed by a physician.

Complications of Nausea

Even routine gastroenteritis can be challenging to manage. As I discussed in the context of prolonged symptoms, it can produce dehydration from excess fluid loss, which, in turn, can result in dizziness, falls, and confusion. In addition to plying your family member with tea and clear juices to make up for the fluid she is losing, you may have to withhold medications such as diuretics, which are intended to promote fluid loss. Other medicines that she takes on a regular basis may also need to be held or the dose adjusted: Insulin or pills to lower blood sugar might need to be cut back and metformin, another medicine often used to treat diabetes, may need to be temporarily discontinued. You will need the advice of the primary physician if your family member has heart failure or diabetes and then begins vomiting.

Much of the time nausea and vomiting is a self-limited, minor nuisance, but sometimes it is more consequential.

That's what makes caregiving so challenging. Your personal experience helps, but only so much: frail older people get the same viral gastrointestinal ailments and food poisoning as everyone else, but they are also prone to other problems. Even if the cause of the symptom is minor, its effects—inability to swallow pills or development of dehydration—can be very serious. You have an important role to play in helping ensure your family member gets the right treatment at the right time and in the right place.

Box 36.1

Causes of Nausea and Vomiting

- Stomach problems
- Inner ear problems
- Central nervous system issues

Treatment of Nausea and Vomiting

- Antacids/proton pump inhibitor medications
- Antihistamines

Complications of Nausea and Vomiting

- Dehydration
- Dizziness

CHAPTER 37

Constipation

Constipation is one of those problems that's usually chronic, although it doesn't make it into the "top ten," and may get worse with age as your family member becomes less active and takes more medications. When constipation develops acutely, your relative may be in considerable distress. Your first challenge, as with other symptoms, is to figure out how serious the problem is.

How Serious Is It?

It helps to know whether constipation has been an issue for your relative in the past. If it's something that's plagued him before, more often than not—though not always—it's a recurrence of his same old problem. If he says he's regular as clockwork and cannot remember the last time he didn't move his bowels in a highly predictable way, you should explore further. One question to ask is how long it's been since his last movement. Many people slow down with age: there's nothing abnormal about going two or three days without a bowel movement, but five days is a long time. You will also want to know if he is having abdominal pain. He probably will feel somewhat uncomfortable if he's very constipated, but actual pain, especially if it's severe, is concerning. You should also ask if he's been having any blood in his stools. Bloody stools can arise simply from straining but can also denote a more serious problem. As cancer of the intestines progresses, for example, it might cause a blockage, preventing your family member from moving his bowels altogether. Checking his weight is also a good idea: if there's an underlying problem such as cancer that's now producing constipation, he may well be losing weight.

What's New That Might Be Causing Constipation?

A sudden change in bowel habits is often due to a new, constipating medication. Unfortunately, many types of medicines slow the bowels. The most common offenders include anticholinergic medications, such as antihistamines and some antidepressants (particularly the tricyclic antidepressants such as nortriptyline and amitriptyline), and opiates, strong pain medications such as morphine and its cousins (hydromorphone, oxycodone, fentanyl, and tramadol). The medicine most often used to treat Parkinson's disease, levodopa, one of the ingredients of Sinemet, is also notorious for inducing constipation. There are also some surprises: the antihypertensive drug, verapamil, which is a calcium channel blocker, often causes constipation.

A change in diet can also trigger constipation. Jews who observe Passover and radically alter their usual diet to substitute matzah for bread products often report they become severely constipated during this eight-day holiday period. If your family member stays with other family members for a few days or a week and is exposed to a new repertoire of foods, he may find he is constipated. Several days in the hospital can produce a similar effect, especially when combined with the lack of exercise associated with illness and hospitalization.

When medications or diet are plausible candidates for triggering constipation, your path is clear: if at all possible, discontinue the new medicine and resume the old diet. While you are waiting for these actions to have an effect, you will probably want to treat the constipation.

Common causes of constipation include

- Depression
- Reduced fluid intake or dehydration
- Side effects of medications
- Low dietary fiber
- Poor mobility
- Muscle weakness
- Disease processes

Treatments for Constipation

Your family member has almost undoubtedly experienced constipation at some point in his life and may have strong opinions about what remedies to use. Some of these old favorites, however, are to be avoided in older individuals. One popular approach, for example, is mineral oil, which works by lubricating the stool, facilitating its passage. Unfortunately, frail older people are at risk of aspirating mineral oil: instead of gliding from your relative's mouth into his gastrointestinal tract, it goes down "the wrong way" and ends up in the lungs, causing pneumonia. Another old standby is milk of magnesia. This product can be toxic to people with some degree of kidney dysfunction. It results in elevated magnesium levels, which are associated with central nervous system problems, muscle weakness, low blood pressure and, as if that is not enough, also with changes on the electrocardiogram. A third type of medication your family member may be familiar with is the stool softener, docusate (Colace). Docusate appears to be safe—it just has not been shown to be effective in treating constipation.

The current recommendation for treating constipation is to begin with a "bulk-forming agent," a fiber-containing medication that works by drawing water from the colon into the stool, increasing its bulk and stimulating contractions of the bowel. Popular bulking agents are bran or psyllium: one formulation is Metamucil, which is a powder available over the counter that is mixed into a glass of water or juice. If a bulk-forming agent is insufficient, the next step is to add an "osmotic laxative." These include liquids such as sorbitol or lactulose and the powder, polyethylene glycol (brand name Miralax), that he will need to add to water. These drugs suck liquid into the colon to make the stool easier to pass. Both sorbitol and polyethylene glycol are sold over the counter. If neither a bulk-forming nor an osmotic laxative does the job, then it's time to turn to a stimulant laxative. These drugs, such as the senna (brand name Dulcolax) or bisacodyl (brand name Senokot) stimulate the muscles in the bowel wall to contract, helping propel the stool. They can, however, cause severe cramping and may lead to loss of fluid and other important body chemicals.

If your family member doesn't have any of the red flags I mentioned earlier—blood in his stools, severe pain, or distension—but says he hasn't had a movement in several days and he's extremely uncomfortable, you may not want to use this stepwise algorithm. Instead, you will want to get things moving promptly with a stimulant and only then revert to the more systematic approach (table 37.1). In fact, your best bet may be to use a single bisacodyl (brand name Dulcolax) suppository, which could work as quickly as within fifteen minutes. Your relative may need an enema—introducing a chemical solution or just plain water directly into the rectum through a lubricated tube. While special enema kits are available at your local drug store, containing whatever you need to administer the enema, this is something you may want a visiting nurse to administer. It's definitely something to discuss with the health-care team.

Table 37.1
Types of Laxatives

Laxative Type	How They Work	Side Effects
Bulk-Forming (Ispaghula husk, Benefiber, fiber gel)	These laxatives add volume to your stool by absorbing water which makes it easier for your bowel to move waste through your colon to create a soft stool.	Gas, bloating, abdominal cramps, constipation if not taken with water
Osmotic (milk of magnesia, Movicol, MiraLax)	These don't add bulk to your stool, but draw water into the bowel by taking it from other areas of the body to soften the stool making it easier to pass.	Nausea, bloating, abdominal cramps, diarrhea, dehydration, increased thirst
Stimulant (Dulcolax, Senokot)	These work by irritating the colon muscles to induce bowel movement.	Dehydration, diarrhea, bloating, abdominal cramps, vomiting, nausea, rectal irritation, lazy bowel, which leads to further constipation (if taken long-term)

Prevention

Once you have dealt with the acute problem, you will want to take steps to prevent the constipation from recurring (see chapter 32, "Prevention"). The key considerations, aside from permanently eliminating any offending medications, are diet and exercise.

The main dietary recommendation is to eat plenty of fiber and drink lots of fluid. The Institute of Medicine suggests 21 grams of fiber for older women and 30 grams for older men. This doesn't have to come in the form of bran cereal—though bran flakes provide about 7 grams of fiber. Other good sources of fiber are

- Split peas (16 grams/cup)

- Lentils (15 grams/cup)

- Black beans (15 grams/cup)

- Lima beans (13 grams/cup)

- Artichokes (10 grams)

- Raspberries and blackberries (8 grams/cup)

- Pears (5 grams/cup)

In terms of fluid, the typical recommendation is to drink eight, 8-ounce glasses of water a day. A more realistic guideline is to drink a full glass of liquid with each meal (and eat three meals a day), plus a supplement of one glass between meals (that is, one between breakfast and lunch and another between lunch and dinner). Your relative will probably want to avoid drinking much after dinner as it may send him to the bathroom during the night.

Finally, how much exercise is enough to prevent constipation? I don't think anyone has the answer, but most physicians believe that getting up and moving around for ten or fifteen minutes several times a day is advisable.

You will probably want to become expert on certain symptoms that afflict many older people, and constipation may be one of those. In the majority of situations, you will be able to remedy the problem, which will be extremely gratifying to both you and your relative.

Box 37.1

Evaluating Constipation

- Ask about bloody stools, abdominal pain, or bloating
- Ask about new medications, dietary changes

Treating Constipation

- Avoid mineral oil, milk of magnesia
- If time permits, start with bulk-forming agent like Metamucil, then add osmotic laxative like Miralax, then stimulant such as Senokot

Preventing Constipation

- Diet: fiber, water
- Exercise: walk 10–15 minutes, several times daily

CHAPTER 38

Confusion

Whatever your family member's mental baseline, whether she is normally sharp as a tack, somewhat forgetful, or afflicted with dementia, she runs the risk of developing acute confusion. The sudden onset of confusion, which sometimes waxes and wanes over the course of a day and which may be associated with an unusual degree of sleepiness, is what geriatricians call *delirium* (see chapter 3, "Thinking like a Geriatrician: Geriatric Syndromes"). As a caregiver, you are likely to be the first to notice that something is not right with your relative. Since delirium is a serious condition, you should be ready to act quickly.

How Severe Is the Problem?

All cases of delirium are serious, but that doesn't necessarily mean you have to take your family member to the doctor or the hospital emergency department immediately. One exception is if you cannot wake your relative up, if she is so sleepy that she can't talk to you, let alone eat something or get up and go to the bathroom. She doesn't have to be in a coma—completely unable to respond—for you to be worried. But if she cannot take fluids or her medications, and if the lethargy does not wear off after an hour or two, she needs to be evaluated promptly.

Another special circumstance is acute confusion shortly after a fall. If your family member fell and hit her head and now she's confused, she needs a neurological examination, probably including a computed tomography (CT) scan of her brain. Even fairly minor trauma can result in a subdural hematoma, bleeding around the brain, sometimes days or even weeks after the initial event. This isn't a problem you can manage on your own, at home.

What Other Symptoms Are Present?

You can look for clues as to the cause of the confusion by probing for other symptoms. Some of the most common causes of delirium are *pain* and *infection*. You can ask your family member if anything hurts. In particular, does it burn when she goes to the bathroom? Are her knees acting up? You may also want to inquire about common infections: Does she have a sore throat, suggestive of an upper respiratory infection? Is she coughing, perhaps indicating pneumonia or bronchitis? Has she been running to the bathroom a lot, possibly indicative of a urinary tract infection? It's also worth asking about a fall, even though she may not remember it. A mnemonic for possible causes of delirium is included in box 38.1.

Is Medication the Culprit?

Medications are a common cause of delirium, accounting for close to half of all cases. Check whether your family member has recently started a new medicine: the main offenders are drugs affecting the central nervous system such as antianxiety drugs, antidepressants, and antiseizure medicine, but drugs used to treat excess stomach acid, anti-inflammatory medications,

Box 38.1

Causes of Confusion

- Metabolic: hyponatremia (low sodium), hypoglycemia (low sugar), hypoxemia (low oxygen)

- Infective: urinary tract infection, pneumonia

- Structural: subarachnoid hemorrhage (brain bleed), urinary retention

- Toxic: drugs (e.g., digoxin, lithium) or poisons

- Environmental: being in the hospital or emergency department

Source: G. Caplan, "Managing Delirium in Older Patients," *Australian Prescriber* 34, no. 1 (2011): 16–18. doi:10.18773/austprescr.2011.012.

and the heart medication, digoxin, are also potential causes of delirium. If any of these medications were recently prescribed, call the doctor right away and make sure your relative does not take another dose unless you have cleared this with him. Also think about over-the-counter medications: antihistamines, for example, which are used against allergies, itching, and sometimes for sleep, can all trigger confusion. So, too, can medications used to treat diarrhea (loperamide, brand name Imodium) and many pain medications, including the over-the-counter nonsteroidal anti-inflammatory drugs (ibuprofen, naproxen, and related medications). All such drugs should be discontinued immediately. If the delirium lifts, which may take a couple of days, you have the answer.

Some medications that cause delirium include

- Anesthetics

- Anticholinergics (e.g., benztropine, atropine, scopolamine)

- Anticonvulsants (e.g., phenytoin, valproic acid, carbamazepine, topiramate, levetiracetam)

- Antidepressants (e.g., amitriptyline, imipramine, doxepin)

- Antiemetics

- Antihistamines

- Antiparkinsonian agents (e.g., levodopa, trihexyphenidyl, amantadine)

- Antipsychotics

- Antispasmodics (e.g., oxybutynin)

- Corticosteroids

- Digoxin

- H2-receptor antagonists (e.g., cimetidine, famotidine, nizatidine, ranitidine)

- Muscle relaxants

- Nonsteroidal anti-inflammatory drugs (NSAIDs)

- Opioids

- Sedative hypnotics (e.g., alcohol, barbiturates, benzodiazepines, chloral hydrate)

Some Simple Tests to Carry Out

Look into your medical bag and pull out the instruments that might shed light on the situation (see chapter 21, "Your Medical Bag"). To start with, you may want to check your relative's *temperature*. Your family member might have an infection even if she doesn't have a fever; but if she does have a fever, an infection is far more likely. Use your watch or your sphygmomanometer (blood pressure cuffs usually have a built-in pulse reader) to measure the *pulse*, or heart rate. An irregular heart rhythm, whether resulting in a very fast or a very slow heartbeat, means that the amount of blood flowing to the brain is reduced, which may result in confusion. Use the sphygmomanometer to check for orthostatic hypotension—blood pressure that falls with a change in position. You will need to take the blood pressure when your family member is sitting and then again after she has been standing for a couple of minutes. A drop of twenty points or more in the systolic blood pressure (upper number) suggests your relative may be dehydrated, resulting in blood chemistries that are out of whack, which can cause delirium. If you find any of these signs, you should alert your relative's primary care physician.

Depending on your family member's situation, you might perform a few other tests. If she has some form of chronic lung disease or pneumonia, she is at risk of hypoxia, or too little oxygen in her system, so you may want to check her oxygen level using an *oximeter*. If she is a diabetic, you should check her blood sugar with a *glucometer* as very low sugars can cause delirium. Very high blood sugars can also cause delirium indirectly, by forcing the body to excrete a great deal of fluid in its effort to get rid of excess sugar, which in turn results in dehydration and other problems.

Your Role in Managing Delirium

The most important task in dealing with delirium is to identify and eliminate whatever triggered the confusion in the first place. But even when the culprit has been dealt with, whether with medication to treat an infection, by discontinuing the drug that triggered the problem, or by giving fluids to reverse dehydration, delirium may take time to resolve. Usually, it begins to clear in a day or two, but you might have to wait a week or longer for it to go away entirely. In some cases, delirium can persist for several weeks. During the period when delirium is improving but is still present, you have an important role to play in easing the symptoms associated with confusion. Your family member might hallucinate (see things that aren't there) or have delusions (believe things that aren't true), either of which can be frightening. Don't even try to correct her perceptions; rather, let her know that you will keep her safe. Being in a familiar environment with someone she knows and trusts is very reassuring. Another common manifestation of delirium is lethargy. If your relative dozes off frequently, she might miss meals and not drink any fluids, which can further exacerbate her confusion. You can help by waking her up regularly and giving her something to eat and drink, sitting with her while she has her meal or her snack to make sure she stays awake enough to swallow safely.

Another strategy for alleviating the symptoms of delirium is to avoid excess stimulation. Your family member may already be disoriented—she's not entirely sure where she is or what's happening around her—so the last thing she needs is a loud or chaotic environment. Rather than having the television on and frequent visitors, you might want to play soothing music on the radio or CD player. Don't try to go for a walk or take your relative on an outing; just sit quietly with her.

In the hospital, physicians may order physical restraints (lap belts, "Posey vests," or side rails) or chemical restraints (typically potent, antipsychotic medications) for your relative if she is delirious. The goal is to keep her safe, but the price is considerable: restraints are an affront to her dignity and some-times result in accidents, for example, if she falls while trying to climb over the bedrails. Antipsychotic medications, while reasonable as a last resort, are associated with a host of side effects, from lethargy to stiffness and even, on rare occasions, death. If you can keep your delirious family member at home and manage her symptoms, you will be doing her a tremendous favor.

As with many other symptoms, sorting out what they mean—their cause and what to do about them—depends heavily on what physicians call the history. By definition, if your relative is confused, she cannot provide much if any history, information about what medications she takes and what else she has recently experienced. By providing that crucial information, you can help with diagnosis. Once there's a diagnosis, your special, intimate knowledge can go a long way to helping resolve your family member's delirium.

Box 38.2

Evaluating Acute Confusion

- Look for evidence of a recent fall
- Check if a new medication was recently started
- See if fever, cough, or frequent urination is present

Managing Acute Confusion at Home

- Remove or treat the cause of confusion
- Ensure adequate hydration

CHAPTER 39

Dizziness

Staying upright is no mean feat. Your family member, like the rest of the species, is precariously perched on two thin, bony sticks we call legs. Many forces conspire to topple him: gravity, uneven terrain, and other moving things in our environment, whether cars, animals, or other people. But he needs to remain vertical in order to walk or run, to be able to see what's going on around him, and to protect his brain from trauma. Not surprisingly, given how important it is to remain erect, humans have evolved a warning system to alert us whenever we are at risk of keeling over. We perceive such a threat as "dizziness."

Because staying upright is so important, we have many different mechanisms that contribute to maintaining our position: we use our visual system (our eyes), the vestibular system (balance organs within the ear), and proprioception (special nerves in the legs that detect where we are in space). Even though more than one system may have to fail for us to actually fall over, a problem in any one domain will trigger the sensation of dizziness and put us on our guard. Two parts of the body serve as coordinating centers: the *inner ear* and the *cerebellum*. The inner ear helps maintain equilibrium with loop-shaped canals (the semi-circular canals) that contain fluid and hair-like sensors. The fluid in the canals flows in response to motion, triggering the sensors, which in turn send a message to the brain. The *cerebellum* is the balance organ of the brain. It controls movement by receiving input from nerves throughout the body that provide information about position and sending messages to the muscles of the body directing motion.

Your first challenge is to pin down what your family member means if he says he feels dizzy. Does he mean he thinks he's going to faint? I'm going to call that "light-headedness." Or does he mean he feels unsteady or that his head (or the room) feels as though it's spinning (vertigo)? I'm going to call unsteadiness or vertigo "balance problems." Figuring out to which category his dizziness belongs is the initial step in getting to the bottom of the problem.

What Other Symptoms Are Present?

If your family member is experiencing light-headedness, he may not be getting enough blood flow to the brain. You will want to find out if he's fallen or come close to falling. You might also ask about palpitations since a rapid heartbeat, or tachyarrhythmia, can result in the heart failing to pump enough blood into the circulation—it's so busy pumping that it doesn't have time to fill up with blood and ejects only small amounts into the circulation. Chest pain is another concerning symptom in this setting: if the heart muscle isn't itself getting enough blood delivered, it may be too weak to pump properly.

On the other hand, if your relative is having a balance problem, you will want to begin to figure out if the source is in the ear (peripheral), or in the brain (central). When the trouble is with the ear, your family member may report he's having trouble hearing. Alternatively, or in addition, he may describe a ringing in his ears (tinnitus). The diagnosis is probably Ménière's disease or acute labyrinthitis, both of which are annoying and treatable, but are not emergency situations. If the trouble is in the brain, your relative may have other neurologic symptoms such as slurred speech (dysarthria) or problems with coordination. Particularly worrisome are nausea and vomiting: these symptoms may accompany a stroke involving the balance center of the cerebellum. The presence of either neurologic symptoms or vomiting is a reason to seek immediate medical attention.

Collecting Other Information

Once you have concluded the situation isn't an emergency and you've learned about other symptoms your family member has along with his light-headedness or vertigo, you are ready to gather a bit more data. If your relative is light-headed (or if he's having difficulty further characterizing his symptoms and just repeats that he's "dizzy"), you should consider taking his blood pressure. Low blood pressure—whether from medication or insufficient fluid intake or loss of blood—is often the reason for light-headedness. If the blood pressure is normal, you will want to check it again after your family member has been standing for a minute or two. When the systolic blood pressure (first number) drops twenty points or more with standing up, your relative has orthostatic hypotension. Low blood pressure, whether at rest or only with standing up, should be reported to the primary care physician promptly. Your family member's blood pressure medication may need to be stopped, at least for a while or, in some cases, he may need intravenous fluids to correct the problem. The right approach will depend on the severity of his symptoms and on the goals of care. If he's woozy but not confused, and if he wants to avoid hospitalization and you're available to provide care, it may be reasonable to put him to bed, stop his blood pressure medications, and ply him with juice and soda. If he's very light-headed and orthostatic but wants to avoid aggressive medical interventions, the best course of action may be to take him to the physician's office or an urgent care center where he can get intravenous fluids over the course of a few hours.

Another easy step for you to take is to measure your family member's pulse. If it is very irregular or either unusually fast or slow, you may have found the cause of his dizziness. You should be aware that a seemingly normal pulse does not prove that an abnormal heart rhythm *isn't* the problem. If your relative's pulse is very elevated, say 150 beats a minute, many of those beats will be too faint for you to detect: you might erroneously conclude that his heart rate is 75 when it's really twice that. The arrhythmia might also be episodic, causing intermittent dizziness, and not detectable at the moment you choose to measure the pulse.

If your family member is light-headed and has diabetes, treated with either insulin or pills, you should do a finger stick blood test to check his sugar. If you do not have access to a glucometer, you may want to go ahead and give him a glass of orange juice to see if his light-headedness improves.

Is Medication the Culprit?

As with so many acute symptoms, medication may be the culprit. Usually it's a new medication, so you should find out if any drugs have been started recently. Sometimes the problem is a medicine your family member has been on for an extended period of time but the amount of drug in his blood has acutely risen, either because he took extra pills, because he's having trouble metabolizing the drug, for ex-

ample, because of a decline in kidney function or because of an interaction with still another medicine.

Many medications produce dizziness by their effect, intentional or incidental, on blood pressure. Drugs that are intended to lower blood pressure are obvious candidates—they can overshoot their target. Various cardiac medications that were prescribed for some reason other than lowering blood pressure can also affect the pressure: beta blockers (such as metoprolol and atenolol) are used to treat angina, as are nitrates (for example, isosorbide). Medications that affect the central nervous system are best known for causing confusion, but in some people, they trigger light-headedness. Examples include opiates (for pain), antihistamines (for itching or allergies), and drugs against anxiety (benzodiazepines such as lorazepam). Medicines that can trigger dizziness if the amount in the bloodstream becomes too high include phenytoin (brand name Dilantin), used to treat seizures, and digoxin, sometimes used to treat heart failure.

Managing Dizziness

If the dizziness seems to have a central origin—vomiting that points to a possible cerebellar disturbance or slurred speech that suggests a stroke—you will not be able to manage the problem without medical input. If the symptoms suggest a peripheral origin—a spinning sensation when your relative gets up from a chair or trouble hearing—the problem is probably not quite so urgent and you may want to try addressing it at home.

Your most basic step will be to advise your family member to get up slowly and to stand still for a moment before walking. He might have "benign positional vertigo," which is just what it sounds like—vertigo on changing from lying to sitting or sitting to standing. Allowing the body time to equilibrate when changing position is the way to deal with this condition.

Another step, if there's any indication that your family member is dizzy because he's slightly dehydrated, is to make sure he gets plenty to drink. He might have an impaired thirst mechanism—most older people do—so he literally does not feel thirsty even when he needs fluid, or he may have developed a way to compensate for difficulty walking to the kitchen to get something to drink by drinking less. You can fill a pitcher with water, juice, iced tea, or whatever beverage he enjoys and keep it close to him. You will want to avoid drinks such as coffee that are diuretics—that will make him go to the bathroom and lose even more fluid. If he has trouble pouring liquid out of the pitcher, you might try giving him a straw. If your relative normally takes a diuretic for heart failure or high blood pressure, you should consult with his physician about holding off on taking that medicine for a day or two.

One medication that is commonly used to treat dizziness is the antihistamine meclizine. This is available by prescription as Antivert or over the counter as the anti-motion sickness drug, Bonine. It can be helpful if the problem is Ménière's disease, a disorder that causes ringing in the ear and progressive hearing loss. You should be aware that antihistamines can cause sedation, dry mouth, and confusion, so they should be used with caution in frail older people. Moreover, while Ménière's may recur from time to time, each episode is self-limiting—the vertigo will go away, usually within days, regardless of whether your relative takes any medication.

Other important ways to manage dizziness do not involve treatment of the condition, but rather prevention of its complications. Using a cane can diminish the chance that your family member will fall because he's feeling dizzy. The same goes for other safety measures such as removing potentially hazardous area rugs and electrical cords. Adequate lighting and a nonskid bath mat are also advisable. Your relative should not put himself at increased risk by driving a car or using a potentially dangerous device such as an iron if he is light-headed.

Dizziness is another of those symptoms that we're all somewhat familiar with. It can indicate a mild, self-limiting problem or a major, life-threatening disorder. In either case, you are the key to figuring out which it is, what to do about it, and how to make your relative comfortable.

Box 39.1

Dizziness

Types of Dizziness

- Balance problem—peripheral (inner ear) or central (brain disturbance)
- Light-headedness—dehydration, irregular heart beat

Simple Management Aids

- Get up slowly
- Drink plenty of fluids
- Question new medications

CHAPTER 40

Bleeding

We are probably hardwired to get at least a little anxious at the sight of blood. Some people faint, others become squeamish, but we are all programmed to regard blood outside the body as abnormal. Blood belongs hidden inside, coursing through our blood vessels; it's not surprising that the sight of blood should trigger an alarm. There's a good reason why a "red flag" is, in fact, red. So, when your family member tells you she's bleeding or you see her bleeding, you will want to be on the alert.

The normal response of the body to bleeding, to the leakage of blood outside of the confines of the arterial or venous systems, is to produce a clot to stop the bleeding. Clotting is actually a sophisticated biochemical process that involves platelets, one type of blood cell, and thirteen different biochemical "factors," substances that are crucial to the coagulation cascade (coagulation is just medical jargon for clotting). If clotting doesn't take place or if the coagulation process is unable to counteract the forces causing bleeding, there's a problem. A large knife wound, for example, is not something that the normal clotting mechanism can handle, although a small nick in the skin usually is. That said, "bleeding" is very different if it is from the skin, if it's from the gastrointestinal tract—the stomach or the colon—if it's from the nose, or if it's hidden away in the brain or the abdominal cavity. Your response will need to vary depending on the type of bleeding.

Bleeding from the Skin

Your family member may discover that her skin has become thin and fragile, that she develops bruises and cuts with only minimal trauma. Usually, small cuts will respond to pressure and the bleeding will stop in a couple of minutes. Sometimes, especially with larger cuts or if your relative takes aspirin or a blood thinner such as warfarin on a regular basis, the bleeding does not stop promptly. If the cut appears very deep or if it's longer than an inch, it may need medical attention. Otherwise, you can try to tend to the wound yourself and only go to the hospital emergency department or urgent care center if your interventions are unsuccessful. The first step is to clean the cut with soap and water and to apply pressure using a clean cloth. If persistent pressure for a good two minutes does not do the trick, you will probably want to get a product such as wound seal powder from your medical bag (see chapter 21, "Your Medical Bag"). Alternatively, you could use steri-strips (figure 40.1), special adhesive tape that holds the two edges of a cut together, much the way stitches do. They are a little trickier to apply than are wound powder or liquid, which turn into a glue-like material when they react with blood.

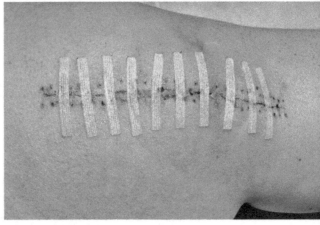

Figure 40.1. Steri-strips

Once the bleeding has stopped, you will need to cover the wound with a sterile gauze dressing. Nonstick gauze is preferable as it is less likely to pull healthy skin off when you remove it. You will secure the dressing with tape, ideally hypoallergenic tape to avoid an allergic reaction. You should make sure that these items are stored in your family member's medicine chest. Once the dressing has been applied, either you or a nurse will need to change it every couple of days and check to be sure there are no signs of infection such as redness, very warm skin, or pus.

You will also want to think about strategies to prevent future bleeding episodes, recognizing that fragile skin is very prone to tearing. For example, you may want to be sure your relative's home is well lit so she can see obstacles in her path. Another environmental modification that may be useful is getting rid of poorly secured throw rugs that slip or slide. Your family member can often decrease the risk of falling if she uses an assistive device such as a walker or cane—even in her home. Avoiding aspirin or other nonsteroidal anti-inflammatory medications (for example, naproxen and ibuprofen) decreases the chance of prolonged bleeding.

Bleeding from the Gastrointestinal Tract

The other major site of bleeding, apart from the skin, is the intestinal tract. Your family member might report that she has just vomited bright red blood. She is understandably very alarmed. This is not a situation for you to manage on your own: you should contact your relative's primary care provider right away and will probably be instructed to go to the emergency department. Even if the focus of care is exclusively on comfort, special steps are needed to halt the bleeding and keep your family member as comfortable as possible.

Bright red blood might also come out the other end of the gastrointestinal tract—your relative may tell you about or show you blood in the toilet bowl. Sometimes the amount of blood seems far greater than it actually is because the blood stains the water in the toilet red. This kind of bleeding also warrants medical attention, first to determine if the bleeding is in fact from the gastrointestinal tract or if it's from the vagina or the bladder. If the bleeding is from the rectum, the physician will want to determine if the problem is something minor, such as hemorrhoids, or major such as cancer, or any of a variety of other problems in between these two extremes. How far to investigate the source will depend on your family member's goals of care and on what procedures she is able or willing to tol-

erate. Figuring out the cause of lower gastrointestinal bleeding may necessitate a colonoscopy (figure 40.2) and, if a malignant tumor is found, major surgery.

Bleeding from the gastrointestinal tract can show up in ways other than bright red blood. Vomiting what looks like coffee grounds typically occurs when there has been bleeding in the stomach, whether from gastritis (an irritation to the stomach lining), an ulcer, cancer, or some rarer problem. If the blood has been around for a while, it reacts with the acid in the stomach and develops the classic coffee grounds appearance. You will want to consult with your relative's primary care physician,

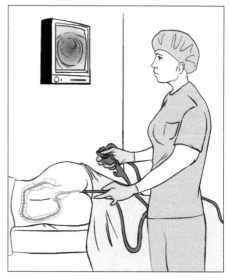

Figure 40.2. Colonoscopy

much as you would if she threw up bright red blood. The appropriate intervention will once again depend on her goal of care: if the focus is on aggressive medical care, an upper endoscopy (figure 40.3) to look into the stomach and small intestine may be warranted, but if the focus is on comfort care, a day or two of resting the stomach by not eating plus a course of anti-ulcer medication (usually a proton pump inhibitor such as omeprazole) and avoidance of aspirin and alcohol may be the way to proceed.

If your relative has bleeding in the stomach that does not trigger vomiting, the blood will make its way out of the body by passing through her intestines and rectum. The result will be black stools rather than overtly bloody stools or blood in the toilet bowl. Time pressure is less intense with this symptom than with bright red blood, but it, too, warrants medical attention. The possi-

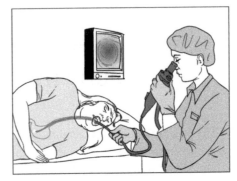

Figure 40.3. Upper endoscopy

ble causes and the options for diagnosis and treatment are much the same, however. Your family member should discontinue potential precipitants such as alcohol or aspirin-type medications, at least temporarily. If her goal is to focus on quality of life, an empiric trial of an anti-ulcer medication may be in order. If her goal is to live as long as possible, regardless of the personal cost, her physician may opt for an upper endoscopy to literally scope out the situation.

Nosebleeds

A third type of bleeding problem is nosebleeds. These are especially common during the winter when the heat is on and your family member's home may be very dry. They also occur in the setting of a cold or allergies if your relative has been blowing her nose very forcefully, or if your relative uses oxygen through nasal prongs. You are probably very familiar with nosebleeds and know that your family member should bend slightly forward, pinch

off the nostril from which the blood is coming, and apply an icepack. Sometimes that strategy is insufficient and your relative will need a physician to pack her nose with gauze to staunch the bleeding. Occasionally, particularly in the setting of recurrent nosebleeds, a blood vessel in the nose is leaking and needs to be cauterized—or sealed off with an electric current. That's a job for an ear, nose, and throat specialist (otolaryngologist).

To prevent future nosebleeds, you will want to remind your family member to blow her nose gently. She can moisten the inside of her nose with a saline mist or gel that is available over the counter. You may also want to set up a cool mist humidifier in her bedroom to keep adequate moisture in the air while the heat is on (see chapter 35, "Cough").

Other Sites of Visible Bleeding

Two other possible sites for visible bleeding are the vagina and the urinary tract. In both cases, your family member might notice blood in the toilet bowl and it may be difficult to figure out the exact source. Is it coming from the bladder? The uterus? The intestines? How urgently your relative needs medical attention will depend on how heavy the bleeding is, but you will need to contact the primary care physician to figure out what's going on.

Internal Bleeding— Brain and Other Sites

So far, I've talked about bleeding that you can see: when blood comes out of the skin, the gastrointestinal tract, or the nose, your family member is obviously having a bleeding problem. Internal bleeding is at least as concerning but much more difficult to detect. Head trauma can result in a *subdural hematoma*, or bleeding under the outer layer of the brain. This may develop weeks after the traumatic event, so you might realize that something is amiss only when or if she becomes progressively confused. If your family member is on blood thinning medication such as warfarin and the amount in her system is too great, she is at risk of bleeding in a variety of sites, including the retroperitoneum, the area behind the gastrointestinal tract. The symptoms of a *retroperitoneal bleed* include back and flank pain; often there is prominent bruising in the groin or flank.

You should think about a possible internal bleed if your family member develops odd symptoms after a fall or if she notices unusual bruises. This is not a problem you can manage yourself: your role is to notice something is amiss and alert your relative's physician.

Bleeding runs the gamut from a small cut requiring nothing more than a band aid to major internal bleeding in the brain or the stomach (box 40.1). If you are alert to the possibilities, you can help manage this condition—whether by dressing a wound, taking your relative to the local hospital emergency department, or discussing with her and her physician how aggressively to pursue the diagnosis.

Box 40.1

Causes and Management of Bleeding

- Skin: have gauze, tape, wound powder in the medicine chest

- Nose: icepack for minor bleed, gauze packing for major bleed, cauterization for oozing blood vessel

- Gastrointestinal tract (stomach, intestines): endoscopy (upper, lower) may be needed to diagnose cause; discuss whether tests are consistent with goals of care

- Brain: serious problem that may develop days or weeks after a fall

CHAPTER 41

Abdominal Pain

Acute abdominal pain is one of those symptoms that can denote a minor nuisance or a life-threatening medical problem, or any of a variety of conditions in between. At the minor nuisance end of the spectrum are disorders such as gas pain; at the dangerous end is a ruptured appendix or ischemic bowel (lack of oxygen to the intestine, causing tissue death). What makes abdominal pain particularly tricky to assess is that older people sometimes experience relatively mild symptoms even though they are in the midst of a medical crisis. Other symptoms that you might ordinarily rely on to help you figure out how serious the problem is, such as fever, may be absent altogether.

Odds are you are going to need medical assistance to address abdominal pain, but you can gather some information that will help guide the decision about whether you should send you relative straight to the emergency room, bring him to the doctor's office, or whether you can wait a day and see how things are going. It's also helpful to realize that abdominal pain usually indicates the problem is in the abdomen, rather than referred pain from some other part of the body, so you may want to begin by thinking about what organs are located in the abdomen. You should remember that the pelvic organs—bladder and, depending on whether your relative is male or female, either the prostate or uterus and ovaries—are right below the abdominal organs, which include the esophagus, stomach, large intestine, small intestine, gallbladder, and liver.

How Severe Is the Pain?

Having just said that sometimes the pain can be mild even in the presence of a major problem, the converse is not true: if the pain is severe, your relative most likely needs medical attention. Being "doubled over with pain" indicates the pain is severe. Experiencing pain with the slightest movement is another indication of severity.

Where Is the Pain Located?

You are probably aware that pain in the lower right side of the abdomen could mean appendicitis (figure 41.1). You may also know that pain in the upper right side of the abdomen suggests a possible gallbladder problem. In fact, the pain may not be easy for your family member to localize precisely. If he does specify just where the pain is, that alone is not enough to make a diagnosis. It may, however, narrow down the possibilities. If the pain is in the lower left, it's almost certainly not a gallstone or an ulcer. If it's in the central upper part of the abdomen, it's probably not constipation.

RIGHT		LEFT
Gallstones Stomach ulcer Pancreatitis	Stomach ulcer Heartburn/Indigestion Pancreatitis Gallstones Epigastric hernia	Stomach ulcer Duodenal ulcer Biliary colic Pancreatitis
Kidney stones Urinary infection Constipation Lumbar hernia	Pancreatitis Early appendicitis Inflammatory bowel Small bowel Umbilical hernia	Kidney stones Diverticular disease Constipation Infammatory bowel
Appendicitis Constipation Pelvic pain Groin pain (inguinal hernia)	Appendicitis Constipation Pelvic Pain Groin pain (inguinal hernia)	Diverticular disease Pelvic pain Groin pain (inguinal hernia)

Figure 41.1. Abdominal pain locations

What Other Symptoms Are Present?

Your family member may have *diarrhea* as well as abdominal pain. This is common in run-of-the-mill gastroenteritis, or what is sometimes referred to as a "stomach bug." The pain in this case is typically crampy and often gets better—transiently—after your family member moves his bowels

Nausea and *vomiting* are other symptoms that may accompany abdominal pain (see chapter 36, "Nausea and Vomiting"). All three may be part and parcel of gastroenteritis, in which case the pain usually abates after your relative has thrown up. If the vomiting is "projectile," the stomach contents come shooting out as though they've been fired by a gun, the problem is usually more serious than simple gastroenteritis. Sometimes your family member cannot keep anything down, which may indicate a blockage between the stomach and the intestine; in other situations, he can keep down liquids and perhaps toast or a banana. If he is vomiting along with having pain and what comes out is bloody or looks like coffee grounds, indicating old blood, he might have an ulcer or gastritis (an inflammation of the lining of the stomach) and you should consult his physician.

Fever is something else to look out for. I mentioned that the absence of fever does not prove anything; however, the presence of fever does. If your relative has a fever, especially if it's 101°F or greater, that's cause for concern. He might have appendicitis, an inflamed

or even a burst appendix. He might have diverticulitis, an inflammation of the diverticula, small outpouchings of the intestines that are very common in older people. Or he might have ischemic bowel, a dangerous condition in which there is lack of blood supply to part of the intestine causing death of tissue, analogous to a heart attack where lack of oxygen causes death of a segment of heart muscle.

Poor appetite is almost universal since most people don't feel like eating when they are experiencing abdominal pain. If your relative doesn't just have a poor appetite, but also has *weight loss,* the combination suggests a more serious problem. Even if the pain is new, weight loss indicates the underlying problem may have been going on for a while. Cancer, for instance, might take away your family member's appetite before the primary tumor has gotten large enough to cause pain.

You should be sure to ask about *constipation* (see chapter 37, "Constipation"). Constipation is another very common issue in older people, especially if they are not very mobile, if they don't drink much, and if their diet isn't rich in fruit and vegetables. Mild constipation results in your relative straining when he goes to the bathroom. More severe constipation results in his not going for days. Very severe constipation can even produce "impaction," or a large mass of hard stool that is stuck in the colon. If your relative has a history of recurrent constipation and his symptoms are identical to what he typically experiences when he gets very constipated, you may feel comfortable going ahead and treating the constipation. If you are unsure or there is a possibility of impaction, he will require medical attention.

Your relative may have *burning on urination* or find he has to go to the bathroom unusually frequently. These are typical signs of a urinary tract infection. This kind of infection is common in older people: your family member may have had such infections in the past and be able to say he feels just the way he did the last time he had a bladder infection. If you transmit this information to the primary care physician, she may be willing to prescribe antibiotics without actually seeing her patient. Some physicians will want to check a urine specimen; others may be willing to treat without a lab test; still others may be willing to make sure you have a supply of the appropriate antibiotic on hand to use whenever such symptoms occur.

Occasionally, abdominal pain will be associated with sweating and confusion. If you check your relative's vital signs, you may discover a rapid heartrate and low blood pressure. This combination is usually indicative of a life-threatening problem such as perforation of the intestine, infection in the bloodstream (sepsis), or a ruptured aneurysm (blood vessel). You will probably want to call an ambulance and take your family member to the nearest emergency room. Even if you have decided that the main focus of his care is comfort, the hospital may be best equipped to make him comfortable. In this situation, you will want to be sure that you bring documentation of his wishes, such as a signed out-of-hospital do-not-resuscitate (DNR) form or a Physician Orders for Life-Sustaining Treatment (POLST) form, along with you.

Duration of Symptoms

We're only talking about acute problems in this section, so abdominal pain that's lasted for weeks or longer would qualify as chronic, not acute. But the pain might have been developing gradually over a couple of days (as with constipation, for instance) or it might have come on with a bang (more typical of gastroenteritis). Some conditions, such as gastroenteritis, usually last two or maybe three days and then start to improve. If your relative shows all the hallmarks of gastroenteritis—crampy abdominal pain, diarrhea, nausea, vomiting, and low-grade fever—but he isn't getting better after three days, you should be asking what's going on. He might have a more serious form of gastroenteritis such as a Salmonella infection and may need a course of antibiotics. Or he might have a condition such as clostridium difficile, an infection that typically results when antibiotics given for some other condition kill off the usual intestinal bacteria (the normal "bowel flora"), allowing clostridium to thrive. This, too, warrants a call to the physician, who will probably want a stool specimen to make a definitive diagnosis. Treatment involves a course of antibiotics.

Is Medication the Cause?

Just as antibiotics can result in abdominal pain if they promote the growth of the clostridium difficile bacterium, other medications can also trigger abdominal pain. The culprit is often one of the nonsteroidal anti-inflammatory medications such as ibuprofen (brand name Motrin) or naproxen (brand name Naprosyn). These drugs may irritate the lining of the stomach, resulting in gastritis—which just means inflammation of the stomach. Nausea and abdominal pain are the most common symptoms of this condition. If gastritis goes unchecked for a long period of time and your family member continues taking the offending agent, he may end up with an ulcer. Ulcers are another cause of abdominal pain. They are usually accompanied by bleeding, either evident as black stools or, if your relative throws up, as material that looks like coffee grounds.

The appropriate approach to treatment will depend on your relative's goals of care. If his goal of care is life-prolongation, the primary care physi-cian may recommend an endoscopy to distinguish between gastritis, an ulcer, or stomach cancer, all of which can cause medication-associated abdominal pain. If your relative's main goal of care is comfort or maintaining his level of function, the primary care physician will probably advocate stopping the offending medication and starting treatment with a proton pump inhibitor such as omeprazole (brand name Prilosec) to promote healing and ameliorate the symptoms. She will need to come up with an alternative treatment for whatever condition prompted the use of an anti-inflammatory medication in the first place.

You can play a valuable role in the initial evaluation of your relative's abdominal pain (box 41.1). By asking how severe it is, where it's located, how long it's been going on, and what other symptoms are present, and by considering his goals of care, you can make sure your family member gets the treatment that's right for him.

Box 41.1

Evaluating Abdominal Pain

- How severe is it?
- Where is it located?
- How long has it been going on?
- What other symptoms are present?
- Have any new medications been prescribed recently?
- What are the goals of care?

CHAPTER 42

Fever

The human thermostat is a very sophisticated, high-precision instrument. Regulated by an important part of the brain, the hypothalamus, it generally maintains body temperature within a very narrow range. An elaborate system is in place to ensure that the temperature stays where it's supposed to: nerves tell blood vessels to constrict, preventing unnecessary exposure to the cold by minimizing the flow to places such as the fingertips and the toes, while other nerves cause shivering, which increases body temperature. Only a major perturbation of the system allows a fever to develop. Because body temperature is so tightly controlled, even a modest elevation, say a temperature of 100°F, feels very uncomfortable.

A few general observations about temperature control in older people before we discuss how you should approach fever. You should be aware that many older people do not respond to situations such as an infection by developing a fever: their ability to have such a response has been blunted by age. Just because your relative *doesn't* have an elevated temperature doesn't mean she cannot have pneumonia or appendicitis or an acutely infected gallbladder. You should also know that an abnormally low body temperature, or hypothermia, is a serious medical problem that is far more common in older people than in younger individuals. In younger people, hypothermia is usually due to prolonged cold exposure—being stranded on a mountain top or swimming too long in the cold ocean—but in older people, it can be a response to infection or to a metabolic abnormality such as an underactive thyroid gland. Most thermometers you will find in a regular drug store do not reliably detect low body temperature; if your device reads 96°F (the normal body temperature is 98.6°F), you should be alerted to the possibility that the true level is actually lower. The third bit of background information about fever deals with the question of what constitutes a high temperature. In hospitals and nursing homes, the conventional cut off is 101°F. A temperature that's greater than 98.6°F but less than 101°F is considered a low-grade fever. A more accurate assessment would rely on your relative's usual baseline. If she almost always runs low, say 97.6°F, then a temperature of greater than that but less than 100°F should be viewed as a low-grade fever; a reading of 100°F or more is high for her.

Suppose your family member says she feels feverish. Perhaps she's already taken her temperature. Or maybe she just says she feels sick, but you touch her (feeling the upper back is a more reliable indicator than the forehead) and she feels warm, so you take her temperature. Now what?

What Other Symptoms Are Present?

Most fevers are due to an infection, so knowing what else is going on with your relative will help pin down the source of the infection. You will want to figure out (either by asking, by observing, or both) whether she has *respiratory symptoms*. Cough or shortness of breath in the presence of fever may indicate a problem in the lower respiratory tract, either pneumonia or bronchitis, while sore throat or a runny nose indicates an upper respiratory tract infection (a cold or other viral illness). Your relative might have *urinary* symptoms such as burning when she goes to the bathroom (the medical term is dysuria) and a frequent urge to go. Alternatively, your family member might have *gastrointestinal symptoms* such as diarrhea, vomiting, or perhaps a stomach ache. Fever and diarrhea typically indicate gastroenteritis (most often due to a virus that's going around or to contaminated food); fever with abdominal pain raises the possibility of a more serious condition such as diverticulitis or appendicitis. In all these situations other than a cold, and particularly in the case of abdominal pain, you will want to consult with a medical professional. As always, it's helpful to provide some information so the physician or nurse can suggest next steps; and as usual, how much you will feel comfortable handling at home depends on your family member's goals of care as well as the potential seriousness of her medical condition.

Your relative might have *skin symptoms*: she may have redness, warmth, and swelling of one or both of her lower legs. This suggests the possibility of cellulitis, a skin infection that warrants treatment with antibiotics. Unless you regularly dress or shower your family member, you will have to ask about this symptom as the redness may well be hidden from view by socks or pants. Occasionally, cellulitis will develop in another part of the body, usually associated with a "foreign body" such as an intravenous catheter.

Fever doesn't always imply an infection. It could be evidence of some other type of inflammatory process. An acutely inflamed joint, what physicians call a "hot joint," often produces localized symptoms only—it's warm to the touch—but may also cause more generalized symptoms, including fever. Autoimmune diseases, any of several diseases with cumbersome names such as systemic lupus erythematosus, rheumatoid arthritis, or polymyalgia rheumatica, often result in fever. Fever can even accompany certain cancers, particularly diseases such as Hodgkin's

lymphoma which is known for producing "night sweats," perspiration
that is so vigorous that the sheets are
thoroughly soaked. Diagnosis and
management of any of these conditions
requires a physician.

What Germs Are "Going Around"?

When there is an outbreak of
influenza (flu) in the area and
your family member comes down with
a fever, sore throat, fatigue, and generalized achiness, she most likely has
what everyone else has—the flu. You
will want to pay attention to what else
may be "going around," especially if
your relative lives in a relatively insular
community such as an assisted living
facility or a nursing home. Norovirus is
a common and highly contagious cause
of viral gastroenteritis. If there's been
an outbreak of norovirus where your
family member lives and she comes
down with vomiting, diarrhea, and a
low-grade fever, she probably caught
the same bug. While most cases of
norovirus are spread through contaminated food, person-to-person spread
occurs as well—apparently, it only takes
a miniscule number of norovirus parti-
cles to transmit the disease.

Potential Complications of Fever

Diagnosing and treating whatever is
causing the fever is a good starting
point, but you will have an important
role to play even after the correct diagnosis has been made and effective treatment initiated. Your family
member probably won't get better
immediately. Her fever may linger for
a while, potentially causing confusion
(delirium) and dehydration.

Whenever physicians analyze potential triggers of confusion (see chapter
38, "Confusion"), infection is high on
the list. Sorting out whether the cause
of the confusion is the underlying infection, the fever, or both is sometimes
difficult. Since many young, otherwise
vigorous people find their thinking is
affected if they have a fever, a problem
that resolves dramatically when their
temperature returns to normal, it is
highly likely that the fever itself is the
culprit. As a result, your best bet is to
bring your family member's temperature down, recognizing that may not by
itself solve the problem. The safest way
to lower the temperature is with a medication such as acetaminophen (brand

name Tylenol). You are best off giving the acetaminophen regularly, typically every four to six hours (but no more than 3 grams a day), at least for a day or two. If you wait until the temperature starts to rise, your relative will experience very uncomfortable fluctuations throughout the day. Once she starts to seem a bit better, when her other symptoms have started to abate, you can try stopping the acetaminophen. If your relative does become confused despite your best efforts, you will need additional help in managing the confusion (see chapter 38, "Confusion").

Dehydration is another potential consequence of fever, especially if the elevated temperature persists for days. Your family member may sweat in response to her fever, losing fluid. She will need to drink more to make up for the loss, but because many older people do not experience thirst as strongly as they once did, she may not respond appropriately. Even if she does feel thirsty, she may not have the energy to get herself something to drink. Excess loss of fluid, as well as the various chemicals contained in sweat, can result in her being dizzy or weak. She may be unsteady on her feet or fall. You will want to try to prevent all these complications by plying your relative with fluid. Leave a pitcher of juice where she can reach it easily and a straw to help her drink it—or make sure someone else provides this for her.

Fever can produce additional side effects, depending on what other medical conditions your relative has. Temperature elevation normally causes an increased heart rate, but in someone with chronic heart failure, this kind of rapid heartbeat can push her over into acute heart failure. A very high temperature can result in seizures. This phenomenon is far rarer in older people than in children, but someone with a seizure disorder who takes chronic medication to prevent seizures may experience a lowering of the seizure threshold with fever.

Protecting Yourself

As a caregiver, you are at risk of all kinds of medical problems yourself, typically because you are so busy taking care of your family member that you neglect yourself. Or you might suffer from depression because you are isolated and alone in your caregiving. Rarely do you have to worry about catching whatever medical problems your relative has. But if your relative has an infection that is contagious—and not all infections spread readily, cellulitis (a skin infection), for example, or cystitis (a bladder infection) are not catching—you should protect yourself. No matter how self-sacrificing you are, remember that you won't do your family member much good if you are sick yourself. Infections that are airborne tend to spread rapidly. You may want to stay away until your relative is no longer infectious, if at all possible. If you feel you need to be around her while she is still coughing or sneezing, and before her fever has clearly gone away ("clearly" is usually defined as being fever free for at least 24 hours), you may want to keep your distance and minimize the time you spend together.

Addressing your family member's fever can go a long way towards making her comfortable and preventing complications (box 42.1). As with other symptoms, you will need to partner with her primary care physician and take care of yourself to be maximally effective.

Box 42.1

Fever

- Get a handle on the diagnosis

- Distinguish between mild and serious illness

- Work with a physician to identify serious problems

- Prevent complications

- Maintain hydration

- Control temperature with acetaminophen

- Protect yourself
  - With good handwashing
  - By staying away

PART VII

Care in the Nursing Home

For years, you may have viewed your job as keeping your family member out of a nursing home. Now that he's being admitted as a long-stay nursing home resident, you may feel like a failure. You're not. In all likelihood, your family member couldn't have remained at home—maybe even in your home—as long as he did if you hadn't been there to help. And despite all the bad press nursing homes received in the past, notwithstanding the fear that many people have of nursing homes, they are often the best possible alternative for the frailest and most vulnerable older people.

In fact, just under 1.4 million people live in nursing homes in the United States today. If your relative is joining their ranks, he is liable to be among the "old-old," those over eighty or eighty-five, and to need help with many of his basic activities. Nursing home residents are disproportionately female, in large measure because women outlive men, leaving them with more disabilities and no caregiver when they reach extreme old age. Because your family member has a high likelihood of having dementia (well over half of nursing home residents suffer from Alzheimer's or a related condition) and of being very dependent, he will need an advocate more than ever before. Your caregiving role will change, just as it changed when he was hospitalized, but you are still a caregiver. In this section, we'll explore your new responsibilities.

CHAPTER 43

Choosing a Nursing Home

Choosing a nursing home for the long haul is a little like selecting a hospital and it's a little like choosing a short-stay skilled nursing facility (SNF), but what it resembles even more is choosing where to live. That's because it *is* choosing where to live. Odds are that if your family member moves into a nursing home, he will stay there until he dies. That might be months but often it is a few years. Figuring out where to spend the rest of one's life, like deciding where to live in middle age or young adulthood, is related as much to the community, the environment, and the location as it is to the physical outlay of the residence.

Because the people who live in a nursing home are dependent on others and those others, principally nurses and nursing assistants, play a major role in their physical well-being, there is a medical dimension to the selection. I'm going to confine my comments to this aspect of the decision-making process—plus a few remarks about "culture change" and how that might contribute to emotional well-being.

Picking a nursing home for your relative, much like selecting a SNF for short-term rehabilitation, is best in-

formed by word of mouth, visits to the various options, and rating systems (see chapter 16, "Choosing a Rehab Facility"). Among rating systems, all of which have their limitations, the most comprehensive in the case of nursing homes is Nursing Home Compare, the site maintained by the Centers for Medicare and Medicaid Services (CMS).

Nursing Home Compare comes up with an overall grade for each nursing home that it evaluates. That grade simultaneously assesses both the short-stay and the long-stay units in the nursing home (many SNFs house both under the same roof) even though it's entirely possible for one site to offer pretty good care and the other to offer care that is mediocre or worse. The grade is a composite measure based on three criteria:

1. Performance on the last state inspection. Annual health inspections assess many aspects of a nursing home including quality of life, food services, and medication management. Star ratings are affected by the scope and severity of any deficiencies and how many visits it takes until it is fixed.

2. Staffing ratios. Staffing is based on the total nursing hours per resident day, which includes registered nurses (RNs), licensed practical nurses (LPNs), and nurse aides, as well as RN hours per resident day. The resident census is also used when determining the staff to resident ratio. Private duty nurses, hospice staff, and feeding assistants are not included.

3. Quality measures. Select measures from Minimum Data Set (MDS) and Medicare Claims Data make up part of the star ratings. These measures differ between short-stay and long-stay residents, and are based on their validity and reliability.

Based on these three areas, CMS assigns between one and five stars.

You may want to look at each of those ingredients individually; I'm going to focus exclusively on the quality indicators because they attempt to measure those aspects of care that directly impact health. Discussing each of them may give you a good sense of what's important in evaluating a nursing home. As of October 2017, there were fifteen quality measures. I mention the date because every couple of years the list is revised, so you should check the latest list. I'm not going to discuss all of them in detail, but I will discuss three to give you an idea of the ways in which the measures are useful—or not so useful.

The first quality measure is *the percentage of residents experiencing one or more falls with major injury.* Obviously,

you'd prefer your family member not fall and you certainly don't want him breaking a hip or wrist or bleeding into his brain. But while there are steps that a nursing facility can take to lower the fall risk, it's impossible to lower the risk to zero. Remember, a fool-proof way of preventing falls would necessitate a combination of handcuffs and leg irons; clearly, there are tradeoffs between safety and autonomy. Moreover, the frailer your relative, the more likely he is to fall, so having a low rate of "injurious falls" can simply mean that the nursing home chooses residents for admission who are in above average condition.

Next, there's *the percentage of residents with a urinary tract infection.* I confess I have a real problem with this one. The majority of frail older people, both men and women but especially women, *chronically* have bacteria and white cells in their urine, a condition that does not require treatment. In fact, treatment promotes the development of resistant bacteria and predisposes residents to the side effects of antibiotics—without conferring any benefit. What Nursing Home Compare presumably wants to know is whether the residents have *symptomatic* urinary tract infections, but I am not certain why this is regarded as a quality measure. The implicit assumption is that a good facility can prevent such infections. True, good hygiene helps to minimize the chance your relative will get a symptomatic infection (by wiping away from rather than towards the opening of the urethra, the tube connecting the bladder to the outside of the body), as does drinking plenty of fluids and going to the bathroom regularly. But many people who wipe properly and drink enough still get a bladder infection.

One measure that I liked, though it was removed from the 2019 revised list, was the *percentage of residents who are physically restrained*. Only rarely should nursing home staff use physical restraints, whether the "Posey vest," which is essentially a chest restraint, or straps around the arms or legs. Once upon a time, nurses and doctors believed that tying people up could prevent them from falling. What we've learned is that the practice seldom works and, moreover, restraints can paradoxically increase the fall risk, particularly of falls resulting in injury. If your family member is tethered to a chair, for example, he might try desperately to rise up and, in the process, fall over head first, chair and all. Patients have been known to vault over the siderails of their bed, another type of physical restraint, again causing far more harm than if they had simply gotten out of bed the normal way or even slid out gently. An intervention that doesn't achieve its intended effect *and* is an assault on individual dignity seems like a really bad idea. Since Congress passed the Nursing Home Reform Act in 1987 (OBRA87), strongly discouraging the use of restraints in the nursing home, the rate of use plummeted, going from 21 percent in 1991 to 5 percent in 2007. Very occasionally some type of restraint may be transiently necessary, for example to prevent a person from pulling out an IV (in use, say, for the treatment of dehydration in someone who is very confused) or removing a bandage (for

instance, a dressing over the eye after cataract surgery). But in general, higher than average restraint use in a nursing home should be a red flag making you wonder what else the facility does wrong.

Another dimension of nursing home life that bears, at least indirectly, on medical issues is the culture of the facility. Culture is difficult to define and hard to measure, but it's important because it reflects how the staff will view your relative, how they will treat him, and the overall spirit of the place. Traditionally, the bedrock of nursing home culture has been a focus on health and safety. That's why restraints were once so popular—they were presumed to be a good way to keep old people secure, especially if their balance was poor or if they were confused and liable to wander off. Residents were lined up in the hall in their wheelchairs so the nurse's aides could keep an eye on them and make sure they weren't doing anything hazardous. Privacy, allowing residents to stay in their own room and putter about, beyond the reach of nursing surveillance, was felt to be inimical to the goal of safety. And consistent with the medical model, a resident's life revolved around taking medications and other types of monitoring, such as weighing or blood pressure measurement. If taking pills three times a day necessitated being on the "unit," as the nursing home wing is often called, for the nurse to administer the medicine, then day trips—to a museum, to a concert, to visit a friend—were frowned upon. *Quality of life* was deemed irrelevant, or assumed to be identical with promoting health and safety.

The culture change movement challenged the idea of the nursing home as dedicated exclusively to health and safety. It's where your family member will live, often for several years, and just because he is old and frail doesn't mean he can no longer have a meaningful life or experience pleasure. But enabling your relative to derive satisfaction from his life over and beyond a sense of security, allowing him to truly experience well-being, isn't so easy. The culture change movement began with the Eden Alternative, a movement created by Bill Thomas, a disillusioned nursing home physician who introduced plants and pets into nursing homes. It took off with the establishment of the Pioneer Network in 1990, a loose collaborative that brought together multiple different institutions seeking to improve the quality of life of their residents. It is embodied in Thomas's newest initiative, the Green House Project, that features small, personal residences instead of large institutions. What all these initiatives have in common is that they seek to be *resident-centered*. That means they focus on your relative as a person rather than as a patient. He will be able to get up in the morning whenever he chooses—not when the nursing assistant says he should get up. Similarly, he can have breakfast when he wishes rather than at a fixed time. The nursing assistants are supposed to help him dress in the clothes he wants to wear or that you've told them he prefers, rather than in what is most convenient for the staff: if your family member doesn't like to wear sweatpants, he won't regularly dress in sweatpants. If your family member needs help turning on

the television and selecting a program, the choice of what he watches will be based on his wishes, often funneled through you. I can't tell you how often I've walked down the long corridors of traditional nursing homes and encountered pop music blaring from each of the rooms even though I'm confident the residents would have preferred ragtime or classical recordings.

Nursing homes that have embraced culture change typically feature private or semi-private rooms rather than the old-fashioned, four-bed style. They also espouse the "universal worker" model in which all staff members perform all or most functions. For example, if your relative needs help getting to the bathroom, instead of expecting him to wait until his assigned nursing assistant is available, which may be too late, any nursing assistant can take him to the bathroom. If no nursing assistant is available, the nurse or social worker or whoever is around will take him to the bathroom. Ditto for getting a snack. Only a few tasks that require specific professional expertise, for example changing a bandage, are restricted to staff members with the requisite license or training. Not only will your family member be better served by this arrangement, the culture change movement believes, but staff members also find their jobs more rewarding because they function more like family members than paid caregivers. Finally, nursing homes that believe in resident-centered care are generally committed to family involvement. They know that you are the key to learning about your relative's habits and interests when he cannot articulate his own preferences.

They understand that you can help troubleshoot if there is a problem with your family member—you may know just what to do if he refuses to take a shower or won't take his medicines.

Ideally, implementation of the culture change model will benefit both your family member's emotional and his physical health. Intended to reduce loneliness and helplessness, it is supposed to decrease depression and anxiety. By keeping residents engaged and active, it should promote physical health and functioning. The evidence that culture change nursing homes achieve these objectives is sparse, both because it's a phenomenon that's difficult to study and because many nursing homes endorse the model but have not fully integrated all the recommended practices. Some nursing homes that make no claim to have become culture change facilities nonetheless have a staff who are supremely caring and competent—which itself has a dramatic effect on the quality of life of the residents. In either case, you should try to assess the culture of any facility you are considering for your family member: it matters as much as the more conventional aspects of care.

Because the medical care in the nursing home is so intimately intertwined with the nonmedical aspects of care, you will need to consider both in choosing a facility for your relative. The medical care is best assessed using word of mouth, formal ratings—such as Nursing Home Compare—and a personal visit. You can begin to get a handle on everything else when you evaluate the model of care endorsed by the facility—traditional or person-centered.

Box 43.1

Quality of Medical Care in Nursing Homes

- Nursing Home Compare
- Focus on falls, restraint use

Person-Centered Models of Care

- The Eden Alternative
- Pioneer model
- Green House Project

CHAPTER 44

Why You Will Still Be a Caregiver

Nursing homes, including the good ones, are a modern form of what Erving Goffman, writing in his book *Asylums: Essays on the Social Situation of Mental Patients and Other Inmates*, called a "total institution." They shape every aspect of their residents' lives. Even facilities that embrace resident-centered care and endorse the "culture change model" (see chapter 43, "Choosing a Nursing Home") are still fundamentally *institutions*. They may try to be homey, they may provide private rooms and give residents a certain amount of autonomy, but they are responsible for all aspects of your family member's life. Because your family member is very dependent—otherwise she wouldn't be in the nursing home in the first place—she *relies* on the nurses and nursing assistants, on the cooks and the orderlies, to survive. This basic fact colors her relationship with these individuals. Unlike the parent/child relationship in which the child is likewise very dependent on her mother or father, the resident/staff relationship is not governed by love. It's a professional or business relationship; even the most caring nursing staff are doing a job. They are paid to do what they do; what you do stems

from affection or a sense of filial responsibility, which is entirely different.

If your family member has dementia, she is going to be particularly hard pressed to articulate her wishes or needs, let alone her dissatisfaction or distress. She will need you to explain what she likes and doesn't like, whether it's dietary preferences, how she combs her hair, or what kind of music she enjoys. It goes without saying that you will be invaluable for the more subtle and complex decisions that will likely have to be made at some point, decisions you will probably be involved in even if your family member doesn't have dementia. She will also need you to speak up if you notice her nails need clipping or her hair needs washing or if you find that she is breathing rapidly or that she is more confused than usual.

I find that the job of caring for someone who is not completely alert—this was as true of comatose patients as it is of nursing home residents with dementia—is much easier if the person providing the care sees her charge as a full person. It's more natural to care deeply about what happens to a person if you have a relationship with her than if you don't. The more advanced her dementia, the harder it becomes to relate to her and the more you need to rely on establishing a sort of vicarious relationship. What helps is learning about the person she has been—her family, her profession, her religion, her ethnic background, her hobbies, her quirks—all the things that make her a unique individual. You are the key to your family member's past. When the staff sees their patient through your eyes, when they can imagine the person she once was, they are more likely to be kind and gentle and to go out of their way to help her.

I remember taking care of a man in a nursing home who was nearly quadriplegic. He had a neurologic disorder that left him unable to do anything as simple as scratching himself if he had an itch. He wasn't fully paralyzed and he could breathe on his own, but his limbs were extremely weak. On his night stand, he kept a photograph of himself when he was in his twenties. He was, I believe, something of a body builder. The picture showed him sporting swimming trunks and flexing his arm muscles. With a little imagination, it was possible to see the continuity between the youthful athlete and the nearly paralyzed, old man. I also knew that he had been a physician and as I listened to him talk about his professional accomplishments and the achievements of his adult children, I began to see him as a full human being, not just a dependent person with a terrible neurological condition. The knowledge of who he had been was useful in helping me develop a sense of what was important to him and what medical treatments were most conducive to achieving his personal goals. But it also made me understand how especially difficult it was for this man who was so used to being in control to have to call for the nurse (we rigged up a special call button that could be speech activated) to relieve his itch.

You will also continue to be key whenever an important decision needs to be made about medical treatment. Even if your family member is sufficiently intact cognitively that she can speak for herself most of the time, when she's acutely ill, her thinking may become fuzzy. Or, she may be too anxious when in the midst of a crisis to reason calmly and clearly about what course of action to pursue. If you are your family member's health-care proxy and if she cannot make decisions for herself, you will be called no matter what time of day or night.

Ideally, you will already have established a relationship with key members of the team and discussed your family member's preferences before you receive that dreaded phone call at eleven o'clock on a Sunday evening. But even if the broad outlines of your family member's preferences have already been recorded in the medical record, translating that general perspective into practice may require some discussion. Suppose, for example, your family member was clear that she wanted her medical treatment to focus on preserving her daily functioning—on keeping her walking or reading or playing the piano or whatever it is that she particularly values. Given that goal, what's the best way to treat the current clinical situation? The answer may be straightforward: if she wants to be able to walk and she just broke her hip, she's going to have to go to the hospital for hip surgery. Or, it may not be so clear cut: She wants to maintain what independence she has and she's just had a major gastrointestinal bleed; should she accept hospitalization, which might leave her very debilitated for a long time, or should she opt for treatment in the nursing home? If she goes to the hospital, should she go to a general medical floor or to the intensive care unit (ICU)? If she goes to a general medical unit, should she receive empiric treatment with fluids and anti-ulcer medication or should she have an upper endoscopy followed by aggressive treatment of whatever condition is identified? You will need to have this conversation with the physician, together with your family member if she's able to participate, and preferably grounded in the advance care planning discussion you held previously.

Speaking of advance care planning, that's another area where you have a critical role to play. Just as short-stay skilled nursing facilities hold care planning meetings after admission and sometimes before discharge, long-stay nursing facilities are also obligated to hold periodic meetings with residents and their family members to discuss how things are going. This is a great opportunity to provide the facility with a written advance directive, if there is one, and to speak more generally about your family member's goals and wishes for future medical care. The rates of advance care planning have risen dramatically in recent years, but usually this means the facility has determined who the health-care proxy is and may have elicited a do-not-resuscitate (DNR) order. Rarely are there more elaborate

advance directives or a medical order set, such as the POLST (Physician Orders for Life-Sustaining Treatment), which asks about cardiopulmonary resuscitation (CPR), but also intubation, dialysis, artificial nutrition, artificial hydration, and other medical therapies. Rarer still is a more general statement of the goals of care—does your family member value, above all else, treatment intended to prolong life? To maximize daily functioning? Or to promote comfort? You will probably need to bring up the subject, ideally well before there is an acute medical problem requiring an urgent decision.

Sometimes the nursing staff finds the advance directive or medical decision made by your relative difficult to understand. They think your family member didn't really mean what she wrote in her advance directive or alternatively, she doesn't fully grasp her current situation. I remember caring for a nursing home resident once who had a skin ulcer on his leg that just wouldn't heal no matter what kind of dressing was used. He was evaluated by a vascular surgeon who felt the ulcer stemmed from poor circulation and that it couldn't heal in light of the inadequate blood supply to the leg. He recommended an amputation. The patient had an advance directive that specifically stated he would never accept an amputation, which the nurses taking care of him found perplexing. They felt he would be far more comfortable if he didn't have a constantly festering wound on his leg. They thought his thought process had been adversely affected by the chronic, low-level infection. Maybe he was worried that he would not be able to walk after his amputation—but in his current condition, he was unable to walk anyway, his leg hurt too much. Finally, we held a family meeting and his health-care proxy explained that our patient had been a marathon runner. Symbolically, his legs were the most important part of his body and he had decided he would rather die or suffer from chronic pain than lose his legs. He knew something about leg amputations because his father, who like him had been a diabetic, had experienced exactly the same problem. The patient had moderate dementia and couldn't explain any of this to us. It was thanks to his health-care proxy, his longstanding caregiver, that we understood our patient better and were able to abide by his wishes.

I can think of still another reason that your ongoing caregiving is important in the nursing home setting. The staff are likely to do a better job caring for your family member if they know someone loves her. Although they are professionally obligated to treat all their patients equally and with respect, that can be difficult. It's especially challenging if your family member is cantankerous or, in their view, "demanding."

It can be particularly difficult if your family member makes racist comments to the nursing assistants, which sometimes happens as older people develop dementia and lose what inhibitions they once had. It's hard to respond with gentleness and kindness to someone who, in nursing home parlance, "resists care," who hits or bites or curses when the aide tries to feed her or give her a shower. Good nursing assistants learn to deal with these situations and continue providing adequate care, but if they see that their patient is loved by her daughter (or son or spouse), suggesting that she was once a lovable person, their job becomes a bit easier. Just as knowing something of who your family member once was—her family, her accomplishments, her background—helps, so, too, does realizing that she is a beloved mother or spouse.

As in so much of caregiving, your role can best be thought of as advocacy (box 44.1). You have special knowledge about your relative and you have a unique relationship with her that transcends the relationship between her and a paid caregiver. These critical functions continue in the nursing home.

Box 44.1

Family Caregiving in the Nursing Home

- Help staff understand who their patient is
- Provide an advance directive
- Assist in translating directive into practice
- Show that you care

CHAPTER 45

Medical Care in the Nursing Home

Medical care in the nursing home is like medical care in the post-acute skilled nursing facility (SNF), but there's even less of it. This should come as no surprise since most long-stay nursing homes and short-stay, post-acute rehabilitation facilities are just different wings of the same building. They may have separate staffs—or they might not. Some short-stay SNFs have no long-stay residents: the reimbursement for a post-acute SNF, which stems largely from Medicare, is much better than that for long-stay care, which is principally from Medicaid (or, in some cases, private pay), so many facilities have converted most, if not all of their beds to short-stay SNF beds.

Your first medical task when your family member enters a nursing home is to find a physician to take care of him. Ironically, when older adults live in their own house or apartment, they are generally expected to travel to a physician's office for medical appointments but, once they move to a nursing home, the physician is required to come to them—even though the nursing home is able to provide door-to-door transportation, a service the home dweller often has difficulty finding. But since few primary care physicians and even fewer specialists will travel to the nursing home to see their patients, your family member will typically need to find a new physician. In the past, the physicians who were willing to take on nursing home patients are themselves getting on in years. They might already be largely retired from practice and decided to maintain a very limited practice in the controlled environment of the nursing home. I've encountered a retired surgeon working in a nursing home and I've run into several eighty-five-year-old physicians working in a nursing home. They may have been competent doctors and compassionate individuals—but they were rarely trained in geriatric issues. While SNF work is growing in interest and prestige—with physicians who see SNF patients now having their own medical society, a medical journal, an annual educational conference, and a certificate exam—many of these physicians primarily or exclusively take care of short-term patients.

Once your family member has a physician, perhaps someone suggested by the facility, that physician must make an initial visit and then either she or her associate must see her new patient once every thirty days for three months. After that period, most state regulations mandate visits every three months. If your family member is hospitalized then the clock is reset: the physician has to come by every month for ninety days before resuming quarterly visits. The problem with this approach is twofold. It only addresses routine medical care, not urgent care. And it says little about what is supposed to happen on the routine visits.

Let's consider the routine visit first. We physicians were trained that whatever else we do during an outpatient appointment, we should check the vital signs (or at least have someone else do that and look at the results), we should listen to the lungs, and perform a heart exam. For patients who have high blood pressure or a diagnosis of heart failure or asthma, this approach is not unreasonable. But for nursing home residents, at least as important—and much more important for the person who doesn't have high blood pressure or heart failure or asthma—is checking the skin for evidence of breakdown (pressure ulcers or, as they are commonly known, bedsores). Your family member should be checked for a dry mouth or poor skin turgor (skin that forms a little tent when you pinch it), both signs of dehydration. He should be monitored for delirium, a state of confusion that may persist for months after hospitalization or that may have arisen from a new medication introduced at the nursing home. Your relative's physician should also spend some time quizzing his nursing assistant and nurse to find out if he's fallen, if he has trouble walking, and if he seems depressed. She should also inquire about pain and whether he is eating well. The conventional model of the office visit in which the physician obtains a history from the patient and performs a physical examination is inadequate in the nursing home setting: it must be supplemented with information gathered from other sources, from the people who provide hands-on care. Geriatric physicians understand this; general internists or retired surgeons sometimes treat the nursing home visit as an office visit— and omit some of the most crucial parts of the evaluation.

Then there's the issue of urgent care. The mandated quarterly visits don't make any provision for problems that arise *between* visits. Your family member may well develop the flu during flu season, diarrhea when there's a bug going around the nursing home, or a bladder infection at any time. Sometimes it will be obvious what's happening, as when there's an infectious outbreak at the facility; the nurse can inform your family member's physician of the situation and she can order the appropriate treatment. But sometimes it won't be clear whether your relative's lethargy is due to an infection or to dehydration or to a medicine he's taking. And with any given diagnosis, your family member may be only mildly under the weather or he may be very sick. Most physicians who care for nursing home patients are not set up to drop whatever they are doing and come out to the nursing home to evaluate one patient. Their knee jerk reaction when the nurse calls their office and reports that your family member has, say, a cough and a fever, is to order that he go to the local emergency department for assessment.

Some nursing homes and some physician practices work with a nurse practitioner or physician assistant who can make urgent visits to nursing home residents. That sort of arrangement can obviate the need to transfer your family member to the hospital every time he has anything more serious than a cold. Ideally, he will be able to receive basic medical care at the facility, both simple diagnostic tests (such as blood tests, a portable chest x-ray, or a urinalysis) and straightforward treatment (oral medications, shots, oxygen, or a nebulizer). At some facilities, he will be able to get intravenous treatment as well, whether fluids or medications. At a handful of nursing homes, you will find an in-house medical staff, physicians hired by the facility to provide medical care to its residents. In those cases, typically large nursing homes that have a teaching mission along with their care obligations, on-site physician treatment is readily available. Whatever professionals come to see your family member at the nursing home are people you should get to know. Make sure they realize your relative has family who care about him, who are involved in his care, and who are eager and available to participate in decision-making about medical issues.

Your family member will almost certainly be less sick when he enters a nursing home as a long-stay resident than he was when he entered a SNF after hospitalization. But as was true when he was living at home, he probably has multiple chronic conditions, any one of which is liable to flare up and cause problems. During the months or years that he will live in the nursing home, odds are he will develop one or more acute problems. It's a good idea to find out at the beginning of your family member's stay what the capacity of the facility is to provide medical care and then to discuss the approach to care that makes sense for him in the event of an acute problem—or, more generally, advance care planning.

If physicians talk about any aspect of advance care planning, it's typically whether you would want attempted cardiopulmonary resuscitation (CPR) if your family member's heart stops. While this is important if your relative goes to the hospital, the likelihood of successful CPR in the nursing home setting is very close to zero. It's not neglecting your family member to decide that the facility shouldn't attempt CPR; it's merely recognizing that when a debilitated eighty-eight-year-old (the average age of nursing home residents) stops breathing and his heart stops beating you can be reasonably certain that nothing can bring him back. To press repeatedly on his chest, apply electric shocks, and force air into his lungs is as close to futile as anything in medicine. It's also not what most people would consider a dignified end.

There's more to discuss with the physician and nursing staff than CPR. In fact, as I've previously mentioned, I prefer to focus on thinking about what is most important to your family member at this juncture in his life, given his overall condition. That means you and—to the extent that he can understand this conversation—your family member need to know just what his overall condition is. You almost undoubtedly realize that he needs a great deal of help with basic functioning—otherwise you would not have opted to move him to a nursing home. You may be aware of his various medical problems and how tenuous they are if, for example, he's been in and out of the hospital a great deal in the past year. But you may or may not have a sense of how these problems are likely to evolve in the ensuing months or years and of how much time he has left. The physician probably isn't going to be able to tell you very accurately whether he has six months or a year or two years—unless he is already in the most advanced stage of a serious disease, it's difficult to be precise. She can, however, answer the "surprise question," namely "would I be surprised if this person is no longer alive in a year?" Based on her response, she can give you some idea of how fragile your family member is (see also chapter 4, "Determining Your Family Member's Health State"). What I say in this situation might be "Mr. S. has pretty severe valvular heart disease, and on top of that, he has Parkinson's and arthritis; he's too frail to have open heart surgery, and while we have medicines that can help the symptoms of Parkinson's and the pain from arthritis, we don't have anything that can stop these conditions from progressing and we certainly don't have anything that reverses them. I'm not sure how much time Mr. S. has, and I'd be happy to be wrong about this, but I suspect it's not very long." Based on this general understanding of your family member's health status, as well as some sense of what the hospital, on the one hand, and the nursing home on the other hand, might have to offer if your family member developed a flare of one of his problems, you can decide if you favor a "do not hospitalize" order (for more on the pros and cons of hospitalization in frail older people, see chapter 10, "The Perils of Hospitalization"). This order, like other medical orders, can always be reversed; the point, however, is to assert that the default strategy if your relative becomes ill is to treat him at the facility.

You should also realize that if your family member has a prognosis of six months or less—as best the physician can tell—then he is eligible for hospice services in addition to the usual nursing care in the facility. This is in contrast to the situation in short-term rehab. The reason is that short-term rehab is generally covered by Medicare Part A (the part of Medicare that also pays for hospitalization) as is hospice care. From Medicare's point of view, having short-term SNF care and hospice care simultaneously is double dipping (there are rare exceptions, but generally this description is accurate). Long-stay nursing home care, by contrast, is not covered by Medicare at all; hence, it's perfectly reasonable to have hospice care (covered by Medicare Part A) on top of nursing home care (covered by Medicaid or paid for privately). Sometimes nurses and doctors, not to mention residents and families, are puzzled by what hospice care would add to conventional nursing home care. The answer is that it can often add quite a bit. Yes, your family member already has a nurse and a nursing assistant in the nursing home but the staff may not be well-versed in managing symptoms that commonly develop near the end of life; they may be accustomed to sending anyone with such symptoms, such as pain or acute confusion, to the hospital. The hospice will provide a hospice nurse who can assess your family member and make suggestions about how best to address his symptoms. Hospices also offer social work and chaplaincy services that may be difficult or impossible to obtain in the nursing home. They are also geared to providing support to you and to other family members, as well as to your relative.

I've been talking about the medical team—the physician and/or advanced practice clinician, physician assistant (PA) or nurse practitioner (NP)—who will deal with any medical problems that arise while your family member is in the nursing home. But the truth is that the most important person in the nursing home for your family member's health and well-being is his nurse. Usually there is a "unit nurse" or a "charge nurse," the person who is principally responsible for your family member's nursing needs. She is the conduit to the medical team (physician, NP, or PA), she's the one who decides whether your family member is sick enough to warrant a call and who reports what she sees so that the clinician can make a judgment about what needs to happen next. In fact, there are typically three shifts of nurses every day (though nurses will sometimes work a ten- or twelve-hour shift) and many facilities have a separate staff on the weekends, so there may be five or six "regular" nurses to get to know. If you start with the charge nurse or the "primary nurse," the person who is supposed to design the care plan for your family member, you've made a good start. If you routinely come in the evenings or perhaps over the weekend, you will tend to get to know the nurses who work at those times best, but it's a good idea to make the effort to meet the main nurse early on in your family member's tenure. Don't hesitate to call the nurse with concerns, issues ranging from "Dad doesn't seem to hear me very well, I wonder if his hearing aid's working?" to "Is Dad on a new medication? He seems more confused to me."

Speaking of medications, you might ask to review your family member's drug list periodically. You no longer have to worry about administering his medications and you probably don't have to worry about paying for them, but nursing homes sometimes start a medicine for a valid reason but don't discontinue it when it's no longer necessary or if it isn't working. A good way to get a handle on your family member's medical situation and keep tabs on the medical care is to ask ever so politely whether you could sit down with the nurse and review the drug list. Or, you might save that task for the interdisciplinary team meeting (see chapter 46, "Team Meetings in the Nursing Home").

Medical care in the nursing home is different from medical care at any other site, both because the specific config-uration of available services is unique and because your relative's needs are different. You will have to adapt, which means getting to know the key professionals and establishing open lines of communication, to continue to serve your all-important advocacy role.

Box 45.1

Medical Care in the Nursing Home

- Find a primary care physician who visits the facility

- Assure that routine care focuses on geriatric issues

- Consider who will provide urgent care: presence of a physician assistant or nurse practitioner can often avoid hospital transfer

- Weigh risks/benefits of hospital versus nursing home care

- Think about supplementary hospice care during the final phase of life

CHAPTER 46

Team Meetings in the Nursing Home

Team meetings in the nursing home, like the care planning or predischarge meetings in the short-stay skilled nursing facility (SNF or what I refer to as "rehab"), are your opportunity to get together with the principal staff members involved in daily care and discuss how things are going. Members of this team may include representatives from primary care, social services, home care, physical/occupational therapy, skilled nursing, pharmacy, recreational therapy, and nutrition, for example. It's a chance to find out who is providing care and what they view as the issues of concern. And it's a chance for you to both shape what will happen in the future and to find ways to help. Ideally, your family member will participate in the meeting along with you, the primary nurse and nursing assistant, and whoever else is actively involved in care, such as a social worker, dietician, or physical therapist. If you're lucky, the physician or nurse practitioner will be there as well.

I can think of a variety of problems that the staff may bring up and you might have additional issues to raise. Consider the social domain—not strictly a medical problem, but it intersects with medical care because isolation or dis-engagement can cause depression. The recreation therapist might report that your family member seldom comes to the groups she organizes—sing-alongs, bingo, current events—and if she does attend, she doesn't say a word and often falls asleep. You might offer a suggestion for how to encourage her to go, such as saying, "It's time for the current events group," instead of asking, "Would you like to go to current events today?" You might propose taking her yourself to make it more palatable. Or, you might tell the staff what kinds of activities your family member enjoys—perhaps she has always liked classical music, especially for the piano, but she intensely dislikes "big band" music and jazz.

Then there's mobility. Perhaps your family member used a walker when she lived at home, but she's increasingly reluctant to get up and walk. The staff aren't sure whether she's finding walking more difficult or she just doesn't want to bother. Perhaps you're appalled that she's hardly walking anymore. You agree to walk with her, at least up and down the nursing home corridors, every time you visit, but you also suggest a physical therapy evaluation. You wonder whether her arthritis is acting up and the real problem is that her knees bother her when she walks. Instead of reporting her joint discomfort, she has taken the path of least resistance and simply opts for the wheelchair.

Next, the staff might bring up nutrition. Your relative has been losing weight—and perhaps she was underweight to start with. She tends to push the food around on her plate and only takes a few bites. The dietician reports she met with your family member to see if there were other kinds of foods she might prefer, but your relative consistently says she doesn't have an appetite. You wonder whether the food is too bland—she's been put on a low-salt diet because she has a history of high blood pressure but maybe it's more important to take in sufficient calories and nutrients than to restrict her sodium intake. Or, you suggest, perhaps her dentures don't fit properly and she has trouble chewing. Then you learn that the speech therapist evaluated your family member's swallowing, concluded she was at risk for aspiration—for food going down the wrong way and ending up in her lungs—so she recommended puréed foods. You are not surprised your family member doesn't have an appetite for baby food. You indicate that you are willing to take the (small) risk that she will aspirate if she has regular food in exchange for the strong likelihood that she will eat better. Maybe you can also share that your family member has always been an ice cream enthusiast and that giving her ice cream every day for dessert or as a snack between meals could be a way to provide some high-calorie nutrition.

When her medical diagnoses are discussed you will find out what the staff members are doing for each of your relative's problems—whether she's getting nebulizer treatments for asthma, whether she uses oxygen for her heart failure, and what medications she's taking. If the drugs are different from what she was on at home, you will want to know the reason for the change. Is it just a matter of what's on the formulary of the pharmacy the nursing home uses? That is, an equivalent medication has been substituted because it's the variant they prefer at the facility? Or was the old medication ineffective? You should have a list of your family member's previous medicines with you to see if anything has been omitted. Is she off her heart medication because she's on a newer medication instead or because she no longer needs it? Or did they simply forget to give it to her? What about any totally new classes of medication? Is she on an antipsychotic medication for "restlessness," even though she is not psychotic or paranoid or delusional? She has an order for a sleeping pill—is that something she takes regularly, or is it on the list "just in case?" If she's taking it consistently, that might be the reason she sleeps half the day or is groggy or confused.

If the nurse and/or social worker don't bring up the question of your family member's mood, you may want to raise it. You know her better than the nurses and nursing assistants. You know whether being quiet and withdrawn is new for her or not and you know whether she has a history of depression. If the staff recognizes that your family member's depressed, have they obtained a psychiatry consultation? Is she on any medicines for depression? If so, how long has she been taking them? Has the dose been adjusted at all? Or maybe you don't think your family member is depressed, you think her dementia is progressing. The team meeting is a good place to discuss her cognitive function.

Such a large proportion of long-stay nursing home residents have dementia that the nursing staff may assume that your family member has dementia, too. Even if it's not listed in her medical record as a chronic condition, they may figure it was simply left out. They're right that dementia is underdiagnosed—many physicians fail to test adequately for dementia. The physician might record only that your family member is "alert and oriented times three," which means she isn't somnolent and she knows her name, where she is, and the date. There's a lot more to normal cognition than just being oriented. You can express concerns about declining cognition, if that's something you've observed, and ask whether your family member has had more extensive mental status testing. If your family member has been evaluated in the past by a neurologist or a geriatrician because of impaired cognition, you might want to share the results of that assessment. If there's any question about whether your relative has dementia, delirium, or depression—and distinguishing the three "D"s can be challenging—you might want the physician to evaluate her. Or you may propose taking her to see the neurologist who examined her previously and who has recorded how she performed on a variety of tests a couple of years ago.

Finally, whether the team brings up advance care planning or not, you may want to raise the issue. Make sure everyone knows what you and your family member decided earlier about the principal goal of care and how that affects decisions such as cardiopulmonary resuscitation (CPR) or hospitalization. Be sure that the nursing home has a copy of your family member's health-care proxy designation on file, indicating that you are the person who is authorized to make health-care decisions if your relative is incapacitated. Depending on whether there's been a major decline in physical or cognitive function since you last engaged in advance care planning, you might want to revise whatever decisions were made previously. If there are any new diagnoses or if any of the leading medical problems are getting worse, you might be able to learn about what to expect over time as those problems evolve further. For example, suppose your family member has Parkinson's disease. So far, that's caused her difficulty walking and made her speech difficult to understand. Your family member's handwriting got very small and is hard to read. But the nurse and/or physician can let you know that patients with Parkinson's disease usually develop swallowing problems as their disease progresses. Eventually, they are at high risk of aspiration, of pneumonia. If that happens, how vigorously should the pneumonia be treated—given that if it develops once, it's likely to develop again and again?

Suppose instead that your family member has heart failure. It's become quite advanced and the only way to enable her to breathe comfortably, given that she's not a candidate for a heart transplant or other invasive therapies, is with higher and higher doses of diuretics, known as "fluid pills." The problem, you learn, is that the result of all these diuretics is that your family member's kidney function, which was previously mildly out of whack, is now approaching the threshold for dialysis. Would you consider dialysis if she reaches that point? You should really be having these conversations with a physician or his representative. If neither is present at the meeting, you might want to set up a phone call or in-person meeting with the physician to talk about problems such as this that surfaced during the team meeting.

I sometimes worried, when I ran interdisciplinary team meetings in the nursing home setting, that family members would feel cowed in the face of multiple staff members. If all the professionals insist that your family member has advanced dementia, or is not depressed, or needs to eat puréed food, you might feel hard-pressed to argue otherwise. After all, you're not a nurse or a doctor. I always try to make the family member feel she is a participant in the process and prevent the meeting from degenerating into an us-versus-them situation. If the team leader doesn't set such a tone, you should nonetheless realize that the choices aren't acquiescence on the one hand and confrontation on the other. The last thing you want to do is become confrontational. You want to indicate that, while you respect the professional judgment of the team, you would feel better if another pair of eyes looked at the situation—a neurologist or cardiologist, or perhaps the staff physician. Or,

in the case of the concern about aspiration, you might say you appreciate that there's a risk but this is something you've thought about and discussed with your family member and you're willing to take the risk of aspiration. You just want to be sure she can take food by mouth as long as possible. Suggest a compromise: you're willing to avoid food like steak that's difficult to chew (odds are, the residents in a nursing home don't get steak very often) and stick to softer foods, like eggplant parmesan or fish, as long as it's not *mush.*

I also sensed, when I ran such meetings, that many of the participants viewed them as a burden, as something required by the nursing home administration (they are required—in fact, they're mandated by the Centers for Medicare and Medicaid Services) and just a waste of time. Again, the team leader can help by emphasizing that by meeting as a group, together with you and your family member, they might be able to *improve* the care plan. But if the team leader doesn't seem to see things this way, you're in a difficult position. What you'd like to do is demonstrate that you can actually make it easier for the staff members to do their jobs because you have valuable information, or that you can work with your family member to persuade her to take her pills or to try walking or whatever it is that the staff feels frustrated about. I understand that's not so easy. Sometimes, the best strategy is to meet one-on-one with the team leader, often the charge nurse, before the group meeting, to try to clear the air. Let her know that you're an ally, not a troublemaker; you just want whatever's best for your family member.

One of the most trying situations that may come up during an interdisciplinary team meeting arises when you or your relative have a problem with a particular staff member, most commonly one of the nursing assistants. The nursing assistant may be a perfectly lovely person but your family member has a racist streak, perhaps unmasked by her dementia, and makes deprecating and insulting comments to her. Or it's your family member who is kind and considerate, but the nursing assistant to whom she has been assigned is impatient with her and handles her roughly. Occasionally there might be a misunderstanding that can be addressed—the nursing assistant didn't understand that patients with Parkinson's disease have "on/off" periods, sometimes they can move well and, at other times, they are frozen and cannot move at all. She thought your family member was malingering, she complained that she wasn't even trying, but she didn't realize she literally couldn't budge. Or the nursing assistant says your family member "resists care," she won't cooperate when it's time to take a shower, but didn't realize that the problem was that the water wasn't warm enough. Maybe the name your family member calls the nursing assistant isn't a racist slur; it's a term of affection from her culture, one that's unfamiliar to the aide. But sometimes the only solution to conflict is a change of personnel. This can be a challenge for the charge nurse—she can work with her staff, but she has to distribute the assignments equally among them. Nonetheless, your role is to be an advocate for your family member, to do whatever you can to improve *her* situation.

Team meetings are almost always scheduled during the daytime to meet the needs of the multiple staff members who must attend—but not necessarily your needs. They are often short: several meetings are typically scheduled back-to-back; your family member may have half an hour or less allotted. They can be boring or feel like they're intended to rubber stamp whatever the staff are already doing or to approve decisions they've already reached about future care. But try thinking about them in a new light: so many people involved in taking care of one person, the person who matters to you! Here's your chance, in less than an hour, to make a difference in your family member's life.

Box 46.1

Team Meetings in the Nursing Home

- Participants: nurse, nursing assistant, physician, social worker, physical therapist
- Topics to discuss: nutrition, mobility, medications, mood
- Opportunity to discuss goals of care

PART VIII

Getting Additional Help

So far in this book, I have focused on you and your family member as he travels through the health-care system receiving care in the doctor's office, the hospital, the skilled nursing facility, and his home. I have talked about the various people, principally health professionals of various kinds, that you will encounter in each of these settings and how best to deal with them so as to ensure the best possible care for your relative. But accessing medical care in the United States today involves more than just people and institutions; achieving excellence requires a good health insurance plan, adequate financial resources, and a network of community resources. You may be involved with many of these aspects of your family member's health care as well as with the people who provide treatment and the facilities where they provide it. And ideally you will share the responsibility for caregiving, at least to some extent, with other family members. This section highlights some of the key issues that you may need to address regardless of the specific medical conditions that afflict your relative.

CHAPTER 47

Choosing a Health Plan

Your relative will probably already be enrolled in a health insurance plan when you start your caregiving role. As you become progressively more involved in his health care, you will find that he needs all kinds of medical services: hospital care, physician visits, skilled nursing facility care, home care, prescription medications, durable medical equipment, glasses, hearing aids—the list goes on and on. You may also become painfully aware of which of these are "covered" by health insurance and which are not. Each year, your relative is free to switch to a different plan during a brief window called "open enrollment." Deciding which one is best, *given his particular circumstances*, is complicated, but a few pointers may help you (figure 47.1).

Perhaps most important, you should realize that a free health benefits counseling service is open to Medicare beneficiaries *and their families or caregivers*. Known as "SHIP" (State Health Insurance Assistance Program), this is an independent program funded by the federal government and is not associated with the insurance industry. The specific name of the program varies from state to state: in Massachusetts, for example, it is known as the SHINE Program (Serving Health Insurance Needs of Everyone). A directory of SHIP programs is available at https://www .seniorsresourceguide.com/directories /National/SHIP/.

Dual Eligibility: Medicare and Medicaid

If your relative is eligible for *Medicaid* (the combined state/federal insurance program for those with low incomes and/or disabilities) and is sixty-five or older, then he is *dually eligible*; that is, he qualifies for both

Medicare and Medicaid. It's actually even more complicated: your relative may not meet the criteria for full-blown Medicaid coverage, but might be eligible for a Medicare Savings Program that pays for part of his health insurance premium (Part A is hospital coverage and Part B is physician and lab test coverage). These programs include

- Qualified Medicare Beneficiary Program, which helps pay for Part A and/or Part B premiums, deductibles, co-insurance, co-payments

- Specified Low Income Medicare Beneficiary (SLMB) Program, which helps pay for Part B premiums

- Qualifying Individual (QI) Program, which helps pay Part B premiums

The options open to your relative if he is dually eligible vary from state to state. In some states, Medicaid is delivered though a managed care plan; in others, Medicaid is exclusively fee-for-service. Your family member may have little choice about what plan to join. A medical social worker may be the best person to help you and your relative negotiate the Medicaid application process. She can also advise you about future eligibility, especially if your relative might one day need nursing home care (paid for by Medicaid if he has used up, or "spent down" almost all of his assets).

Traditional Medicare versus Medicare Advantage

If your relative is not on Medicaid, you will need to decide whether he should enroll in "traditional" (fee-for-service) Medicare or a Medicare Advantage plan. Traditional or usual Medicare has the advantage of providing the greatest amount of choice—of physicians, hospitals, and whatever else your family member might need. On the other hand, to obtain comprehensive coverage and limit out-of-pocket expenditures, your relative will need Medicare Part A (hospital care) *and* Medicare Part B (physician and lab test coverage) *and* Medicare Part D (drug coverage) *and* a supplemental plan (to cover the co-pays and deductibles from Parts A, B, and D, which can be considerable).

By way of illustration, there is a $1,364 deductible for each "benefit period" under Part A in 2019, so the cost of the first hospital stay of the year will be $1,364 plus $341 co-insurance per day for a stay longer than sixty days. Medicare does not cover several services such as dental care, vision care, and hearing aids, some or all of which are provided by select Medicare Advantage plans. Finally, case management and other systems of coordinating care are limited in traditional Medicare plans. By contrast, Medicare Advantage plans generally come with hospital, physician, and drug coverage bundled together. No supplementary plan is necessary as the deductibles and co-pays are modest. Your family member will not receive an itemized, incomprehensible report each month with the heading, "this is not a bill," and then other statements that are bills, as is customary with Medicare. He may be able to get glasses, dentures, and a hearing aid through the Medicare Advantage plan. At the same time, his choice of physicians and hospitals will likely be restricted by the plan. If your relative is thinking of switching to a Medicare Advantage plan but is happy with his current physician, you should check whether that doctor accepts the new plan.

As of 2018, about 30 percent of older people are opting for a Medicare Advantage plan. Individuals who are sicker and with greater needs tend to dis-enroll from Medicare Advantage and choose fee-for-service Medicare, though the extent of this phenomenon varies markedly from plan to plan.

How to Select a Medicare Advantage Plan

In areas of the country with multiple Medicare Advantage plans, you will have to figure out which one is best for your relative if you choose to go this route. One place to start is with national ratings. Medicare uses a five-star system to rate plans. In addition to a summary rating of plan quality, Medicare provides a rating for the plan's effectiveness in keeping patients healthy (how often its patients receive screenings, tests, and vaccines), another rating for how well they manage chronic conditions, a third one for "member experience," a fourth based on member complaints, and a fifth based on "customer satisfaction," which is presumably closely linked to "member experience."

Another alternative is to use a private rating system such as the one offered by *U.S. News*, which combines Medicare's star rating system with other measures of quality (figure 47.2).

Some Medicare Advantage plans offer a "special needs plan" (SNP) that covers extra services such as coordination of care. Your relative may be eligible for this type of plan if he lives in a nursing home, if he is enrolled in both Medicare and Medicaid, or if he has a severe chronic condition.

Once you have identified a couple of good prospects, you should look up whether your relative's physicians and usual hospital are in their "network." Most plans allow you to receive care out of network but charge much more for these services. Ideally, you should also look at what physicians are covered whom your relative doesn't currently see but might benefit from—such as geriatricians or palliative care doctors.

This process should narrow down your selection considerably. In some states (Massachusetts, where I live, is one), a given company may offer several variants: one plan has more generous

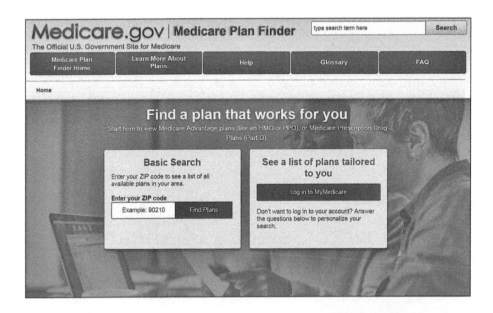

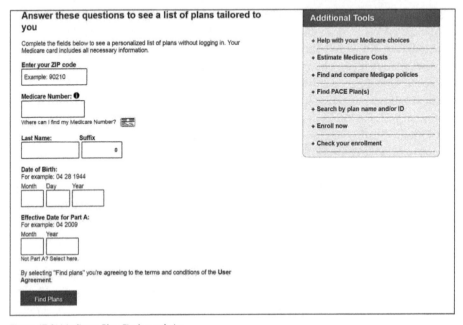

Figure 47.1. Medicare Plan Finder website

drug coverage (or covers a particular expensive medication that your family member takes regularly) and another one lets him see physicians out of network with minimal or no penalty. Each comes with a different monthly premium. You will need to figure out whether your relative is likely to be better off with a bare-bones plan that has no monthly premium or a more comprehensive plan that has a monthly premium.

Choosing a Traditional (Fee-for-Service) Medicare Plan

The main choices here are whether to select a prescription drug plan (and, if so, which one) and whether to get a Medigap policy (and, if so, which one). With respect to a prescription drug plan (covered by Medicare Part D), the average monthly cost in 2018 was $34. You should be sure that the plan

STATE	COMPANIES
	US.News Best Insurance Cos. for Medicare Advantage 2019
ALABAMA	CIGNA-HEALTHSPRING
ARIZONA	CIGNA
ARKANSAS	CIGNA-HEALTHSPRING
CALIFORNIA	KAISER PERMANENTE ANTHEM BLUE CROSS CHINESE COMMUNITY HEALTH PLAN SCAN HEALTH PLAN
COLORADO	KAISER PERMANENTE
DISTRICT OF COLUMBIA	KAISER PERMANENTE
FLORIDA	CAREPLUS HEALTH PLANS, INC. FLORIDA BLUE HMO HEALTHSPRING OF FLORIDA, INC. HEALTHSUN HEALTH PLANS, INC. CAPITAL HEALTH PLAN FREEDOM HEALTH, INC. OPTIMUM HEALTHCARE, INC. ULTIMATE HEALTH PLANS
GEORGIA	KAISER PERMANENTE

Figure 47.2. *U.S. News and World Report* Medicare Advantage ratings from *U.S. News* website

covers whatever drugs your relative is taking on a regular basis. Some plans charge different amounts for various drugs depending on what "tier" they are in, with cheap generic drugs in the lowest tier and expensive, brand name drugs in the highest tier. It's also important to realize that, until 2020, all prescription drug plans have a "donut hole," the time between when your family member has consumed more than $3,000 but less than $4,700 worth of medication. During that period, he will be charged a much larger amount for prescription medications. When he emerges from the donut hole, he enters the period of "catastrophic coverage," during which he will pay 5 percent of the cost of his medications—until the end of the calendar year, at which point the clock resets and the process starts all over again. You should also know that if your family member meets certain income limitations, he may qualify for the "Extra Help Program" that pays part of the cost of premiums, deductibles, and co-payments. Once your relative signs up for a Medicare Part D plan, he can switch plans during the open enrollment period; however, if he fails to sign up right away when he becomes eligible, he may be charged a penalty when he does enroll.

As for Medigap policies, these are designed to cover whatever traditional Medicare charges by way of deductibles and co-payments. Ten different supplemental plans (labeled A, B, C, D, F, G, K, L, M, and N) are available in most states, with varying coverage and cost (figure 47.3).

The average monthly premium for an F plan, which offers the most comprehensive coverage, is $321 and for the K plan, which offers less extensive coverage—for example, it pays only 50 percent of the cost of a rehab stay—is $124. There is also a high deductible plan, referred to as "high F," which costs much less (an average of $72 per

Medigap Plans	A	B	C	D	F*	G	K	L	M	N
Part A coinsurance and hospital costs up to 365 days after Medicare benefits are used up	✓	✓	✓	✓	✓	✓	✓	✓	✓	✓
Part B coinsurance or copayment	✓	✓	✓	✓	✓	✓	50%	75%	✓	✓₁
Blood (First 3 pints)	✓	✓	✓	✓	✓	✓	50%	75%	✓	✓
Hospice Care coinsurance or copayment	✓	✓	✓	✓	✓	✓	50%	75%	✓	✓
Skilled nursing facility care coinsurance			✓	✓	✓	✓	50%	75%	✓	✓
Part A deductible		✓	✓	✓	✓	✓	50%	75%	50%	✓
Part B deductible			✓		✓					
Part B excess charges					✓	✓				
Foreign travel (up to plan limits)			80%	80%	80%	80%			80%	80%
Out-of-pocket limit +							$5,120	$2,500		

+ When you meet your out-of-pocket yearly limit and your Part B deductible, the Medigap plan has 100% of covered services for the rest of the calendar year.

* Plan F offers a high-deductible plan. This means you pay for medicare-covered costs up to the deductible amount of $2,200 in 2017 before your plan pays anything.

1 Plan N pays 100% of the Plan B coinsurance, except for a copayment of up to $20 for some office visits and up to $50 copayment for emergency room visits that don't result in inpatient admission.

Figure 47.3. Medicare Supplement Insurance (Medigap) comparison chart from unitedmedicareadvisors.com

month) but doesn't kick in until out-of-pocket costs have reached a specified amount, which in 2018 was $2,240.

If this seems complicated, it is. To choose wisely, you need a crystal ball to foresee whether your relative will run up a large physician bill or be admitted to a skilled nursing facility in the coming year. It's simpler and often cheaper to enroll in a Medicare Advantage plan which, once you select the company offering the insurance, offers a "prix fixe" rather than an "à la carte" menu of choices. But remember your family member can change plans during the annual open enrollment period.

Box 47.1

Choosing a Health Insurance Plan

- Medicare Advantage plans are all-in-one plans that often cover hospital care, outpatient care, and drug costs

- Frail elders using traditional Medicare should generally enroll in Part B, Part D, and Medigap

- Choices for dually eligible elders, who qualify for Medicare and Medicaid, vary by state

- State Health Insurance Assistant Programs (SHIP) can help guide the selection

CHAPTER 48

Paying for Health Care

I f you are involved in your family member's health care, you may well be concerned with her finances. Paying for food and rent plus other basic necessities, not to mention concert tickets or television repairs or travel, is beyond the purview of this book. But paying her medical expenses is not—you simply won't be able to arrange for services, such a private home health aide, if your relative cannot afford them. The decision whether to opt for a brand name drug or to ask for a generic alternative may depend on how much her prescription drug plan charges for each. You may also be involved in choosing which physician, hospital, or health insurance plan your family member selects. To make a wise choice, you will at the very least want to know what her current plan pays for and what it does not. You should also realize that for the frailest, oldest individuals spending on health care takes a big bite out of their budget: the Kaiser Family Foundation calculated that people over age eighty-five spend 22 percent of their per capita total income on out-of-pocket health-care costs.

Paying for a Health Insurance Plan

A lmost everyone who is over age sixty-five is entitled to Medicare but that doesn't mean it's free. There are no premiums for Medicare Part A, the component covering hospital care, but everything else comes at a price—where everything else means physician fees and lab tests (covered by Medicare Part B), medications (covered by Medicare Part D), and co-pays and deductibles (covered at least in part by Medigap). The cost of a Medigap plan depends on where you live and on how extensive the coverage you select is, the cost of a Medicare D plan depends on which drugs are included, and the cost of a Medicare Part B plan varies depending on your relative's income (table 48.1).

Table 48.1

Cost of Medicare Part B (2018)

Individual tax return with income	Joint tax return with income	Income-related surcharge	Total monthly premium amount
Less than or equal to $85,000	Less than or equal to $170,000	$0.00	$134.00
More than $85,000 and less than or equal to $107,000	More than $170,000 and less than or equal to $214,000	$53.50	$187.50
More than $107,000 and less than or equal to $133,500	More than $214,000 and less than or equal to $267,000	$133.90	$267.90
More than $133,500 and less than or equal to $160,000	More than $267,000 and less than or equal to $320,000	$214.30	$348.30
More than $160,000	More than $320,000	$294.60	$428.60

If your family member opts for a Medicare Advantage plan instead of conventional fee-for-service Medicare, she will still need to pay for Medicare Part B. In addition, your family member will need a Medicare Part D plan to pay for prescription medications unless she enrolls in a Medicare Advantage plan that includes medications. The average monthly cost in 2018 for Part D coverage was $34 although there is variability depending on just what plan you choose.

Because most health plans require co-payments and deductibles, many people also pay a separate premium for a Medigap policy (or opt for a Medicare Advantage plan that is equivalent to Medicare Parts A, B, and D as well as Medigap insurance all rolled into one). The average cost for the most popular Medigap policy is $1,813 per year, or about $150 per month (for information about choosing a health insurance plan based on what's covered rather than cost, see chapter 47, "Choosing a Health Plan"). Frail older people generally have sufficiently complex medical needs to warrant a comprehensive health plan.

Medication

The cost of prescription medications varies enormously. Without insurance coverage, the cost of a thirty-day supply of a commonly prescribed generic drug such as hydrochlorothiazide (the lowest dose, 12.5 mg) in my area is about $14. But the cost of a thirty-day supply of a typical dose of the targeted chemotherapy drug Tarceva (150 mg) is $9,000 a month, again without insurance. You can see why having drug coverage (either a Medicare Part D plan or a Medicare Advantage plan that includes medications) is so important for your family member.

Even with health insurance your relative can run up a substantial bill based on the co-payments. Many plans today use a tiered system that classifies drugs as in one of three (or sometimes four or five) levels, with the monthly co-payments in one popular plan running at $4 for tier 1, generic drugs (such as hydrochlorothiazide), $38 for tier 3, brand name drugs, and a charge of 33 percent of the cost for tier 5 specialty drugs (such as Tarceva). Choosing the best plan for your relative requires adding up the costs of the premium plus the co-pays for the medications she is *already taking*. What makes selecting a plan so tricky is that you cannot possibly predict what medications she will require in the future. However, you can make an educated guess about whether she will benefit from a plan that provides generous coverage: if she has multiple medical problems or one complex, serious illness *and* her overriding goal of care is to prolong life, there's a good chance she will be taking one or more expensive medications.

It is also a good idea to ask your family member's physician about the cost of any new medication that he prescribes. You may be shocked to learn that he has no idea about drug costs in general and almost certainly not about the cost with your relative's plan in particular. You may want to inquire about the availability of a generic medication. At the very least, when you go to the pharmacy to fill the medication you should inquire about the cost when you present the prescription and *before* it's actually filled.

Physician Visits

A major component of medical care for your family member is apt to be physician visits. Assuming that she has Medicare Part B and that she's enrolled in a fee-for-service plan, she will pay 20 percent of the Medicare-allowable charge for a physician visit after she has met the yearly deductible ($185 in 2019). If her physician "accepts assignment," she cannot be charged an additional fee by the physician, even if what Medicare pays is less than what the physician charges. If her doctor does not "accept assignment," he can charge up to 15 percent above the Medicare-approved amount. Most Medigap plans will cover these additional charges—but premiums for such policies range between $124 and $423, depending on just what they cover.

The situation is quite different if your family member is enrolled in a Medicare Advantage plan. Many of these plans have no deductibles but do have a modest co-pay for a physician visit: a typical Medicare Advantage plan in Massachusetts, for example, features a $10 co-pay for primary care visits and a $25 co-pay for a visit to a specialist. If you are interested both in keeping things simple and keeping costs low, a Medicare Advantage plan has a great deal to recommend it. Provided there is a high-quality option in your area, one that allows your family member to see whatever physicians she is already going to, you might want her to switch to such a plan during the next open enrollment period.

Your family member will face a very different set of health-care costs if she opts for a concierge practice. In this arrangement, she pays a retainer fee to her physician, regardless of how often she sees him. The retainer averages $1,500 a year but there is significant variability, with some practices charging less and some charging considerably more. In most cases, this fee is what the physician gets on top of his usual Medicare reimbursement—ostensibly covering things that Medicare does not provide for, such as twenty-four-hour access to the physician and extensive coordination of care. In some models, the physician opts out of the Medicare program entirely. In this variant, also called "direct primary care," the physician does not bill an insurance company: the retainer fee covers doctors' visits and there are no co-pays or deductibles—or claims to be filed. It's important to underscore that while the physician might not be part of the Medicare program, your family member should continue to be enrolled in Medicare. Your relative needs insurance so as to have access to hospital care, specialist care, and skilled nursing facility care as well as diagnostic tests, none of which is included in the concierge physician's retainer fee.

Because concierge practices allow physicians to do well financially despite a relatively small number of patients (typical concierge practices keep the size of the "patient panel" at four hundred to six hundred rather than the usual two thousand for conventional physicians), your family member may get more individual attention with such a plan. More time is usually allocated per visit and physicians are more accessible than with standard care. However, no studies to date have demonstrated that the quality of care is superior with this kind of arrangement. Since your relative will need to purchase health insurance on top of paying the concierge fee, it's an expensive way to get a few extras.

Nursing Visits

Nursing care in the home is principally one of two types: ongoing primary care in which a registered nurse or nurse practitioner is the main person providing service, or transitional care basically after an acute illness. Your relative will have a nurse who comes to the home on a continuing basis if she is part of a primary care program that provides this service or if she is enrolled in hospice. A small but growing number of primary care programs have a home visit component (table 48.2); most of them are participants in Medicare's "Independence at Home" demonstration program, an offshoot of the Affordable Care Act. These practices cater to a small subset of the two million Americans who are essentially homebound and the five million additional Americans who can only get to a physician's office with difficulty.

Hospice, by contrast, is utilized by far more people. In 2016, 1.43 million Medicare beneficiaries were enrolled in hospice at some point during the year. Hospice is generally fully covered by Medicare, although your family member can be charged up to $5 for each medication prescribed by the hospice physician. If your relative was enrolled in a Medicare Advantage and then opts for hospice care, coverage of treatment related to her terminal illness will be covered by the Medicare hospice benefit. The Medicare Advantage plan can continue to provide coverage for all medical problems *unrelated* to her hospice diagnosis.

A far more common reason for your relative to receive nursing visits than either home hospice or primary care at home is post-acute care. Sooner or later, your family member is likely to receive care through a home health agency such as the Visiting Nurse Association. The most common version of this service is transitional care arranged by the hospital or skilled nursing facility at the time of discharge after an acute illness. In this situation, a nurse will provide whatever monitoring or direct care the physician ordered: checking blood pressure, dressing wounds, and reviewing that medications are being taken correctly are several common examples. The nurse will usually visit a few times, after which your relative is regarded as stable or as having recovered from her acute illness and no longer deemed to need a visiting nurse. This service is covered by Medicare Part A and is administered by an agency certified by Medicare.

Your family member might also have nursing visits for a short time while she is being treated at home for an acute problem instead of going to the hospital. If she is taking a course of antibiotics for bronchitis or pneumonia and her condition is a bit tenuous, her primary care physician can arrange for a visiting nurse to make sure she is improving with treatment. To qualify for coverage, whether after hospitalization, after a stay at a rehabilitation facility, or during acute home treatment, your

Table 48.2
Sample Home Visit Programs

Practice	Doctors Making House Calls	House Call Providers	MedStar Health*	Penn Medicine*	Visiting Physicians Association**	Landmark Health
Year founded	2002	1995	1999	1994	1993	2012
Organization type	For-profit medical group	Not-for-profit medical group	Academic medical center	Academic medical center	For-profit medical group	For-profit, risk-based medical group that contracts with Medicare Advantage plans
Location	Headquartered in Durham, NC; serves most of the state	Headquartered in Portland, OR; serves three Portland-area counties	Headquartered in Washington, D.C.; serves patients in D.C. and Baltimore	Philadelphia	Headquartered in Troy, MI; serves patients in 12 states	Headquartered in Huntington Beach, CA; serves patients in six states
Number of patients	8,000 currently served	Average daily census of 1,400 to 1,450	Average daily census of 620	Average monthly census of 210	Average daily census of 37,000	45,000 currently served

Source: S. Klein, M. Hostetter, and D. McCarthy, "An Overview of Home-Based Primary Care: Learning from the Field," *The Commonwealth Fund*, last modified June 7, 2017, https://www.commonwealthfund.org/publications/issue-briefs/2017/jun/overview-home-based-primary-care-learning-field.

* MedStar and Penn Medicine participate in the Independence at Home Demonstration as part of the Mid-Atlantic Consortium, which also includes Virginia Commonwealth University (not profiled).

** Visiting Physicians Association works closely with its management services organization, U.S. Medical Management, to assess and meet patients' needs.

family member needs to be under the care of a physician who is required to periodically review her care. She is also supposed to be homebound and to need services intermittently or for a short time. If your relative meets these conditions, Medicare will pay in full for the nursing visits.

If your relative does not meet these criteria, or if you feel she needs skilled nursing care for a longer period of time or more hours a day than Medicare will provide, you can arrange privately to hire a nurse to come to the home. Most people find a nurse through a home health agency that vets their employees and can make alternate arrangements if the nurse you have been using is unable to come as scheduled. You can also hire someone directly but will need to inter-view that person, check references, and make do without a backup. Your family member will only rarely need a licensed practical nurse (LPN) or registered nurse (RN) at home outside of what Medicare provides; she is far more likely to need supplementary home health aide services. Medicare covers the cost of an aide, someone who helps with personal care, but typically for only a very limited number of hours a week, over a short period of time, and only if she qualifies for nursing care. If your family member is enrolled in Medicaid, she may qualify for a home health aide, though in many parts of the country there is a long wait for such services. If you need to arrange for more hours, beyond what Medicare or Medicaid provides, you will find rates averaging $22 per hour.

Physical Therapy

Physical therapy is another modality that is usually covered by Medicare, whether provided at home or in a physical therapy center. The same home health agency that is your family member's source for a visiting nurse—and a home health aide, if she needs one—will also provide a physical therapist to come to the house. Coverage is usually limited to a few visits. If you feel your relative needs ongoing physical therapy, you can choose to pay privately. It's expensive: the average cost of a one-hour visit is $41. Instead, you might try asking the physical therapist to supply your relative with a list of exercises she can do on her own at home. Or, she may decide to join a gym.

Dental Care

Good dental care is a long-neglected aspect of geriatric health care. Your family member needs her teeth to speak clearly and to chew her food thoroughly. Poor dentition and unhealthy gums are a breeding ground for bacteria that sometimes make their way into the lungs, causing pneumonia. Shockingly, fee-for-service Medicare does not cover dental care. In fact, the 1965 legislation authorizing the Medicare program specifically *excluded* dental care from the list of covered services. A few Medicare Advantage programs are the exception to the rule and do provide limited dental coverage. Extensive dental work, such as a set of dentures, is almost never covered.

Dental insurance is available on the private market, but the offerings for older people are limited. Curiously, dental insurance tends to work according to the opposite principle of most insurance—instead of providing cata-strophic coverage, it pays principally for preventive care and perhaps simple fillings. In other words, it pays for predictable but relatively inexpensive care, leaving your family member at risk of substantial bills if she has unanticipated, major needs. Complete, permanent dentures can cost anywhere from $300 to $5,000 per plate, and your relative will likely need both an upper and a lower plate. The cheapest dentures are made using standard molds rather than being custom fitted for your family member. Less expensive dentures are made with lower quality materials that are prone to breakage and that look artificial. A reasonably good quality set of dentures will cost at least $1,600 and probably closer to $3,000. You should realize that to be fitted for dentures, your family member may also need to have one or more residual teeth extracted, adding further complications to the procedure—and additional costs.

Durable Medical Equipment

Your family member may benefit from a variety of devices that Medicare calls "durable medical equipment," including a cane or walker, a wheelchair, a hospital bed, or a bedside commode (figure 48.1). She may need a cane or walker to maintain her mobility and decrease the risk of falling. For longer distances, or if she has a greater degree of impairment, a wheelchair might be more appropriate. If she has difficulty sitting up in bed or getting in and out of bed, an electric bed such as is used in the hospital might be essential to maintain some degree of independence. If walking from the bed to the bathroom is too far for your relative, a commode might allow her to maintain her dignity—and to avoid the need for a night time personal care attendant.

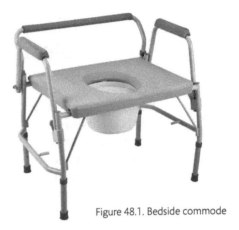

Figure 48.1. Bedside commode

Mental Health Care

Mental health is a critical, if often neglected, component of medical care. Coverage under Medicare is principally short-term and may not suffice for ongoing psychotherapy. Moreover, finding a geriatric-oriented therapist can be challenging: geriatric psychiatry is a small specialty. You may find that a clinical psychologist, clinical social worker, or clinical nurse specialist meets your relative's needs. Medicare Part B pays for any of these clinicians, although co-pays and deductibles apply. Medicare Part D pays for psychiatric medications. Finally, Medicare Part A pays for mental health hospitalization.

Other mental health services specifically covered by Medicare include an annual *depression screen* by your family member's primary care physician, *group therapy*, and *family counseling* if needed to help with ongoing treatment.

Other Services

Your family member may wish to belong to a gym in order to participate in a regular exercise program. Gym membership is not covered by traditional, fee-for-service Medicare but some Medicare Advantage plans offer discounted rates.

If your relative has difficulty taking in sufficient protein and calories to maintain her weight, or to gain weight if necessary, she may benefit from nutritional supplements. Over-the-counter supplements such as Ensure can provide between 8 and 16 grams of protein in 8 ounces. Neither Medicare Part B nor Medicare Part D covers oral supplements of this type. The cheapest way to obtain nutritional supplements is to buy in bulk from online suppliers. For example, in the fall of 2019, Amazon offered a case of sixteen bottles of Ensure Plus (each 8-ounce bottle includes 13 grams of protein) for $24.97. You can also purchase a six-pack at your local drug store or supermarket, where the cost of a six-pack is in the range of $11.

Overall Expenditures

If you add up all of your relative's out-of-pocket health-care costs—that is, all the premiums, all the deductibles and co-payments, and all the expenses that are not covered by health insurance at all—you may be shocked. The more chronic conditions she has and the more limitations she has in her daily activities, the higher the cost. An estimate of costs from 2014 can be seen in table 48.3, where "median annual out-of-pocket costs" give you an idea of the typical expenditure, recognizing that half the people spent more than that and half spent less. The "highest tier of spending" lists what the costs were for the top 10 percent of spenders.

Table 48.3
The Cost of Chronic Illness

Condition	Median Annual Out-of-Pocket Costs	Highest Tier of Spending*
No chronic conditions	$2,127	$6,004
1–2 chronic conditions	$2,959	$7,414
5+ chronic conditions	$3,751	$9,397
3+ limitations in activities of daily living**	$4,192	$20,611

Source: Kaiser Family Foundation report, 2014.

Those with chronic conditions such as diabetes, cancer, Parkinson's, arthritis, high blood pressure, osteoporosis, and pulmonary disease pay less over a lifetime but more annually than healthier retirees.

* Based on the top 10 percent of health-care consumers.

** Activities of daily living are eating, bathing, dressing, mobility, continence, and toileting.

You may not have bargained on playing a role in your family member's finances when you took on your caregiving role. Perhaps your family agreed on a division of labor and someone else is responsible for paying the bills and making fiscal decisions. You can see from the discussion of medical expenses in this chapter, expenses that range from paying for an insurance policy to gym membership, with everything from medications, private nursing and home health aides and dentures in between, that the medical and the financial are often inseparable. Working together with whoever does handle your relative's money, whether that is your relative herself, a sibling, or a paid professional, is crucial for promoting her health.

Box 48.1

Major Out-of-Pocket Medical Expenses

- Health insurance premiums
- Co-insurance and co-payments for services
- Medications
- Physician visits
- Nursing visits
- Physical therapy
- Dental care
- Mental health care
- Medical equipment

CHAPTER 49

Planning for Future Medical Care

As a caregiver, you may be so busy dealing with today that you have a hard time thinking about tomorrow. Because so much about the future is unpredictable, I don't advocate an enormous amount of planning, but laying the groundwork for future illness seems prudent. After all, since your family member already has significant problems—otherwise you wouldn't need to be a caregiver—odds are that he will develop additional problems in the future, or at the very least will experience an acute worsening of some of his symptoms. You can predict which problems are most likely to act up and have a plan in place for dealing with those issues: if your relative has chronic heart failure, his lungs are very likely to fill up with fluid at some point; if he has chronic lung disease, his breathing is probably going to get worse, especially if he has the flu or pneumonia; if he has early Alzheimer's disease, he's going to get progressively more advanced dementia over time.

When I suggest thinking about what to do in each of the situations that's most likely to occur, recognizing that your relative may develop an entirely new problem that you had not prepared

for, I mean specifying the broad outlines of an approach. Would he want to go to the hospital? If so, would a stay in the intensive care unit (ICU) be acceptable? Would he be willing to undergo major surgery? Would he want attempted cardiopulmonary resuscitation? To help think about these questions, it's useful to begin with reviewing your family member's goals of care, once he has a clear idea of his overall health (for more on the relationship between health state and goals of care, see chapter 4, "Determining Your Family Member's Health State"). Ideally, his primary care physician will then help you translate those goals into a treatment plan.

While your relative may have all kinds of goals, all sorts of things he'd like to do, ranging from seeing the birth of a new great-grandchild to writing his memoirs, from a *medical perspective*, there are only a few major goals. Your family member may want to live as long as possible, regardless of how uncomfortable or risky the treatment. He might want to focus exclusively on his physical and emotional comfort. Or he might want something in between these two extremes, such as treatment that gives him the chance to remain as independent and able to function as he is currently. Clarifying with you and with his physician what his goals are is the first step in planning for the possibility of future illness. The "Starter Kit" of the Conversation Project (theconversationproject.org) offers suggestions for ways to help you start a conversation about wishes. Other programs, such as Prepare (https://prepareforyourcare.org/welcome) and My Directives (mydirectives.com), provide more comprehensive advance care planning tools.

Your relative may want to put in writing what is most important to him. He can do that in the form of a letter, or he can make an audiotape or, if you're really ambitious, you could make a videotape of him talking about his goals. To actually translate those goals into practice, many people find it helpful to prepare an *advance directive* or a *medical order* governing future care.

Let's start with advance directives. The first type of directive spells out *who* has the legal right to make decisions for your family member if he's not able to make decisions for himself. It says nothing about *what* decisions his surrogate (or agent or health-care proxy, as the person is also called) should make. I strongly believe, and most ethicists and physicians agree, that *everyone* should appoint a health-care surrogate. It's especially important for older people who are at high risk of finding themselves in a situation where they cannot speak for themselves; it's important for the physicians to know with whom they should speak about medical decisions. Every state has its own official form, which you should use. Typically, your relative has to sign the form and his

signature must be witnessed by two adults. You don't need a lawyer, though in some states the form has to be notarized. Here's an example of a typical form (figure 49.1).

The second type of advance directive, which generally supplements choosing a health-care proxy, is a *living will* (figure 49.2). This is a document that spells out in greater or lesser detail what your relative would want if he became seriously ill and could not speak for himself. Most states have their own living will forms; some states, such as Massachusetts, do not technically recognize a living will, though any statement of this form that your family member signs and shares with his physician and his health-care surrogate will carry moral weight. Most living wills only apply to someone who has "an incurable and irreversible illness, disease, or illness judged to be a terminal condition," and many are restricted to situations where "death is imminent." In those limited circumstances, the document generally indicates that the person would want treatment only if it promoted "comfort care."

Other advance directives are more detailed and specific. They list a variety of scenarios, of possible situations in which your family member might find himself, and ask what approach to care he would want in each one. An example of this kind of directive is contained within the Five Wishes, a comprehensive advance care planning document (figure 49.3). Wish number two is "My Wish for the Kind of Medical Treatment I Want or Don't Want."

Instead of using an advance directive, your family member might opt for a *medical order.* You can think of advance directives as wish statements: they attempt to spell out in advance what your relative thinks he would want in certain circumstances. A medical order, by contrast, is signed by a physician, as well as by your family member (or by you, acting as his representative), and is like any other medical order in a hospital—it is supposed to dictate what actually happens. Most states let patients sign an out-of-hospital do-not-resuscitate (DNR) order, which is one form of a medical order. It deals exclusively with whether or not to attempt cardiopulmonary resuscitation (CPR). If your relative doesn't want CPR tried if he is found by emergency medical technicians (EMTs) to have stopped breathing and his heart is not beating, then he will want to sign such a form and tack it onto his refrigerator door—EMTs are trained to look there for just such a form.

Finally, the last few years have seen the rise of a new kind of medical order which is similar to scenario-driven directives in enumerating a variety of possible treatments, but it's an order, not an advance directive, and it is applicable in the event of any acute illness. The original such document, which was developed in Oregon, is called a POLST form (Physician Orders for Life-Sustaining Treatment). Many but by no means all other states have developed similar forms that are targeted to frail and chronically ill patients living in their own home, in assisted living, or in a nursing home. West Virginia calls its form the MOST (Medical Orders for Scope of Treatment) and Massachusetts has the MOLST (Medical Orders for Life-Sustaining Treatment). Often, the beginning of the form deals with the direst emergencies—what to do if your relative isn't breathing or his heart isn't beating—and then addresses other situations, such as infections (would he want antibiotics?) or the inability to swallow (would your relative want a feeding tube?). Ideally, completing a POLST should take place only after your relative has discussed his prognosis and goals of care with you and his physician. The beauty of the POLST approach is that the form can travel with your relative as he goes from home to the office, to the hospital, or to rehab, and should be recognized as valid everywhere (figure 49.4).

Physicians are much better than they used to be at asking you and your family member to think about your wishes in the event of a serious medical problem. But it never hurts to be proactive. Explain to your relative that you want to be able to advise his physician appropriately if he is unable to speak for himself and the best way to achieve this goal is to discuss, together, his preferences. Then raise the issue with his physician and make sure his wishes are documented. And if his situation changes—if he develops a new serious illness or his ability to function independently declines—bring the subject up again. In the long run, this strategy will help both of you.

YOUR BIRTH DATE (m/d/y)
___/___/___

MASSACHUSETTS HEALTH CARE PROXY

1 I, _____, residing at
(Principal: PRINT your name)

_____
(Street)   (City/town)   (State/ZIP)

appoint as my **Health Care Agent**: _____
(Name of person you choose as Agent)

of_____
(Street)   (City/town)   (State/ZIP)

Agent's tel (h) _____ (w) _____ E-mail _____

OPTIONAL: If my agent is unwilling or unable to serve, then I appoint as my **Alternate Agent**:

_____
(Name of person you choose as Alternate Agent)

of_____
(Street)   (City/town)   (State/ZIP)   (Phone)

2 My Agent shall have the authority to make all health care decisions for me, including decisions about life-sustaining treatment, subject to any limitations I state below, if I am unable to make health care decisions myself. My Agent's authority becomes effective if my attending physician determines in writing that I lack the capacity to make or to communicate health care decisions. My Agent is then to have the same authority to make health care decisions as I would if I had the capacity to make them **EXCEPT** (here list the limitations, *if any*, you wish to place on your Agent's authority):

I direct my Agent to make health care decisions based on my Agent's assessment of my personal wishes. If my personal wishes are unknown, my Agent is to make health care decisions based on my Agent's assessment of my best interests. Photocopies of this Health Care Proxy shall have the same force and effect as the original and may be given to other health care providers.

3   **Signed:**_____ **Date:** ___/___/___ (mo/day/yr)

Complete only if Principal is physically unable to sign: I have signed the Principal's name above at his/her direction in the presence of the Principal and two witnesses.

_____   _____
(Name)   (Street)

_____
(City/town)   (State/ZIP)

4 **WITNESS STATEMENT:** We, the undersigned, each witnessed the signing of this Health Care Proxy by the Principal or at the direction of the Principal and state that the Principal appears to be at least 18 years of age, of sound mind and under no constraint or undue influence. Neither of us is named as the Health Care Agent or Alternate Agent in this document.
In our presence, on this day ___/___/___ (mo / day / yr).

Witness #1 _____   Witness #2 _____
(Signature)   (Signature)

Name (print) _____   Name (print) _____

Address _____   Address _____

_____   _____

Figure 49.1. Massachusetts health-care proxy form

Statements of Health Care Agent and Alternate Agent (OPTIONAL)

Health Care Agent: I have been named by the Principal as the Principal's **Health Care Agent** by this Health Care Proxy. I have read this document carefully, and have personally discussed with the Principal his/her health care wishes at a time of possible incapacity. I know the Principal and accept this appointment freely. I am not an operator, administrator or employee of a hospital, clinic, nursing home, rest home, Soldiers Home or other health facility where the Principal is presently a patient or resident or has applied for admission. But if I am a person so described, I am also related to the Principal by blood, marriage, or adoption. If called upon and to the best of my ability, I will try to carry out the Principal's wishes.

(Signature of **Health Care Agent**)_____

Alternate Agent: I have been named by the Principal as the Principal's **Alternate Agent** by this Health Care Proxy. I have read this document carefully, and have personally discussed with the Principal his/her health care wishes at a time of possible incapacity. I know the Principal and accept this appointment freely. I am not an operator, administrator or employee of a hospital, clinic, nursing home, rest home, Soldiers Home or other health facility where the Principal is presently a patient or resident or has applied for admission. But if I am a person so described, I am also related to the Principal by blood, marriage, or adoption. If called upon and to the best of my ability, I will try to carry out the Principal's wishes.

(Signature of **Alternate Agent**)_____

* * * * *

Figure 49.1. Massachusetts health-care proxy form

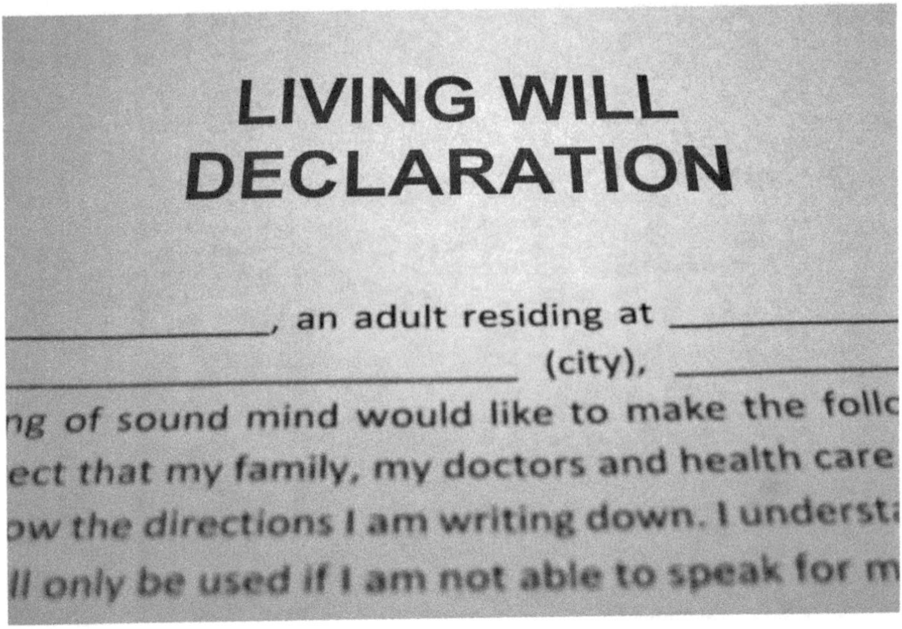

LIVING WILL DECLARATION

_____, an adult residing at _____

_____ (city), _____

ng of sound mind would like to make the follo

ect that my family, my doctors and health care

ow the directions I am writing down. I underst

ll only be used if I am not able to speak for m

Figure 49.2. Sample living will

Here is the kind of medical treatment that I want or don't want in the four situations listed below. I want my Health Care Agent, my family, my doctors and other health care providers, my friends and all others to know these directions.

Close to death:

If my doctor and another health care professional both decide that I am likely to die within a short period of time, and life-support treatment would only delay the moment of my death (Choose *one* of the following):

❏ I want to have life-support treatment.

❏ I do not want life-support treatment. If it has been started, I want it stopped.

❏ I want to have life-support treatment if my doctor believes it could help. But I want my doctor to stop giving me life-support treatment if it is not helping my health condition or symptoms.

In A Coma And Not Expected To Wake Up Or Recover:

If my doctor and another health care professional both decide that I am in a coma from which I am not expected to wake up or recover, and I have brain damage, and life-support treatment would only delay the moment of my death (Choose *one* of the following):

❏ I want to have life-support treatment.

❏ I do not want life-support treatment. If it has been started, I want it stopped.

❏ I want to have life-support treatment if my doctor believes it could help. But I want my doctor to stop giving me life-support treatment if it is not helping my health condition or symptoms.

Permanent And Severe Brain Damage And Not Expected To Recover:

If my doctor and another health care professional both decide that I have permanent and severe brain damage, (for example, I can open my eyes, but I can not speak or understand) and I am not expected to get better, and life-support treatment would only delay the moment of my death (Choose *one* of the following):

❏ I want to have life-support treatment.

❏ I do not want life-support treatment. If it has been started, I want it stopped.

❏ I want to have life-support treatment if my doctor believes it could help. But I want my doctor to stop giving me life-support treatment if it is not helping my health condition or symptoms.

In Another Condition Under Which I Do Not Wish To Be Kept Alive:

If there is another condition under which I do not wish to have life-support treatment, I describe it below. In this condition, I believe that the costs and burdens of life-support treatment are too much and not worth the benefits to me. Therefore, in this condition, I do not want life-support treatment. (For example, you may write "end-stage condition." That means that your health has gotten worse. You are not able to take care of yourself in any way, mentally or physically. Life-support treatment will not help you recover. Please leave the space blank if you have no other condition to describe.)

7

Figure 49.3. Five Wishes document. © Aging with Dignity. All rights reserved.

Physician Orders for Life-Sustaining Treatment (POLST)

First follow these orders, then contact Physician/NP/PA. A copy of the signed POLST form is a legally valid physician order. Any section not completed implies full treatment for that section. **POLST complements an Advance Directive and is not intended to replace that document.**

EMSA #111 B
(Effective 4/1/2017)*

Patient Last Name:	Date Form Prepared:
Patient First Name:	Patient Date of Birth:
Patient Middle Name:	Medical Record #: (optional)

A

Check One

CARDIOPULMONARY RESUSCITATION (CPR): *If patient has no pulse and is not breathing.*
If patient is NOT in cardiopulmonary arrest, follow orders in Sections B and C.

☐ Attempt Resuscitation/CPR (Selecting CPR in Section A <u>requires</u> selecting Full Treatment in Section B)

☐ Do Not Attempt Resuscitation/DNR (Allow Natural Death)

B

Check One

MEDICAL INTERVENTIONS: *If patient is found with a pulse and/or is breathing.*

☐ <u>Full Treatment</u> – primary goal of prolonging life by all medically effective means.
In addition to treatment described in Selective Treatment and Comfort-Focused Treatment, use intubation, advanced airway interventions, mechanical ventilation, and cardioversion as indicated.

      ☐ *Trial Period of Full Treatment.*

☐ <u>Selective Treatment</u> – goal of treating medical conditions while avoiding burdensome measures.
In addition to treatment described in Comfort-Focused Treatment, use medical treatment, IV antibiotics, and IV fluids as indicated. Do not intubate. May use non-invasive positive airway pressure. Generally avoid intensive care.

      ☐ *Request transfer to hospital <u>only</u> if comfort needs cannot be met in current location.*

☐ <u>Comfort-Focused Treatment</u> – primary goal of maximizing comfort.
Relieve pain and suffering with medication by any route as needed; use oxygen, suctioning, and manual treatment of airway obstruction. Do not use treatments listed in Full and Selective Treatment unless consistent with comfort goal. *Request transfer to hospital <u>only</u> if comfort needs cannot be met in current location.*

Additional Orders: _____

C

Check One

ARTIFICIALLY ADMINISTERED NUTRITION: *Offer food by mouth if feasible and desired.*

☐ Long-term artificial nutrition, including feeding tubes. Additional Orders: _____

☐ Trial period of artificial nutrition, including feeding tubes. _____

☐ No artificial means of nutrition, including feeding tubes. _____

D

INFORMATION AND SIGNATURES:

Discussed with: ☐ Patient (Patient Has Capacity) ☐ Legally Recognized Decisionmaker

☐ Advance Directive dated _____, available and reviewed →   Health Care Agent if named in Advance Directive:
☐ Advance Directive not available   Name: _____
☐ No Advance Directive   Phone: _____

Signature of Physician / Nurse Practitioner / Physician Assistant (Physician/NP/PA)
My signature below indicates to the best of my knowledge that these orders are consistent with the patient's medical condition and preferences.

| Print Physician/NP/PA Name: | Physician/NP/PA Phone #: | Physician/PA License #, NP Cert. #: |
| Physician/NP/PA Signature: (required) | | Date: |

Signature of Patient or Legally Recognized Decisionmaker
I am aware that this form is voluntary. By signing this form, the legally recognized decisionmaker acknowledges that this request regarding resuscitative measures is consistent with the known desires of, and with the best interest of, the individual who is the subject of the form.

Print Name:	Relationship: (write self if patient)
Signature: (required)	Date:	Your POLST may be added to a secure electronic registry to be accessible by health providers, as permitted by HIPAA.
Mailing Address (street/city/state/zip):	Phone Number:	

SEND FORM WITH PATIENT WHENEVER TRANSFERRED OR DISCHARGED
*Form versions with effective dates of 1/1/2009, 4/1/2011,10/1/2014 or 01/01/2016 are also valid

Figure 49.4. Sample POLST form. Forms are available through a number of websites, including www.acpdesigns.org.

HIPAA PERMITS DISCLOSURE OF POLST TO OTHER HEALTH CARE PROVIDERS AS NECESSARY

Patient Information

Name (last, first, middle):	Date of Birth:	Gender: M F

NP/PA's Supervising Physician	**Preparer Name** (if other than signing Physician/NP/PA)	
Name:	Name/Title:	Phone #:

Additional Contact   ☐ None

Name:	Relationship to Patient:	Phone #:

Directions for Health Care Provider

Completing POLST

- **Completing a POLST form is voluntary**. California law requires that a POLST form be followed by healthcare providers, and provides immunity to those who comply in good faith. In the hospital setting, a patient will be assessed by a physician, or a nurse practitioner (NP) or a physician assistant (PA) acting under the supervision of the physician, who will issue appropriate orders that are consistent with the patient's preferences.
- **POLST does not replace the Advance Directive**. When available, review the Advance Directive and POLST form to ensure consistency, and update forms appropriately to resolve any conflicts.
- POLST must be completed by a health care provider based on patient preferences and medical indications.
- A legally recognized decisionmaker may include a court-appointed conservator or guardian, agent designated in an Advance Directive, orally designated surrogate, spouse, registered domestic partner, parent of a minor, closest available relative, or person whom the patient's physician/NP/PA believes best knows what is in the patient's best interest and will make decisions in accordance with the patient's expressed wishes and values to the extent known.
- A legally recognized decisionmaker may execute the POLST form only if the patient lacks capacity or has designated that the decisionmaker's authority is effective immediately.
- To be valid a POLST form must be signed by (1) a physician, or by a nurse practitioner or a physician assistant acting under the supervision of a physician and within the scope of practice authorized by law and (2) the patient or decisionmaker. Verbal orders are acceptable with follow-up signature by physician/NP/PA in accordance with facility/community policy.
- If a translated form is used with patient or decisionmaker, attach it to the signed English POLST form.
- Use of original form is strongly encouraged. Photocopies and FAXes of signed POLST forms are legal and valid. A copy should be retained in patient's medical record, on Ultra Pink paper when possible.

Using POLST

- Any incomplete section of POLST implies full treatment for that section.

Section A:

- If found pulseless and not breathing, no defibrillator (including automated external defibrillators) or chest compressions should be used on a patient who has chosen "Do Not Attempt Resuscitation."

Section B:

- When comfort cannot be achieved in the current setting, the patient, including someone with "Comfort-Focused Treatment," should be transferred to a setting able to provide comfort (e.g., treatment of a hip fracture).
- Non-invasive positive airway pressure includes continuous positive airway pressure (CPAP), bi-level positive airway pressure (BiPAP), and bag valve mask (BVM) assisted respirations.
- IV antibiotics and hydration generally are not "Comfort-Focused Treatment."
- Treatment of dehydration prolongs life. If a patient desires IV fluids, indicate "Selective Treatment" or "Full Treatment."
- Depending on local EMS protocol, "Additional Orders" written in Section B may not be implemented by EMS personnel.

Reviewing POLST

It is recommended that POLST be reviewed periodically. Review is recommended when:

- The patient is transferred from one care setting or care level to another, or
- There is a substantial change in the patient's health status, or
- The patient's treatment preferences change.

Modifying and Voiding POLST

- A patient with capacity can, at any time, request alternative treatment or revoke a POLST by any means that indicates intent to revoke. It is recommended that revocation be documented by drawing a line through Sections A through D, writing "VOID" in large letters, and signing and dating this line.
- A legally recognized decisionmaker may request to modify the orders, in collaboration with the physician/NP/PA, based on the known desires of the patient or, if unknown, the patient's best interests.

This form is approved by the California Emergency Medical Services Authority in cooperation with the statewide POLST Task Force. For more information or a copy of the form, visit **www.caPOLST.org**.

SEND FORM WITH PATIENT WHENEVER TRANSFERRED OR DISCHARGED

Figure 49.4. Sample POLST form. Forms are available through a number of websites, including www.acpdesigns.org.

Box 49.1

Steps in Advance Care Planning

- Clarify the underlying health state
- Elicit and prioritize goals of care
- Designate a health-care surrogate (proxy)
- Complete an advance directive
  - Living will
  - Scenario-based directive
- Complete a medical order
  - Out-of-hospital do-not-resuscitate (DNR) form
  - Physician Orders for Life-Sustaining Treatment (POLST) form

CHAPTER 50

Community Resources

D epending on where your family member lives, she may have other services available to facilitate her medical care. Transportation to medical appointments, access to home-delivered nutritious meals, flu shots, and free blood pressure checks are examples of resources that you may find useful to know about. These services are underwritten either by the federal government, local govern-ment, or private organizations. Some are unique to your family member's community and you will have to learn about them from friends, neighbors, your relative's primary care practice, or the relevant Area Agency on Aging (the local branch of the federal agency, the Administration on Aging). Others are universal or at least widespread and I will mention some of them here.

Home-Delivered Meals

G ood nutrition is an essential part of your relative's medical care. One way to promote good nutrition, especially for frail older people who have difficulty doing their own food shopping and food preparation, is through home delivered meals. The largest and best-known program that provides this service is Meals on Wheels America, a not-for-profit organization that has a presence in over five thousand American communities. With some support from the federal Older Americans Act, it supplies hot meals to people in their homes. The charge is based on a sliding scale, with the 2019 cost of one full meal a day set at $7.10. The program, which is staffed to a great extent by volunteers, also serves a social purpose: the person who delivers the food will interact with your family member.

Alternatives to Meals on Wheels include a number of plans that are meant for busy working people, not just for older individuals. An example that has been around for several years and has received good reviews is "Personal Chef to Go." This service advertises that it uses locally sourced vegetables and whole grains; it also prepares fresh meals that are shipped on Thursdays for delivery Friday or Saturday. The meals are individually wrapped in sealed, microwaveable trays to guarantee freshness. The cost depends on the number of meals delivered (between five and ten per week) and starts at $78. The service requires online ordering so you may have to help your relative arrange for it. It also does not include the added social component of the personal delivery of Meals on Wheels.

Finally, many if not most urban areas now feature companies such as GrubHub that pick up meals from restaurants and deliver them to your family member's door. There is a $10 fee for the service and a $50/meal minimum, so it's not a reasonable strategy for most single people. If your relative is able to cook but cannot go grocery shopping, home delivery of groceries is an option (see chapter 32, "Prevention," for specific home delivery services).

Transportation

Transportation is often the key to maintaining independence and to a satisfactory social life, but it also plays a role in medical care: your relative often needs to travel to her physician's office or to the hospital, and she needs to pick up prescription medications from the pharmacy. Your family member may be able to drive herself or, more rarely, take public transportation, or you may be the chauffeur, but there are alternatives. Many cities offer a paratransit program—in Massachusetts, it's known as "The Ride"—that provides door-to-door service using wheelchair accessible vans. Appointments must be booked at least twenty-four hours ahead of time and many people complain that the service is slow since it makes multiple stops. Another option, available in some towns, is subsidized taxi service. Instead of relying on paratransit vans,

the community contracts with a local taxi company to provide vouchers, at a discount, for taxi rides. In some cases, these taxis are handicapped accessible and the drivers may even have received special training, but other programs rely on conventional cabs and drivers.

If your family member does not drive but uses a smartphone and if she lives in an urban or, in some cases, a suburban area, she can take advantage of a rideshare service such as Uber or Lyft. In certain locations, such as the San Francisco Bay Area, these cars are so pervasive that your relative will be able to get virtually anywhere at any time. The service is cheaper than regular taxis—but only a minority of frail older people have a smartphone. Because of this limitation, a handful of intermediaries have sprung up. Sporting names such as GoGoGrandparent, these companies allow your family member to call in using a conventional cell phone and then the company forwards the request to Uber or Lyft. This adds an additional fee, it is not widely available, and your relative may not be comfortable with the user interface, but it's an option to explore.

Adult Day Health Centers

Your image of "adult day care" may be a nursery school for old people—and both you and your family member may accordingly be skeptical of the idea. The good centers, however, provide an opportunity for meaningful social interactions for adults with physical or cognitive impairment. Moreover, while some operate on a strictly social model, others use a medical model and provide nursing, case management, and other medical services. These other services can include physical therapy and social work consultation. Fully 80 percent of adult day centers have a nurse on site, at least part of the day, who can administer medications, monitor blood pressure, and take other vital signs. Adult day centers also typically serve lunch. If they are part of the Program of All-Inclusive Care for the Elderly (PACE), physical therapy and nutritional counseling are also available. Adult day health programs that are specifically tailored to individuals with dementia feature activities appropriate for the cognitive capacity of the attendees.

Medicare does *not* cover adult day health care but Medicaid does. The Veterans Administration will pay for the medical but not the exclusively social model of adult day care. If your family member is not on Medicaid and is not eligible for VA benefits, most programs offer a sliding scale. The average daily cost, without adjustment for income, across the United States is $70, ranging from a low of $20 in Alabama to a high of $100 in Alaska.

If your family member would benefit from more individual attention and social interaction than she usually gets at home *and* stands to gain from the medical services offered, then you should consider adult day health.

Senior Centers

Community senior centers vary dramatically in what they offer, so you will need to explore the center in your relative's area. In terms of medically oriented activities, many have exercise classes, yoga classes, and/or Tai Chi classes that focus on balance. They often provide periodic screening tests for various conditions, from high blood pressure (probably the most common) to diabetes and hearing loss. Many senior centers invite physicians, nurses, or other clinicians to give lectures on topics such as advance care planning, dementia, or falls.

Senior centers often work with the local Area Agency on Aging to provide a hot lunch on site. This is another opportunity to improve your family member's nutrition as well as to socialize with her peers.

Legal Services

Lawyers often offer their assistance with advance care planning. While your relative can designate a health-care proxy and fill out a living will without legal counsel, you may choose to take care of completing the necessary paperwork at the same time that you tend to other legal matters such as a will. If you decide to avail yourselves of the services of a lawyer, you should discuss any limitations of care that you and your family member decide on with her primary care physician and be sure that the doctor has a copy of any forms signed in the lawyer's office.

Legal services are necessary if your relative is sufficiently impaired that she cannot choose a health-care surrogate and instead needs a guardian. Guardianship entails more than the right to make medical decisions on behalf of your relative, although courts can also limit the role of a guardian, depending on the type and extent of the disabilities. Obtaining guardianship is a judicial process that requires going to court and presenting evidence of incapacity, to which two physicians must usually attest.

Housing

At some point, your family member may need more help, either personal, medical, or both, than can be provided in her home or yours. One possibility is a nursing home, which I discuss in part VII, "Care in the Nursing Home." Another option is assisted living. Such facilities are *not* medical institutions. As defined by the National Center for Assisted Living, they are part of a continuum of long-term care that provides a combination of housing, residential care services, and limited health-care facilities to people in need of some assistance with their normal daily activities.

Faith Communities

If your family member belongs to a local church, synagogue, or mosque you may find that organization a source of support. Most commonly, the assistance is in the form of friendly visitors, but it may include concrete services such as running errands or providing meals. If the faith community helps your relative derive a sense of meaning and engagement, it can also play an important role in staving off loneliness and depression.

Resources for Finding Resources

To find out about other resources in your family member's community, you can consult any of several offices, many of which are the local branch of a national organization. The Area Agencies on Aging are an offshoot of the Older Americans Act (OAA), legislation passed in 1965 as part of the "Great Society" program. The OAA's mission is to help older Americans live in the community "with dignity and independence" as long as possible. The Area Agencies on Aging were added in 1973 to be the "on-the-ground organizations" that carry out the mandate of the OAA. They provide information and referral, home-delivered meals, health and wellness programs, elder abuse prevention, transportation, adult day care, in-home care and caregiver support, either directly or through outsourcing to a private organization. The National

Association of Area Agencies on Aging works with the local branches and develops resources for their use. Recently, for example, it created a toolkit of information for caregivers about dementia.

The Administration on Aging has an Eldercare Locator website (figure 50.1) that enables you to find services in your area.

The National Center on Caregiving, a subdivision of the Family Caregiver Alliance, is another repository of valuable information. It is a not-for-profit organization that focuses on services, educational programs, and other resources to help family caregivers. The Family Caregiver Alliance has developed an online site with information for caregivers called FC CareJourney. It also has a resource online called "Family Care Navigator" that can help you identify support services in your state.

You should also feel free to ask the staff of your relative's primary care practice for suggestions. If the practice includes a social worker, she should be able to help you identify the health-care resources you need and how to find

them. If the practice does not have its own social worker and if your family member is eligible, the physician might make a referral to the local Visiting Nurse Association for both nursing and social work services.

The World Health Organization defines health as a "state of complete physical, mental, and social well-being, and not merely the absence of disease or infirmity." This definition implicitly categorizes almost all human activities as contributing to health. While perhaps excessively broad, it nonetheless gets at a fundamental truth that you as a caregiver have undoubtedly already recognized: just as you will have difficulty providing for your relative's medical needs if she cannot afford medications or a comprehensive health insurance plan, you will be much better equipped to care for her medical needs if you can access assorted services such as nutrition programs, subsidized transportation, and adult day care. Learning about what's available in your community can make your job considerably easier—and improve your family member's health.

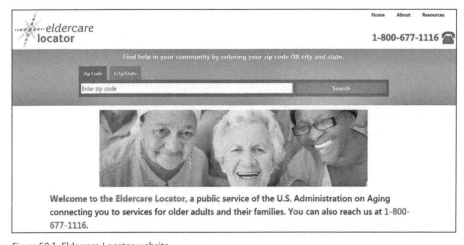

Figure 50.1. Eldercare Locator website

Box 50.1

> ## Community Services
>
> - Home-delivered meals (Meals on Wheels, private services)
> - Transportation (paratransit, taxi vouchers, Ride Share)
> - Adult day centers (health, socialization, meals)
> - Senior centers (education, blood pressure checks, flu shots)
> - Legal services (advance care planning, guardianship)
> - Housing (assisted living, congregate living, nursing homes)
> - Faith communities (friendly visitors, spiritual care)
> - Resources to find resources (Agency on Aging, Eldercare Locator)

CHAPTER 51

Home Hospice

In the section on hospital care, I began with the perils of hospitalization before I talked with you about how to advocate for your family member during a hospital stay. That strategy might have seemed backwards or biased, but I chose this approach because I thought you needed to know about the potential hazards so you were in the best position to avoid them. Similarly, I'm going to start this chapter with a discussion of what home hospice is like, what demands it will place on you, and its potential benefits *before* addressing what might seem like the prior question, how to decide about enrolling in the first place. I think you need to have a good grasp of what hospice care actually entails—both for you and for your family member—before you try to decide about participating (figure 51.1).

Most hospice care takes place at home, though some regions have residential hospices and hospice services can also be provided to long-stay nursing home residents. By definition, with home hospice your family member remains at home and hospice services come to him. But what you should realize is that means at most a few hours of home health aide assistance each day

(and often a few hours a couple of times a week) and a visit from a nurse one or a few times per week. Hospices also provide episodic social worker involvement, a volunteer to sit with your family member periodically, a chaplain if you are interested and, occasionally, physical or occupational therapy. Even if all those people are involved in your family member's life and if he has a home health aide for four hours a day, seven days a week (and this much help is unusual), that still leaves a good many hours of the day. Think about it—for eighteen hours each day and often

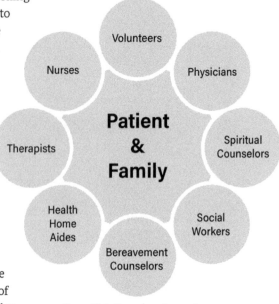

Figure 51.1. Home hospice services

more, care falls on the shoulders of friends and family. That doesn't mean you have to be there all that time, but you probably need to make sure that someone is. Many hospice programs will not accept a patient unless there is a live-in caregiver or the equivalent. The equivalent can be multiple people and it can include caregivers who are paid for privately. What you need to ask yourself is, can you manage your family member's needs without additional assistance, beyond what's provided by hospice care? If not, is there a viable alternative source of help?

Just what your family member will need once he is enrolled in hospice depends on his clinical situation and on how much he can do for himself. Ideally, he will enroll in hospice well before he is dying so he has the chance to derive maximum benefit from home medical care. He may still have months, sometimes many months, before the end comes: he has simply decided that he doesn't want to spend his time going to doctors and hospitals; he'd rather have medical care come to him. He may be able to go out—he just doesn't want to use up his limited energy on medical appointments. If your family member started out in hospice at a point in his illness when he is able to handle at least some of his basic daily functions (activities of daily living, or ADLs), he probably won't need—or be eligible for—home health aide services more than a few hours a week. You may find you don't need to do much more than you did before. Maybe you will do a bit less if you were formerly in the habit of taking your family member to frequent physician appointments.

If your family member enrolls in hospice when he has extensive needs—or if he's been in hospice for some time, but now has taken a turn for the worse—you may be called upon to perform all sorts of medical tasks. Perhaps the most common is administering strong pain medications. Many people with advanced illness experience pain and require potent medicine such as opioids (the technically correct name for what are often popularly referred to as narcotics). Usually these medicines can be taken orally, but adjusting the amount of drug your family member takes to adequately deal with his pain while minimizing side effects may be challenging. The hospice nurse and her backup physician can help you determine a good regimen and the nurse can coach you through implementing the regimen, but a good deal of discretion is required. Since most patients benefit from round-the-clock pain medication, many take a long-acting or "extended release" medication once or twice a day—in the case of a patch applied to the skin, once every two or three days—to simplify the schedule and assure a steady level of medication. While the goal of long-acting medicines is to fully control pain, patients often have break-through pain, defined as significant pain before the next scheduled dose of medicine, and benefit from a "rescue dose" of medication. If your relative's pain is consistently poorly controlled and frequent rescue doses are needed, then his hospice nurse needs to be notified so she can orchestrate an increase in the dose of the long-acting medication.

You may worry about whether you are giving your family member too much medication. You don't want to harm him and you know that excessive amounts of opioids can cause constipation, confusion, or even death. Your relative may himself be reluctant to take sufficient medication because he is worried he will become addicted or that he will overdose. At the same time, you want to avoid suffering. The hospice nurse will tell you and I will reiterate—the proper use of opioids in the setting of advanced illness does not generally lead to addiction and the benefits of pain control greatly outweigh the risks. Gradual increases in the dose are entirely appropriate and are not associated with problems breathing (respiratory depression). What's critically important to remember is that as your family member approaches the end of life, his breathing is likely to become weak. That's part of the dying process. The last thing you want to do in this situation is withhold the medication that is keeping him comfortable. It *is* legitimate to worry about "diversion," the use of your family member's opioid medication by others—many cases of addiction have been facilitated by illicitly obtaining drugs in this way.

That said, administration of very strong medication is a weighty responsibility. If your family member has difficulty swallowing, perhaps because he is not very alert, you may be asked to give him highly concentrated liquid morphine under the tongue. This entails figuring out the right dose, filling a dropper with that amount, gently opening your family member's mouth, and squeezing the drops out under his tongue. You are not likely to be asked to give a shot—physicians avoid use of painful injections when medication is used over an extended period of time—but you may need to check on a continuous drip that the hospice nurse has set up. Unless you are a trained nurse, these will be new roles for you and not always ones with which you feel comfortable. It's perfectly acceptable to express your anxieties to the nurse and get the training and support you need to do a good job. Unfortunately, licensed home health aides are not authorized to administer medications, so unless you hire a full-time nurse, you will either need to give medications yourself or hire and train a private aide. If you remain very uncomfortable with carrying out medical treatment, and if enlisting the help of friends, family, or a professional nurse is not a realistic possibility, then your relative will need to enter a nursing home or a residential hospice. You might want to think about whether you are likely to be able to do what's necessary to manage pain *before* your family member actually enrolls in hospice.

Other common tasks for caregivers near the end of life focus on basic bodily functions such as eating, urinating, and defecating. These are intensely personal activities and you may not feel comfortable relating in this way to your family member. Men are particularly likely to have difficulty with these tasks, although plenty of women find them challenging as well. At least as important is whether you are the same gender as your family member: many women are uncomfortable playing the role of nursemaid for a man and conversely. A special awkwardness arises when an adult takes care of a parent in this intimate way—it emphasizes the role reversal that many caregiver/family member pairs find troubling. The number of permutations of diseases are many: Your family member may be the one who doesn't want you tending to these functions, because he feels embarrassed or ashamed; or your family member may not want anyone other than you engaged in these activities. In any case, you should expect that someone may have to tend to such matters, you should realize that hospice will provide only a limited amount of the care that's apt to be required, and you are going to have to decide whether you are up for the responsibility.

Feeding your family member if he is unable to feed himself is symbolically fraught—you will inevitably draw the analogy to caring for an infant—but many caregivers find feeding another person deeply gratifying. In fact, and here's a potential problem that might not have occurred to you, many caregivers are troubled when their family members will not or cannot take anything by mouth, even if they are handfed. Providing nourishment is a way to show love, to demonstrate that you care, and many caregivers experience their relative's inability or unwillingness to take nutrition as rejection. You may want to discuss these feelings with the hospice nurse and/or social worker: she might be able to find ways for your family member to take in some nutrition or for you to demonstrate your love in another way.

Excretory functions present their own challenges. If your family member is bedbound but continent, then the problem is to feel comfortable supplying a urinal or bedpan. Incontinence is difficult for many caregivers to deal with, whether in the setting of care near the end of life or far earlier in your family member's trajectory, but it is uniquely challenging with someone who is not mobile. In that case, we're talking about adult diapers, use of rubber sheets, changing the sheets and, hardest of all, cleaning your family member's most intimate areas. One clinical pearl that may help you ever so slightly: as your family member gets closer to the end, as he eats less and drinks less, there's going to be correspondingly less waste. Another clinical tidbit: normally, clinicians do not recommend chronic use of a Foley catheter, a catheter inserted into the bladder to continuously drain the urine, except for people who are unable to pass their urine. An indwelling catheter, as it's called, is associated with an increased risk of infection. But for someone who is dying, a catheter is entirely reasonable if it is the best way to promote comfort.

If your family member's needs are more than you can manage, you will need outside help. The hospice can help you find reliable home health aides to supplement the hours it provides. Home health aides cost less than nurses, but they're not cheap: if you hire someone through an agency (probably a good idea unless you happen to have a personal connection to a good home health aide), you will pay on average $20 per hour, more in some geographic regions and less in others.

The hospice team has the potential to make all the medical tasks bearable by offering you psychosocial support. Unlike much of medical care, hospice care is focused on the family unit. Yes, your family member is at the center of what hospice does, but the nurse and social worker understand that they need to work with the entire family. This may mean letting you vent when you are exasperated with your siblings or others because they're leaving the tough parts of the job to you. It might involve asking them to speak with your spouse or children, who are feeling neglected as you spend so many hours with your family member. It may involve sitting down with those siblings or other family members and exploring their concerns, reservations, and anxieties. It may mean mediating between you and those others—making sure that they understand your feelings and you understand theirs.

Whether you are in this alone or are sharing responsibility for your relative with multiple family members, you can still benefit from psychosocial support. Acknowledging your emotions is important for your well-being and even for your ability to carry out medical tasks. You might experience emotions ranging from deep satisfaction at being able to help at such a difficult time in your family member's life, frustration that your family member doesn't adequately appreciate you, or even dismay that your family member hasn't died yet. Just as it is helpful for you to have knowledge and skills to be able to function as a good caregiver, it is also very helpful for you to receive encouragement and understanding as you undertake your new responsibilities.

Home hospice will offer you a number of other services that you should know about and take advantage of. I'll mention three. First, hospices are required by law to train volunteers to spend time with your family member. Many caregivers find that they need a mental health break—they'd like to visit the hairdresser's or go for a run or do some shopping. Having someone who will stay with your family member for a few hours, perhaps reading to him, listening to music together, talking to him, or just being with him, can make these breaks possible. Second, many hospices have a contract with a local pharmacy and will deliver prescription medications. You need to conserve energy and not devote endless time to performing errands, so if the hospice can arrange for prescriptions to be delivered to the home, that means one less errand for you. You'd be surprised how often physicians will order new medications as your family member's illness evolves. Third, after your family member dies, the hospice will provide bereavement support. You are so busy focusing on his day-to-day needs that you may not even be able to imagine that there will come a day when your family member is gone, let alone that you will continue to be involved with him, albeit through memories, sadness, and a sense of loss. Physicians typically drop out of your life once their patient is gone; the hospice maintains a relationship of sorts for the next year.

Now, at last, I can address whether to enroll in hospice. Your relative is eligible for Medicare hospice (assuming he is enrolled in Medicare) if he has a prognosis of six months or less, assuming his disease follows its usual course. Many private insurers have less stringent prognostic criteria for enrolling in hospice. They focus more on what I think is the important question: Does your family member want to concentrate his medical care on comfort or is he still interested in pursuing potentially life-prolonging treatment? He might choose comfort as his overriding goal when he realizes he has only days remaining or he might choose comfort far earlier in the course of his illness if he feels the burdens of treatment outweigh their possible benefits.

Opting for hospice care does not mean forgoing *all* medical treatment. Not only is symptomatic treatment a key part of hospice (medications and other interventions designed to alleviate uncomfortable conditions such as pain, shortness of breath, nausea), but so too is treatment of infections with oral antibiotics and treatment of internal bleeding with antacids or proton pump inhibitors. The key issue is whether the proposed medical treatment comes at a cost in terms of your family member's comfort. Enrolling in hospice only makes sense if your relative is at a point where he does not want treatment that may cause suffering, which usually means forgoing hospitalization, intravenous medication, and other approaches that most people find burdensome. If hospice care seems like the best way to achieve your family member's goals, then you need to think about whether the services it provides will work for you. Hospice is an excellent option for many people—provided it is a good match, given their needs and their preferences.

Box 51.1

Hospice

What Hospice Offers

- Home medical care, mainly RN-delivered
- 24-hour, on-call availability
- Social work, limited home health aide time
- Medications
- Volunteer service
- Bereavement support

What Hospice Does Not Provide

- Fulltime home health aide
- Regular home visits by an MD
- Coverage for treatment intended to prolong life

CHAPTER 52

Involving the Rest of the Family

I have been addressing my comments to you as though you are the sole caregiver, alone in the lonely business of caring for your relative. My hope is that if you know enough about your family member's medical conditions, if you've talked with her about what's important to her, and if you are well-equipped to navigate through the doctor's office, the hospital, and the skilled nursing facility, you can be a superb caregiver. Your relative will benefit and you may find caregiving rewarding. Even if all this is true, you will probably find you are generally happier and do a better job helping your family member if you don't do it alone. While community resources and caregiver support groups are important sources of strength for you, family participation is especially meaningful for all concerned.

Ways Family Can Help

You will quickly figure out that different family members can contribute in varying ways, given their circumstances, where they live, their expertise, and their personalities. In some cases, you will have a willing and able sibling or in-law or family friend with whom to split caregiving responsibilities. More often, you will jointly decide on a division of labor: maybe you handle the medical and personal care side and your sister takes care of the legal and financial aspects. Or you may discover that your brother who lives out of state and has a demanding job and a family of his own cannot regularly participate in caregiving, but is willing to take over for you when you go on vacation or for occasional weekends. This kind of family respite may be more acceptable to you and your relative than institutional respite—moving your family member to assisted living or another facility for the time you are unavailable. You probably will want to have open lines of communication when momentous decisions must be made: Should mom have surgery? Should she move to assisted living? Should she enroll in hospice? If your siblings see your relative frequently and you share information about her physical, emotional, and cognitive situation, you are less likely to have major disagreements about her care and are more apt to be able to work through whatever differences you do have.

Family members can help just by listening. When you are overburdened or exasperated, whether with your family member or with the health-care system, when you are discouraged or just saddened by your relative's decline, venting to someone who has shared childhood memories of your common parent can be very useful.

Your siblings may be able to contribute to the cost of caring for your relative. Someone may have to pay privately for home health services that exceed what Medicare provides. If your family member enrolls in home hospice, she may need more assistance than the maximum that the hospice offers. The only way to keep her at home may be to pay for supplementary personal care attendants. If your relative goes to adult day care, a supervised social/medical program that she can attend up to five days a week, she may be charged based on a sliding scale, but that amount could still be more than she can afford. Ideally, she will have the financial wherewithal to pay for these things herself as there's nothing like disputes about money to sow discord within families. But if she doesn't have the personal resources, you and your siblings may decide to split the cost, perhaps in accordance with your own financial situations.

Strategies for Working with Your Family

You will find that clear communication is the key. You already have a host of caregiving responsibilities; you don't want to rely on your brother, only to find that he meant something different by "being available as backup." You had in mind, say, that he would come over and provide personal care while you go away for the weekend. If he turns to you and asks, "What do you mean, you want me to give her a shower?" after you explain that personal care does indeed mean toileting and bathing, the two of you may be well on the way to having a major blow-up. Keeping track in writing, if necessary, with a spread sheet, of who will do what and when can help build a strong working relationship.

Periodic family meetings to update everyone on your relative's condition and her needs can also help. You may want a health-care professional, whether the primary care physician, nurse practitioner, or social worker, to facilitate such a meeting. Alternatively, you might opt for more informal gatherings that serve the same purpose, for example, talking about mom when you are all together for Thanksgiving dinner or Mother's Day.

Sharing medical reports is another way you can help your siblings or others to remain engaged in your family member's care. Many primary care physicians hand their patients an "after visit summary" that reviews the problems addressed and the plans initiated during the visit. Hospitals and emergency departments give out similar documents at the time of discharge. If your relative agrees, you may wish to distribute these to your siblings to help keep them up to date on the latest medical developments.

Why Family Support Matters

I started this chapter by suggesting that you will find the support of others, especially your family, personally helpful to you as a caregiver. You may also discover that if you don't involve your family, you will feel angry and resentful toward them. Longstanding family conflicts tend to blossom under the stress of caring for a parent. Even good relationships can turn sour if the responsibilities of individual family members are inequitably distributed or the roles are ill-defined.

Physicians are very familiar with family conflict, especially in the setting of end-of-life care. We on the east coast call it the "daughter from California syndrome" (and presumably our counterparts on the west coast speak of the son or daughter from Massachusetts): an uninvolved family member shows up during a crisis and insists on a particular course of action that is at odds with what you, the primary or sole caregiver, advocate. Motivated by guilt,

ignorance, or a strong belief that she is acting in her mother's best interest, the visiting sibling can severely disrupt the decision-making process. In this scenario, a family meeting, sometimes convened by the hospital ethics committee (if your relative is in the hospital), may be the best way to resolve the conflict.

Ideally, you will prevent this situation from developing by keeping your siblings in the loop throughout your caregiving journey. During a period when your family member is able to speak for herself, you may want to make a record of her goals of care and specific treatment preferences. She might complete an advance directive or a POLST (Physician Orders for Life-Sustaining Treatment) form in which she specifies, with some degree of precision, what she wants and why. Or you may want to tape record your family member talking about the kind of care she favors for herself. Even more compelling would be a video in which she discusses her wishes. At the very least, you can try to guard against the daughter from California successfully throwing a wrench into end-of-life discussions by making sure you are the designated health-care surrogate.

Spouses and Children

We've been talking about involving your siblings, if you have any, or other close friends or relatives. But what about your spouse? What about your children? They are going to be affected by your caregiving responsibilities, whether or not they participate in performing concrete caregiving tasks. And what if you are the caregiver for one parent and the other parent is still alive but is unable to function as the primary caregiver?

Because we are living longer today than ever before and because many women defer childbearing until they are in their late twenties or their thirties, nearly half of all middle-aged Americans (people in their forties and fifties) are members of the "sandwich generation." They have dual, sometimes conflicting, caregiving responsibilities. It's worth pointing out that in surveys of life satisfaction, adults who are involved in caring for both the younger and the older generation are no less happy with their lives than their counterparts with fewer responsibilities. But the older and sicker your aging family member—and the needier your children—the more challenging the role becomes. Dual caregivers experience stress because of the demands on their finances, their emotions, and their time. A few key strategies can make an enormous difference: most important is setting your priorities. This will help you let go of some tasks and postpone others.

We've talked a great deal about establishing and then prioritizing the goals of care for your family member; it turns out that you will have to do something analogous if you are to successfully balance your various caregiving tasks. You cannot be in two places at once: if your daughter happens to be in the emergency room of one hospital with a broken arm and your mother is in the emergency room of another hospital with pneumonia, you are going to have to choose. On the other hand, if your daughter has an appointment with her pediatrician at the same time that your mother has an appointment with her geriatrician, you might opt to postpone one of those appointments. Or, you might arrange for your spouse to go wherever you cannot be. More generally, you will have to learn to delegate. How important is it really for you to be at every one of your daughter's soccer games? Maybe you should select the most important ones and set aside those times as sacrosanct. And maybe you should have a heart-to-heart chat with your daughter about whether she wants you to attend her games and speak with your spouse about his degree of involvement. Similarly, you can identify those elder care responsibilities that can readily be handed off to another family member or to a paid caregiver such as a geriatric care manager.

To avoid generating resentment from your spouse and your children of your caregiving, you may want to involve them in ways they find pleasurable. Rather than seeing every activity as a duty that someone needs to perform and simply slotting in various interchangeable individuals to carry out the necessary function, you may be able to figure out alternative strategies. If your family member is lonely—or anxious or depressed—and needs companionship, maybe your ten-year-old would enjoy playing Scrabble with her. Perhaps your family member can teach your child how to knit or crochet, or

they can jointly do an art project. And remember that if you model good caregiving for your child, you may one day be the beneficiary yourself.

You may sometimes feel as though you and your family member are like a binary solar system: two stars orbiting around each other, drawing each other with a strong gravitational field. You are so busy experiencing the pull and the brightness of your co-star that you might at times forget that circling both of you are a multitude of planets and that other celestial objects such as meteors and asteroids are nearby. Those planets are part of your family and you need to remember that you are linked together, just as you should remember that the other objects in the neighborhood are, like community services, resources on which you can draw as a caregiver.

Box 52.1

Strategies for Involving Families

- Divide the responsibilities to each according to his abilities
- Vent your frustrations to family members
- Update family on your relative's medical condition
- Set up a family meeting to make joint decisions
- Don't shortchange your children; prioritize your caregiving

CHAPTER 53

Caregiver Support

The basic perspective underlying this book is that knowledge is a major source of support for you as a family caregiver. Much of what caregivers find burdensome is the time spent on caregiving and the emotional stress that derives from seeing someone you care about decline to the point that he needs you to help care for him. But you may feel woefully unprepared for your new role. Knowledge, in this situation, really is power. This volume offers one type of support: understanding and guidance about the medical problems your family member is likely to face. To do your job well, you will also need other kinds of support. Fortunately, much has been written about these other kinds of support—for example, respite programs and support groups. What I will focus on, in the spirit of this book, is the medical information you may find helpful that relates to *your* health and well-being. Remember that if you are not in good shape, both you and, indirectly, your family member, will suffer. Caregiving is a demanding job—you need to be strong and healthy to do your best.

You may have heard that caregiving takes its toll. You might come across all sorts of dire predictions about what will happen to you: you will develop heart disease, you are going to start drinking heavily or taking drugs, your marriage will be ruined, you may die. My goal in talking about your health and well-being is not to scare you; rather, it's to highlight some of the potential pitfalls of caregiving that *could* lead to adverse health outcomes and to point out what you can do to avoid them. It's also important to remember that not everyone who is a caregiver experiences strain. Moreover, even when caregiving is stressful it can simultaneously be rewarding. But the longer you spend as a caregiver (we're usually talking about years, not weeks or months) and the more hours each week you devote to caregiving, the more likely you are to find it stressful. In addition, the greater your relative's physical impairments, the more burden you may feel. If your family member has cognitive impairment, you are at high risk of feeling caregiver strain. Let's begin with the *physical* hazards associated with caregiving.

Signs of Burnout

Experts in caregiving point out that *all* forms of chronic stress have health effects and caregiving has all the characteristics of chronic stress. It causes both psychological and physical strain over an extended period, it is often unpredictable, and it can interfere with work and with family relationships. Because burnout is so common among family caregivers, you need to be vigilant for telltale signs in yourself.

Many of the signs are identical to the symptoms of depression: losing interest in the activities you previously found enjoyable, feeling irritable or hopeless, sleeping poorly, and either gaining or losing weight. One sign specific to caregiving is the feeling that you want to hurt the person for whom you are providing care.

You may find it useful to score yourself on the short version of the "Burden Scale for Family Caregivers" (figure 53.1). The short version is a ten-item questionnaire, where you get a score of 3 for the answer "strongly agree," a score of 2 for the answer "agree," a score of 1 for the answer "disagree," and a score of 0 for the answer "strongly disagree." The total score is from 0 to 30, with higher scores denoting higher degrees of caregiver burden.

Caregiving and Your Physical Health

Your family member may require substantial physical assistance to get by on a day-to-day basis: he may need help getting up out of a chair and walking, or he may need help climbing into the bathtub or shower. If you try to help, you could strain your back or other muscles you didn't even realize you had. You may want to avoid providing this kind of assistance and leave the heavy lifting to home health aides.

Caregiving can also adversely affect your health if you neglect your own health care. Postponing screening tests such as mammograms or colonoscopies because you are too busy is a risky strategy. You might also be tempted to skip your annual physical. That could mean nobody notices that your blood pressure is elevated or your blood sugar is too high. Untreated or inadequately treated high blood pressure predisposes you to a stroke or heart attack. A high sugar may indicate diabetes which causes all sorts of problems.

Short version of the Burden Scale for Family Caregivers in 20 European languages

With this scale, valid assessment of subjective burden among family caregivers is possible all over the United States and Europe using the same questionnaire.

Background

The burden experienced by family caregivers is the most important caregiver-related variable in care at home of a chronically ill person. The extent of subjective burden has significant impact on the emotional and physical health of the family caregiver, and even influences the mortality of spouse caregivers. It affects the way the family caregiver deals with the care-receiver and determines the time of institutionalization.

Burden Scale for Family Caregivers BSFC-s

We are asking you for information about your *present* situation. The present situation comprises the caregiving you provide because of the illness of your family member (or friend).

The following statements often refer to the type of your assistance. This may be any kind of support up to nursing care.

Please draw an "X" for the best description of your present situation. Please answer every question!

	Strongly agree	Agree	Disagree	Strongly disagree
1. My life satisfaction has suffered because of the care.	☐	☐	☐	☐
2. I often feel physically exhausted.	☐	☐	☐	☐
3. From time to time I wish I could "run away" from the situation I am in.	☐	☐	☐	☐
4. Sometimes I don't really feel like "myself" as before.	☐	☐	☐	☐
5. Since I have been a caregiver my financial situation has declined.	☐	☐	☐	☐
6. My health is affected by the care situation.	☐	☐	☐	☐
7. The care takes a lot of my own strength.	☐	☐	☐	☐
8. I feel torn between the demands of my environment (such as family) and the demands of the care.	☐	☐	☐	☐
9. I am worried about my future because of the care I give.	☐	☐	☐	☐
10. My relationships with other family members, relatives, friends, and acquaintances are suffering as a result of the care.	☐	☐	☐	☐

Scoring

Give yourself the the following number of points for each response.

Strongly agree: **3** points   Agree: **2** points   Disagree: **1** point   Strongly disagree: **0** points

Figure 53.1. Burden Scale for Family Caregivers

You might also find yourself cutting back on other important activities such as exercise because you are busy taking care of your family member. Giving up regular exercise has a variety of potentially unfortunate consequences. You might gain weight—making it harder to be a good caregiver and possibly triggering diabetes. You might develop heart disease, especially if you have other risk factors such as an elevated cholesterol level. You might find yourself depressed. Caregiving itself can result in depression, so the last thing you want to do is to stop whatever measures you are already taking to treat or stave off depression.

Finally, you might try to treat your caregiver stress by smoking, drinking, or even taking drugs. Obviously, these strategies are not good for your overall health. They certainly won't make you a better caregiver, and they are unlikely to be effective in achieving your goal of stress-reduction. Women are especially prone to putting themselves in jeopardy by pursuing one of these potentially harmful approaches. If you are a caregiver for your spouse, you are also at particularly high risk. Just remember the instruction on airplanes to put on your oxygen mask *before* attending to your child. You cannot help anyone else if you don't take care of yourself first.

Caregiving and Your Emotional Health

Many of the same symptoms that signal depression when they occur in your family member also indicate depression when you develop them (see chapter 31, "Depression"). Are you developing trouble sleeping? Have you lost your appetite? Do you find you're apathetic, that you have trouble getting enthusiastic about things? Is your libido diminished? As many as 70 percent of family caregivers develop symptoms of depression at some point during their work with their relative, and about one-quarter of these experience major depression, an illness requiring treatment. If your family member has dementia,

you are at particularly high risk; ditto if your relative has severe limitations in her ability to function independently. The best approach to preventing depression is to preserve some semblance of your old social life, to exercise regularly, and to be sure to get periodic breaks—take the weekend off, go on vacation, or arrange for someone else to take over your caregiving responsibilities for a few days or a week.

If you do develop symptoms, you shouldn't medicate yourself, whether with alcohol or sleeping pills. Instead, seek medical attention—sooner rather than later. When depressive symptoms persist over time and interfere with your life they may spell "major depression," a serious but treatable disease.

Even if you do not have symptoms of depression, you might suffer from a high level of stress or frustration. Many caregivers report feeling drained, helpless, guilty, or angry in response to caregiving. Women are particularly prone to these feelings, especially if they are caring for a spouse. As with the symptoms of depression, it's important for you to recognize what you are feeling and to cut back on your caregiving activities, attend a support group, or seek psychiatric help—or all three.

Physicians are just beginning to recognize the importance of asking about caregiver stress. Ideally, both your family member's doctor and your own primary care physician will be aware of your role and will ask you how you are doing, but the reality is that you may need to take the initiative to find help if caregiving is affecting your mental health.

Caregiving and Your Financial Well-Being

Caregiving can adversely affect your well-being by interfering with your physical or mental health, but it can also exert a deleterious effect by negatively impacting your financial situation. This typically occurs if you are working and find you have to change jobs or reduce your hours at work. About 60 percent of caregivers make changes in their work situation at some point during their caregiving journey. If you are working outside the home and are not self-employed, you may find yourself taking sick days or needing flexible hours to accommodate caregiving. Many family caregivers take early retirement, choose to go into business for themselves, or cut back on their hours, all of which have significant financial consequences.

The other way to incur financial strain is by paying directly for some of the costs of caring for your family member (see chapter 48, "Paying for Health Care"). If you live with your relative or spend many hours a week on caregiving, you might very wisely decide to substitute paid help for some of what you do. Ideally, your family member will have the resources to pay for whatever help he needs, but if not, you should discuss with him how much you can reasonably contribute. A home health aide to provide hands-on care might be covered by Medicare or Medicaid, but the number of hours will be limited.

The financial burdens of caregiving do not directly impact your health, but they clearly can have an indirect effect. If you are paying for some of your relative's medical needs, that money has to come from somewhere. You might choose to draw on the discretionary component of your family budget—but you should be careful not to define elective surgery (scheduling your own hip replacement operation) or psychotherapy as optional.

Many people are not entirely comfortable with the idea that promoting their own health is a means of helping their family member; it sounds a bit self-serving. But think of caregiving as analogous to long-distance running: you need to be in top notch physical condition, and you will require both mental preparation and stamina to perform at the highest possible level.

Box 53.1

Taking Care of Yourself

- Watch for signs of burnout
- Prioritize: you cannot do everything
- Maintain your physical health
- Attend to your emotional health
- Don't let caregiving bankrupt you

Rest in Peace

When you recognize that your family member is approaching the end of her life, you will probably experience mixed emotions: you may start to mourn her loss, but you might also find yourself looking forward to a time when your caregiving responsibilities are over. If you anticipate experiencing a sense of relief, you will probably feel guilty for harboring such thoughts. But what you may not realize is that even after your relative dies, you will have a few remaining medically related responsibilities. You may be asked about performing an autopsy. Or, if your relative previously requested that her body be donated to a medical school after death, you will be expected to facilitate that process. If your family member registered as an organ donor, you will be asked to authorize any donations she is eligible to make. How can you possibly think about any of these matters? And if you are able to think clearly, how should you decide what to do?

Almost immediately after your relative dies, her physician might ask if you are interested in an autopsy. You may be a bit taken aback by the question, but it is routine at the time of death. An autopsy, or post-mortem examination, is conducted by a pathologist certified in forensic medicine and involves systematic and careful examination of the outside of the body as well as of the contents of the chest, abdomen, and head (although you can request a limited autopsy that involves only some of these areas). Often, the pathologist will take small tissue samples to examine under the microscope. Unless you have previously discussed an autopsy with your family member, your initial reaction will probably be that you want your relative left alone—so no autopsy. But, as always with medical decision-making on behalf of your family member, you should ask yourself what she would want.

Your relative might have held the view that she wished to be buried with dignity, and perhaps what that meant to her was not cutting into her body after death. More likely, she never gave the matter any thought. You should know that an autopsy is recommended by the College of American Pathologists for *everyone* because it provides feedback to physicians about the quality of their medical care during life and it may be beneficial to future patients by enhancing medical science. In rare circumstances, an autopsy will be legally required—if, for example, there is suspicion of foul play surrounding the death—in which case it will be performed by the local medical examiner, an official whose job it is to perform a forensic autopsy.

You might also find that an autopsy can help *you* by clarifying the cause and circumstances of death. An autopsy can also reveal the existence of previously undiagnosed genetic disorders that may have implications for you or other relatives. Remember that your relative can no longer suffer; when presented with the possibility that an autopsy would help you or other people, she might have been interested. Moreover, the pathology lab should assure you that your family member will be treated with the same respect as you expect from a funeral home. After the post-mortem examination is complete, the body will be sent to the funeral home of your choice.

In making the decision, you should be aware that Medicare and private insurance do not pay for an autopsy, though if it is required for legal reasons, you will not be charged. However, most teaching hospitals and some other hospitals provide autopsies for their patients free of charge. Sometimes, the hospital will do an autopsy for your relative even if she died at home or in a nursing home, provided she has been a patient at the facility in the past.

The process for obtaining permission to do an autopsy varies from state to state. In Massachusetts, by way of illustration, the health-care proxy is the person who gives consent for an autopsy. If no one has been designated as the proxy, then authorization is required from the next of kin. This is defined as the spouse or, if there is no spouse or the spouse is unavailable, adult children; if there are no children,

the responsibility falls to parents. An autopsy should be conducted within the twenty-four hours following death. The report will be available to you within a few weeks.

If your family member dies in the hospital, you may be asked about tissue or organ donation. The health-care proxy or next of kin is typically the person who can authorize this procedure. In making this decision, you should know that all the major religions approve of organ donation as a means of saving lives; this imperative generally trumps any religious precepts regarding maintaining the integrity of the body at death. In some instances, your relative will have filled out a donor registration card indicating she wanted any eligible organs to be used for transplant. According to the Uniform Anatomical Gift Act, a model statute for regulating organ donation that has been accepted by all fifty states and the District of Columbia, a properly witnessed donor registration card should be sufficient for the donation to proceed, even without your input.

The United Network for Organ Sharing (UNOS) is the private, not-for-profit organization in the United States that manages the nation's organ transplants. It is under contract with the federal government and has standards in place to ensure that organs are matched and distributed in a fair and equitable way. Factors including tissue type, organ size, medical urgency, and geographic location are fed into a national computer system to match potential donors and recipients. In principle, there is no age beyond which organs such as kidneys, heart, or liver become unusable. In practice, UNOS will determine if your family member's organs are eligible for transplantation based on her medical conditions at the time of death. But even if she cannot donate a solid organ because of one or more of her medical disorders, she may well be able to donate her corneas. The cornea is the outermost layer of the eye; it is a thin, clear tissue that covers the lens and helps the eye focus. A variety of diseases cause profound injury to the cornea, in some cases leading to blindness. A corneal transplant in these situations can literally restore sight.

The process of organ and tissue donation begins when the local organ bank is notified of a potential donor. Within a day, and often sooner, arrangements will be made to evaluate your relative's eligibility to donate. This involves a review of her medical records and may involve physical inspection as well as taking a blood sample to look for HIV or other infectious agents that are a contraindication to transplantation. If approval is granted, the organ bank will move quickly. Removal of an organ entails a major surgical procedure performed by a surgeon in an operating room and will only be arranged if a suitable recipient has been identified. Removal of the cornea, by contrast, can be done by a technician using sterile technique at the bedside. Corneas, moreover, can be preserved for several weeks and no specific recipient has to be identified in advance of removal.

If your relative has already willed her body to "science," which usually means she has agreed to donate it to a medical school, then neither autopsy nor transplantation is appropriate.

The medical school will use the body to teach anatomy to medical students or to teach new operative techniques to surgeons. This option has become increasingly popular in recent years, especially in light of the rising cost of conventional funerals—the recipient medical school will cremate the body after it is finished with it and provide the cremains to the family, all without charge. We are a long way from the days when medical students raided cemeteries at night to obtain cadavers! Your role here is simply to inform the medical school that your family member has died, an institution with which she already has an agreement, and let the school know they can pick up the body. Obviously, you need to know about your relative's plan in order to implement her wishes.

You will have plenty of other tasks to attend to after your family member passes away, ranging from making funeral arrangements to notifying financial institutions of her death. You will also need to grieve your loss and to adjust to the dramatic changes in your life. Suddenly you won't have to make appointments or take her to the doctor, you won't be measuring her blood pressure or rushing over to check on her when she calls to tell you she is short of breath. On average, caregivers spend over twenty-four hours a week providing care, and nearly a quarter of all caregivers spend upwards of forty hours a week helping out. If you are anything like the norm—and the older and frailer your relative, the more likely you are to be at the higher end of the range—there is now an enormous hole in your life. But your *medical* responsibilities are over. You have performed a remarkable service: you've straddled the roles of physician, nurse, home health aide, and social worker. If there were such a thing as a degree in caregiving, you would have earned it, with distinction.

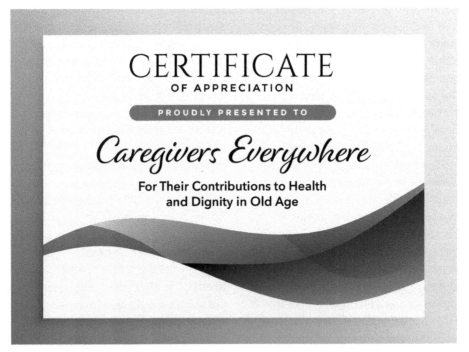

Figure E.1. Certificate of appreciation

Acknowledgments

This book is based on years of experience taking care of older patients in the various settings discussed in the book: the doctor's office, the hospital, the rehabilitation facility, the family home, and the nursing home. I am indebted to those patients and their family caregivers for helping me understand what they needed to know to function effectively. While I consulted numerous medical journals and other publications to make sure the medical information is up to date, I have not included a bibliography as the book is meant to be a guide for family caregivers, not a textbook. I benefited enormously from the thoughtful comments of a number of readers. My profound thanks to my physician colleagues, Susan Kalish, Deborah Levy, Rick Lane, and Mark Yurkofsky, who read many of the chapters on chronic disease management. And I am grateful to my nurse practitioner colleagues, Debbie Nolan, Sarah Penyack, and Gisela Perkins, for their insights on the chapters on acute symptom management.

As always, my biggest thank-you goes to my husband, Larry, whose encouragement and support kept me writing.

Index

do-not-attempt-resuscitation (DNAR) order, 141

do-not-hospitalize (DNH) orders, 311

do-not-resuscitate (DNR) orders, 104, 135, 141, 149, 208, 341

drug-drug interactions, 90, 172

drugs. *See* medications

dry air and cough, 254–55

dry mouth, 234

dual eligibility for Medicare and Medicaid, 321–22

durable medical equipment, 335–36. *See also* assistive devices

dying: assessment of status, 17; conversations about, 208–9; end-of-life care, 357–59, 364–65; and notification about approaching death, 15; as underlying health state, 45. *See also* hospice care

ECT (electroconvulsive therapy), 228–29

edema, 198

Eden Alternative, 302

educators, nurses as, 66

Eldercare Locator website, 354

electroconvulsive therapy (ECT), 228–29

electronic medical records, 75, 77

emergency rooms/departments: abdominal pain and, 288; accidents, bleeding, and, 163, 280, 281, 284; advanced practice clinicians as alternatives to, 64; availability of primary care physicians and, 56; decision to go to, 246, 251, 285; delirium or confusion and, 32–33, 269; IV placement in, 108; nursing home referrals to, 309–10; quality of medical care and, 129

emotional health: of caregivers, 370–71; of family members, 25–27, 315–16. *See also* mental health services

emotions of caregivers: at end of life of family members, 373; hospice care and, 360; support for, 68, 364, 365. *See also* stress of caregiving

emphysema, 218–19. *See also* chronic obstructive lung disease

end-of-life care, 357–59, 364–65. *See also* hospice care

enemas, 267

environmental modifications: for arthritis, 180–81; to prevent falls and injuries, 35–36, 280

excretory functions, 359

exercise: for arthritis, 176; for caregivers, 370;

dementia and, 216; finding place for, 236–37; for high blood pressure, 167; to prevent constipation, 268; types of, 235–36

eye exams, 36

faith communities, 353

falls: causes of, 37–38; confusion after, 269; in hospitals, 87, 89, 90; internal bleeding from, 283; low blood sugar and, 75; in nursing homes, 300; prevention of, 34–37, 71, 236, 280

false positive test results, 88–89, 112

families: in nursing home team meetings, 317; physicians partnering with, 58; support from, 68–69, 362–65

Family Caregiver Alliance, 354

Family Caregiving for the Elderly (Merck manual), 5

family member, use of term, 3

fans, blowing, and shortness of breath, 252

federal government hospitals, 95

feeding issues, 359

fevers: complications of, 293–94; confusion and, 271; diabetes and, 191–92; germs "going around" and, 293; overview of, 291–92; symptoms with, 259, 287, 292–93

fiber in diet, 267–68

financial issues. *See* out-of-pocket medical expenses

financial well-being of caregivers, 371–72

fires and smoking, 237

first aid supplies, 163–64, 280

Five Wishes document, 340, 345

fluid, daily intake of, 268

fluid pills. *See* diuretics

Foley catheters, 108, 359

Folstein Mini-Mental State Exam (MMSE), 24

food, obtaining, 233–34

footwear and falls, 35–36

for-profit hospitals, 97–98

for-profit rehabilitation facilities, 131

frailty: ACE units and, 113–18; comprehensive home care for, 155–56; CPR and, 141; health-care costs for, 328; oral health and, 235; technological interventions and, 107–12; as underlying health state, 13–14, 16–17, 49–51

frontotemporal dementia, 211–12

functional decline from hospitalization, 90, 109, 113–18

functional incontinence, 39

hospital care: advance care planning after, 153–55; benefits of, 91–92; complications during, 89–90; delirium and, 32, 89–90, 105; frailty and, 14; functional decline from, 90, 109, 113–18; geriatric assessments during, 81; goal of, 135; for heart failure, 204; home care compared to, 1–2; ICUs, 105, 110, 117–18; medications and, 103; mid-level practitioners in, 63; multiple tests during, 88–89; perils of, 87–88; primary care physicians and, 59–60; readmission to, 152–53; rehab facilities as alternatives to, 144–46; risks of, 85; technology use in, 107–12; transfer from rehab care to, 141–42; transition to home from, 67. *See also* hospitalists; hospitals; palliative care

Hospital Elder Life Program (HELP), 117

hospitalists: clarifying baseline state with, 103–4; engagement and communication with, 101–2; geriatric, 116–17; goals of care and, 104–6; role of, 96, 100–101

hospitals: ACE units of, 82, 113–18; in networks or systems, 59, 98; ownership of, 97–98; quality ratings of, 93–95; types of, 95–96. *See also* hospital care; hospitalists

housing, 353

humidifiers, 254–55, 257, 283

Huntington's chorea, 111–12

hydrophilic medications, 42

hygrometers, 256–57

hypertension. *See* blood pressure

hypothermia, 291

IADLs (instrumental activities of daily living), 27–29

ibuprofen, 200

ICDs (implantable cardioverter defibrillators), 188

ICUs (intensive care units), 105, 110, 117–18

impaction and abdominal pain, 287–88

implantable cardioverter defibrillators (ICDs), 188

incontinence, 38–40, 359

infection: catheter-associated, 107–8; confusion and, 270; cough and, 253; delirium and, 31–32; fevers with, 292; gastroenteritis, 258, 259, 262, 287, 288; protection from, 294–95; shortness of breath and, 249; of skin, and diabetes, 195; urinary tract, 89, 288, 300–301

influenza (flu), 238–39, 293

informed consent, 109

inhalers, 219

inner ear: dizziness and, 274; nausea and, 261, 262

inpatient comprehensive geriatric assessments, 81

instrumental activities of daily living (IADLs), 27–29

insulin, 190–91, 192–93

insurance. *See* health insurance plans

intellectual stimulation and dementia, 215–16

intensive care unit (ICU) psychosis, 89–90, 105

intensive care units (ICUs), 105, 110, 117–18

interdisciplinary teams. *See* teams

intermediate care, 105–6

internal bleeding, 283–84

interns, 97

intravenous catheters (IVs), 107–8

irritability and dementia, 213

ischemia, 166, 182

ischemic bowel, 105, 287

IVs (intravenous catheters), 107–8

Johns Hopkins Hospital at Home program, 144

Katz Activities of Daily Living scale, 22, 23, 27, 138

kidney disease, 197–203

kidney function and aging, 42–43

knee replacement surgery, 177–78

Lawton Instrumental Activities of Daily Living Scale, 27–29

laxatives, 266, 267

Leapfrog Group Hospital Safety Grade website, 93–95

legal services, 352

lethargy, 269, 272–73

Lewy body dementia, 211

licensed practical nurses (LPNs), 66

life expectancy, 9, 36, 121, 165, 175, 194

light-headedness, 274. *See also* dizziness

lighting and falls, 35, 71

lipophilic medications, 42

liver function, 43, 177

living wills, 216, 217, 340, 344

LPNs (licensed practical nurses), 66

lung cancer, 255

malignant hypertension, 166

MCI (mild cognitive impairment), 24

Meals on Wheels, 143, 195, 233, 349

Medicaid: application for, 135; dual eligibility for Medicare and, 321–22; nursing homes and, 308; SNFs and, 127–28

medical bag for chronic conditions, 159–64

medical caregiving, focus on, 3–4

medical care in nursing homes, 308–13

medical competence, 57

medical decision-making. *See* decision-making, medical

medical expenses. *See* out-of-pocket medical expenses

medical orders, 340–41. *See also* do-not-resuscitate (DNR) orders; Physician Orders for Life-Sustaining Treatment (POLST) forms

medical records: electronic, 75, 77; permission to access, 58, 101–2; problem-oriented, 11–12, 20

medical reports, sharing with family members, 364

medical social workers, 68

medical specialists: coordination of care from, 77; evaluating need for, 76–77; as members of teams, 59; organ-specific views of, 73–76; training of, 61–62; types of, 73–74

medical teams. *See* teams

Medicare: choosing plan for, 325–26; dual eligibility for Medicaid and, 321–22; durable medical equipment under, 181; health benefits counseling service for, 321; hospice care coverage in, 360; Hospital Compare website, 93, 94, 95; joint replacement surgery and, 178; Plan Finder website, 324; Nursing Home Compare website, 127–28, 299–300; Part A, 311, 322; Part B, 322, 328–29; Part D, 41, 326, 328–29; Readmissions Reduction Program, 152; rehab facility coverage in, 142; SNFs and, 126; supplementary oxygen and, 222; visiting nurses and, 67

Medicare Advantage: choosing plans, 323–25; costs of, 331; dental care coverage in, 335; gym memberships and, 336; "three-day rule" and, 145; traditional Medicare compared to, 322–23

medication management, 40–41

medication reconciliation, 67

medications: abdominal pain and, 289; in ACE units, 114, 116; antipsychotic, 129; for arthritis, 176–77; for blood pressure, 165, 167–68; blood pressure rise due to, 169;

for cholesterol, 172–74; choosing health plans and, 325–26; for COLD, 219–21; compassionate use of, 123; constipation and, 265; for coronary heart disease, 183–84; cost of, 326; costs of, 330; for delirium, 33; delirium due to, 31, 89, 270–71; delivery of, 360; dementia and, 14, 212–13; for depression, 227–28; for diabetes, 192–93; dizziness and, 276–77; falls and, 37; for heart failure, 206–7; hospital care and, 103; kidney disease and, 200, 202; for nausea and vomiting, 262; over-the-counter, 164; for pain, 177, 357–58; and polypharmacy, 40–43, 90; to quit smoking, 238; reviewing, in nursing homes, 312, 315; for specialty care, 75–76. *See also specific medications*

Medigap policies, 326–27, 329

Ménière's disease, 275, 277–78

mental health services, 68, 229–30, 336

mental status examinations, 24–25

metabolism: delirium and, 32; excretion of medications and, 42–43

Metamucil, 266

methylxanthines, 220–21

mild cognitive impairment (MCI), 24

milk of magnesia, 266

mineral oil, 266

Mini-Cog, 46–48

mixed incontinence, 39

MMSE (Folstein Mini-Mental State Exam), 24

mobility issues: from arthritis, 176; canes and walkers for, 70–71, 178–79; in nursing homes, 314–15; in rehab facilities, 129

Montreal Cognitive Assessment, 24

multimorbidity, definition of, 50

multi-specialty group practices, 59

National Coalition for Hospice and Palliative Care, 120

nausea and vomiting: abdominal pain with, 287; causes of, 260–61; complications of, 262–63; dizziness with, 275; seriousness of, 258–59; symptoms with, 259; treatment of, 262; vomiting blood, 281–82

nephrologists, 201, 203

neuropathy, 74, 195

nicotine patches, 238

nitrates, 183, 206

nonsteroidal anti-inflammatory medications, 169, 280, 289. *See also* acetaminophen

norovirus, 293

nosebleeds, 282–83

not-for-profit hospitals, 97–98
not-for-profit rehabilitation facilities, 131
NPs. *See* nurse practitioners
nurse practitioners (NPs): costs of, 332; in nursing homes, 310; role of, 59, 63–64; training of, 62–63
nurses: in hospitals, 91; in nursing homes, 312; in rehab facilities, 131, 133–34; as team members, 66–67; visiting, 64, 67, 332–34
nursing assistants: in nursing homes, 299, 302, 318; in rehab facilities, 135, 145
Nursing Home Compare website, 127–28, 299–300
Nursing Home Reform Act of 1987, 301
nursing homes: advance care planning and, 305–7, 310, 316; caregiving related to, 304–7; choosing, 299–303; culture of, 301–3; hospice care in, 311–12; interpersonal conflicts in, 318; medical care in, 308–13; residents of, 297–98; team meetings in, 314–18; as total institutions, 304
nutritional supplements, 337
nutrition and diet, 231–34

occupational therapists (OTs), 70–72, 134
offices of physicians: accessibility of, 55–56; nurses in, 66–67
open enrollment, 321, 327
opioids, 177, 252, 255–56, 358
oral health, 234–35, 335
oral hypoglycemics, 192–93
organ donation, 374–75
orthostatic hypotension, 167–68, 271–72, 275–76
osteoporosis and falls, 36–37
otolaryngologists, 282
OTs (occupational therapists), 70–72, 134
out-of-pocket medical expenses: dental care, 335; durable medical equipment, 335–36; financial well-being of caregiver and, 371–72; health insurance premiums, 328–29; medications, 330; mental health care, 336; nursing visits, 332–34; overall, 337–38; physical therapy, 334; physician visits, 330–31; splitting with family, 363
overflow incontinence, 38–39
ownership: of hospitals, 97–98; of rehab facilities, 131
oxygen, supplementary, 208, 221–22, 237
oxygen saturation, monitoring, 162, 244–45, 249, 272

PACE (Program of All-Inclusive Care for the Elderly), 155–56, 351
pacemakers, 187–88
pain: abdominal, 259, 264, 285–90; arthritis, 176; breakthrough, 357; chest pain, 182–83, 243–47; confusion and, 270; medications for, 177, 357–58; palliative care consultations for, 122–23, 149; rating, 244; ratings for quality of care and, 128–29
palliative care: availability of, 120–21; consultations for, 121–23; overview of, 3, 119–20; in rehab facilities, 148–49
Parkinson's disease: advance care planning for, 316; dementia in, 212; falls and, 37; medication for, 75
partnering with physicians, 53, 58
PAs. *See* physician assistants
patient-centered care, 114
patient drug assistance programs, 123
PCI (percutaneous coronary intervention), 185, 186
PCSK9 inhibitors, 173–74
pelvic organs, 285
percutaneous coronary intervention (PCI), 185, 186
peritoneal dialysis, 201
permission, obtaining: for autopsies, 374; to communicate with hospitalists, 101–2; to review medical information, 58
personal care, provision of, 39–40, 358–59
Personal Chef to Go, 350
pharmacology, geriatric, 41–43
physical function, in underlying health state, 21–23
physical health of caregivers, 368, 370
physical therapists (PTs), 70–72, 134, 138–39, 334
physician assistants (PAs): in nursing homes, 310; role of, 59, 63–64; training of, 62–63
Physician Orders for Life-Sustaining Treatment (POLST) forms, 104, 135, 149, 306, 342, 346–47
physicians: cardiologists, 188–89, 205; costs of visits to, 330–31; coverage group of, 59; geriatricians, 30, 57, 78; in health plan networks, 323–24; hospital privileges of, 93; nephrologists, 201, 203; nurses as liaisons to, 66; in nursing homes, 308–9; otolaryngologists, 282; podiatrists, 195; psychiatrists, 229–30; in teaching hospitals, 97–98; training of, 61–62; underlying health state

and, 11–12. *See also* hospitalists; primary
care physicians
pill dispensers, 207
planning. *See* advance care planning; advance
directives; health-care proxies; living wills
plaques in blood vessels (atherosclerosis),
183, 184–85, 198, 215, 237–38
pleural effusion, 250, 255
pleuritic pain, 245
pneumonia vaccines, 239
pocket talkers, 57
podiatrists, 195
POLST (Physician Orders for Life-Sustaining
Treatment) forms, 104, 135, 149, 306, 342,
346–47
polypharmacy, 40–43, 90
portable oxygen containers, 222
potassium, 167–68, 197–98, 200
pressure ulcers, 129–30, 309
prevention: of chronic conditions, 231–39; of
complications of dizziness, 278; of constipation, 267–68; of delirium, 117; of falls and
injuries, 35–37, 71, 236, 280; of infections,
294–95; of progression of dementia, 215–16
preventive strategies: dental hygiene, 234–35;
exercise, 235–37; nutrition and diet,
231–34; quitting smoking, 237–38; vaccinations, 238–39
primary care physicians: ability to communicate of, 56–57; accessibility of offices of,
55–56; availability of, 56; coordination of
care by, 77; follow-up visits to, 153; geriatric assessments by, 57–58; hospital care
and, 100; as members of teams, 59–60;
partnering with, 58; types of, 53
priorities, setting for caregiving, 365–66
problem-oriented medical records, 11–12, 20
procedures. *See* tests; treatment
prognosis, 9. *See also* life expectancy
Program of All-Inclusive Care for the Elderly
(PACE), 155–56, 351
projectile vomiting, 258, 287
proton pump inhibitors, 246, 254, 262, 289
psychological factors. *See* emotional health
PTs (physical therapists), 70–72, 134, 138–39,
334
pulse, taking, 206, 244, 271–72, 276
pulse oximeters, 161–62, 244, 249

quality of care: in hospitals, 93–95, 100–101;
in nursing homes, 299–301; in rehab
facilities, 127–30

questions to ask: of medical specialists,
76–77; of physicians, 45, 311

ratings: of hospital quality, 93–95; of Medicare Advantage plans, 323, 325; of pain,
244; of rehab facility quality, 127–30
registered nurses (RNs), 66
regulators for oxygen tanks, 222–23
rehabilitation facilities: acute medical
problems in, 140–42; admission to, 90,
125–26, 133, 140; advance care planning in,
147–48; as alternative to hospitals, 144–46;
caregiver involvement in, 137, 138–39;
choosing, 127–28; discharge from, 142–43;
functional decline from hospitalization
and, 90; geriatric assessments in, 83,
146–47; goal and function of, 135–37;
nurses in, 131, 133–34; palliative care
consultations in, 148–49; ratings of quality
of, 127–30; readmission after stays in,
152–53; visits to, 130–31. *See also* skilled
nursing facilities
relationships, importance of, 69
relative, use of term, 3
relaxation techniques for shortness of breath,
252
resident-centered nursing homes, 302–3
residential environment and underlying
health state, 10
residents, 97
resistance exercise, 235, 236
respirators, 223–25
respiratory rate, 205–6
respiratory symptoms and fever, 292
respiratory system, 218
respite, 68, 362
restraints, 108, 273, 301
retinopathy, 74–75, 195
retroperitoneal bleeds, 283
rhinitis, allergic, 254
risks: of diversion of opioids, 256, 358; of
having chronic conditions, 157; of high-
tech procedures, 109; of hospital care, 85;
of low-tech procedures, 107–8; of readmission to hospital, 152–53; of tests, 87
RNs (registered nurses), 66
robustness, 13, 51
rugs and falls, 35, 71

salt, intake of, 167
sandwich generation, 365
scales, bathroom, 152, 163, 205